Supervisory Management For Health Care Institutions

Theo Haimann
The Mary Louise Murray Professor
of Management Sciences
Saint Louis University

D1412157

The Catholic Hospital Association
St. Louis, Missouri 63104

Library of Congress Catalog Card No. 72-92380
ISBN 0-87125-004-7

To
Ruthie
Lyn and Mark

This book is intended for department heads and supervisors engaged in all types of health care facilities be they hospitals, extended care facilities, nursing homes, homes for the aged, rehabilitation centers, long-term care facilities, or other institutions of this type. Most department heads and supervisors in such facilities were placed into their supervisory positions primarily because they did an outstanding job in their chosen health care fields. Their previous experience and education, however, rarely included the area of supervision *per se*. Thus, these supervisors who rise from the ranks often find themselves in increasingly demanding positions having precious little or no familiarity with the managerial aspects of their newly attained rank. Suddenly they are confronted with the need to be an effective manager of a department, to stay on top of a more sophisticated job, to gain new perspectives and insights into human relationships. Their position may have changed from being a good nurse, for example, to becoming an efficient head nurse, supervisor of nursing, or whatever the title may be. The primary function changes from doing things oneself to getting things done through and with employees by motivating them so that they enthusiastically go about achieving departmental and institutional objectives.

This text is intended to aid people in the health care field who are faced with such a task. Its purpose is to demonstrate to the supervisor that proficiency in supervision will better equip him to cope with the ever-increasing demands of getting the job done, will contribute more effectively to the over-all goals of his institution, and at the same time will make him more valuable to the facility's administrator.

This book is introductory in the sense that it assumes no previous knowledge of the concepts of supervision on the part of the reader. Although the book does include material of a sophisticated nature, this material is explained in terms that can easily be understood by the inexperienced supervisor. The book will help such a newly appointed supervisor become acquainted with the many problems which he will face, and it offers practical advice for their solution. For the experienced supervisor, this book is intended to refresh thinking and widen horizons by taking a different and challenging look at both his own position and that of his employees.

Even though the text is written for supervisors, not for administrators, most of its content would be of great interest to the latter also. The common denominator of all levels of supervisors is the part that they play as managers within the administrative hierarchy of the institution. Without going into the technical details of specific supervisory positions, the book discusses the managerial aspects common to every supervisory job whether it is in nursing, medical records, medical social work, housekeeping, dietary, laboratory, x-rays, inhalation therapy, laundry, maintenance, engineering, or any of the numerous other specialities found within the health care field.

It is important to realize that the supervisory position in any field is the most critical point in the entire organizational structure. It involves the management of people in the day-to-day running of a department within an institution. In hospitals and other health care facilities, the supervisor's position is exceptionally strategic since in most cases the recipient does not elect to receive the services provided, nor does he understand them. The supervisor in a hospital or related health facility must contend with emotional factors involved in the care of the patients and their relatives under conditions which make effective supervision unusually difficult. In addition to this, the supervisor is often torn between considerations of a professional nature and those of an administrative nature. But above everything else, the supervisor's activities must ultimately reflect the welfare of the patient. All of these internal factors make it imperative for the supervisor to be a capable manager of his department.

Moreover, external factors also affect the supervisor's role. It is an established fact that hospitals and related enterprises comprise one of the largest activities in the United States today. Provisions for health care services will become more complex due to rapidly expanding areas of concern, growing government support, increasing population, and advances of medical science and technology. In addition, it is essential for all health care facilities to keep pace with the social and environmental progress of civilization. This again means an ever-increasing challenge for efficient management capable of coping with more sophisticated problems, whether they are of an economic, professional, scientific, or educational nature.

Thus, the focus of this book is on the managerial process, more specifically on the managerial functions of planning, organizing, staffing, influencing, and controlling and their relation to the daily job of the supervisor. Connecting these functions together are the decision-making process and communication. In reality, all of the managerial functions are closely related and such a distinct classification is not always discernible in practice. But this type of academic separation does make possible a methodological, clear, and complete analysis of the managerial functions of a supervisor.

Of course, the supervisor's job of getting things done with and through people has its foundation in the relationship between the supervisor and the people with whom he works. For this reason the supervisor must have considerable knowledge of the human aspects of supervision, of the behavioral factors that motivate his employees.

This book attempts to integrate such behavioral factors into the conceptual framework of managing. Although it is obviously not an all-comprising text on management, the book does try to present a balanced picture. Thus, human relations and behavioral aspects are kept in proper perspective in relation to the other aspects of the supervisory job.

Material for this text has come from the writings and research of scholars in the areas of management, behavioral and social sciences, as well as from the practical experience of numerous supervisors, managers, and administrators. In addition, this text also reflects the author's own experiences in teaching management, in consulting, in conducting many supervisory development programs, and in giving lectures to administrators and supervisors at different levels in the managerial hierarchy of hospitals and related health care facilities.

In writing the book, the author fully realized that most people working in health care facilities are women, and he was seriously tempted to refer to supervisors as "she" and to use the female gender throughout the book. However, current authoritative publications, including government publications, continue to use the male reference. Therefore, instead of referring to "her" employees, the author speaks of "his" employees, etc. He hopes that those readers who are sensitive to such terminology will forgive him and not interpret this stylist device as prejudicial to the vital managerial role of women in the health care field.

Finally, in writing a book such as this the author is indebted to so many persons that it is impossible to give them all due credit. Special thanks go to Mrs. Janice Adleman for her skillful editorial assistance. The author also wishes to acknowledge with thanks the help and encouragement given by The Catholic Hospital Association and especially by their Department of Publications and its director, Mrs. Mary Krieger. Last but by no means least, thanks go to Miss Valda Tuetken who skillfully transcribed many challenging notes into readable manuscript. To all these the author extends his grateful appreciation while bearing full responsibility for any sins of omission or commission.

Theo Haimann

CONTENTS

PART ONE

Stepping Into Management

CHAPTER 1

The Job of Supervisor

The *delivery of health care* is a term which is becoming increasingly common in the daily press, in magazine articles and in conversations in the United States. What is generally meant by this term is the problem of providing adequate health care services of all types, preventative and curative, to all people regardless of age, color, where they live, or their ability to pay. The reason that health care delivery systems are receiving such attention in the United States is that the cost of health care has risen more steeply than any other item in our national economy. Not only have the total expenditures in the field of health services risen by leaps and bounds, but these expenditures have also become an ever-increasing percentage of our over-all economy, as expressed in our gross national product. Hence, it is understandable that the delivery of health care has become a major national issue and that the institutions which are engaged in this service such as hospitals and related health facilities are receiving continuous and increasing scrutinization. Moreover, since the delivery of health care largely means providing a service, it is understandable that from sixty to seventy per cent of the total expenditures within the field are for wages and salaries. Therefore, many attacks have naturally centered around the clamor for increased employee productivity to justify such large wage and salary expenditures. What is needed, in other words, is better and more effective administration of health care centers, that is, better supervision throughout. This is the case because in the final analysis it is the supervisor of a department, regardless of his title, who is in the best position to see that his department functions smoothly and efficiently. It is essential therefore that due emphasis be paid to the need for the further development of effective supervisors within all phases of the health care field.

THE DEMANDS OF A SUPERVISORY POSITION

The job of a supervisor or department head in a health care center, hospital, or in any other related medical facility is a demanding one. You have probably learned this from your own experience or by observing supervisors in hospitals and related institutions as they go about their daily tasks.

If we look carefully at the job of almost any supervisor, regardless of what he supervises, we can see that it involves four major dimensions. First, the supervisor must be a good boss and a good manager of the employees who work under him. He must have the technical, professional, and clinical competence to run his department smoothly and to see that his employees carry out their assignments successfully. Second, the supervisor must also be a competent subordinate to the manager above him. In most instances, this manager would be an administrator, an associate administrator, or a director of a service. Here we see that the supervisor needs to be a good employee and follower of his own boss.

In between these two dimensions of the supervisor's role, there is a third area in which he acts as a connecting link between the employee and the administration. In fact, to his employees the supervisor represents the administration of the institution. He is usually the only contact they ever have with any member of the administrative group. The supervisor is in effect that part of the administration who must make certain that the work gets done.

The fourth and final part of the supervisor's role is that he must maintain satisfactory working relationships with the heads of all other departments and services in the medical center. The relationship to these other department heads must be that of a good colleague who is willing and eager to coordinate his department's efforts with those of the other departments in order to reach the over-all objectives and goals of the institution.

We might be able to visualize the four dimensions of the supervisor's job more clearly if we look at a diagram such as that shown in Figure 1-1. By examining this figure, we can see the direction of the relationships that the supervisor must maintain. He must be successful in his vertical relationships downward with his subordinates and upward with his superior. In addition, he must be skillful in handling his horizontal relationships with other supervisors as this will facilitate getting his own job done.

Partly because of the complexity of these relationships, it is commonly acknowledged that the role of the first line supervisor in any industrial or commercial undertaking is a most difficult one. It is even more difficult for supervisors within a health care facility because their activities directly or indirectly affect the quality of patient care and the smooth over-all functioning of the institution. In addition to their many professional obligations, hospital supervisors must always bear in mind the needs and desires of patients and their relatives who, at the time, are physically and emotionally upset people. Thus, the supervisor should be continuously aware of the problems of human relations among medical staff members, other hospital

FIGURE 1-1

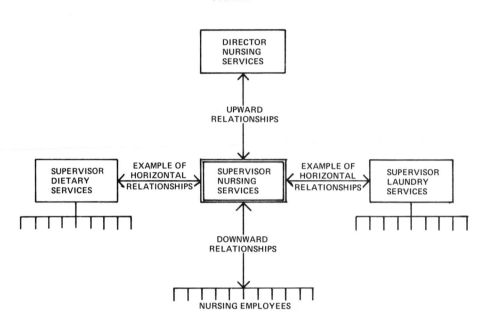

personnel, and patients. This is necessary in order to accomplish the primary objective of any health care center, namely, providing the best possible patient care. All of these considerations make the job of the hospital supervisor a particularly demanding and challenging one.

Let us be more specific and look at the demands made on a head nurse in charge of a nursing unit. It is her duty to provide for and supervise the nursing care rendered to the patients in her unit. She does this partly by delegating a certain amount of her authority for the care of patients and the supervision of personnel to team leaders within her area. But the head nurse must still plan, direct, and control all activities within the nursing unit. She must make the rounds of her unit with medical and nursing staff. She also is expected to make rounds for personal observation of the condition and behavior of patients and to assess the need for continued nursing care. She may even have to assume general nursing functions in the care of those patients who have complex problems.

Furthermore, the head nurse must interpret and apply the policies, procedures, rules, and regulations of the hospital in general and of the nursing services section in particular. She must provide coverage of the unit for twenty-four hours by making out schedules to have the unit properly staffed at all times. She is to communicate and report to her nursing supervisor (assuming that the nursing supervisor is the immediate superior of a number of head nurses) all pertinent information regarding patients in her unit. She must orient new personnel to the unit and acquaint them with the general philosophies of the hospital. She is also concerned with continued in-service education in her unit, in other words with teaching personnel. Likewise, she participates in the evaluation of her subordinates. In addition, it is part of the head nurse's job to coordinate the activities of her unit with unit managers if these are available. She also must coordinate her patient care with other departments throughout the hospital. Moreover, she is involved in the design and regular re-evaluation of the budget. She serves on a number of committees in addition to attending all head nurses' meetings. She might also be expected to help in the supervision and instruction of student nurses when necessary. In all likelihood there are many other duties which are assigned to a head nurse, depending what the particular health care facility specifies in its description of this very demanding position.

We might also look at the work which is required of another supervisory position in a hospital, that of the supervisor of the housekeeping department, often called the Executive Housekeeper. Generally, a job description will tell you that it is this supervisor's job to maintain the hospital in a clean and orderly condition. She must continuously study new cleaning methods and new cleaning equipment, and recommend changes of layout and location of equipment, if necessary, to facilitate the cleaning of various areas of the hospital. She also plans and directs the work schedule for the housekeeping staff, taking into consideration visiting hours, traffic, and the amount of work to be done. She is expected to write instruction sheets and training manuals for housekeeping procedures and she must be able to teach her staff members both prevailing and new methods and demonstrate these with equipment. Furthermore, she must periodically inspect their completed work for quality of service. In addition to this, she will plan and select furnishings for the various rooms, considering serviceability, decorative appeal, and other factors.

Moreover, the housekeeping supervisor must develop and maintain effective working relationships with the professional, administrative, and maintenance personnel of the institution. She is also expected to interview and make the final selection of applicants who have been referred to her by the personnel department. And it is her job to dismiss unsatisfactory employees and to take disciplinary action whenever necessary. In addition to these, there may be many other duties connected with the job of Executive Housekeeper, making this another demanding supervisory position in a medical facility.

With our growing, complex society and with the increasing demands for more and better health care, the job of any hospital supervisor is likely to become even more challenging. This is true whether the title is head nurse, supervisor of medical records, operating room supervisor, director of maintenance, chief inhalation therapist, laboratory supervisor, chief technologist of radiology, food service supervisor or supervisor of any one of the many other activities necessary for the smooth functioning of a health care center.

THE MANAGERIAL ASPECTS OF SUPERVISION

The job of a supervisor can be somewhat simplified, however, if we think of it in terms of two main requirements. First of all, the supervisor is required to have a thorough knowledge of the job to be performed and must be technically and clinically competent to do the job in question. The second aspect of the supervisor's job is that he must also be a manager of his department. It is this managerial aspect which will significantly determine the effectiveness of a supervisor's performance.

You may have observed various supervisors on different occasions and noticed that some of them are usually harassed, disorganized, and overly involved in doing the job at hand. They are muddling through and are knee-deep in work. Such supervisors put in long hours and are never afraid of doing anything themselves. They are working exceedingly hard, but they never seem to have enough time left to actually supervise. On the other hand, you may have observed supervisors who seem to be on top of the job and whose departments function smoothly and orderly. They have found time to sit at their desks at least part of the day and keep their desk work up to date. Why is there such a difference you may ask. Of course, some supervisors are basically more capable than others. But if you compare two chief engineers in two hospitals to try to discover why one is on top of his job and the other is continuously fixing things himself, you will probably find that the reason is that the one understands his job better than the other. Let us assume that both are equally good mechanics, that both have similar equipment under their care, and that the conditions under which they perform are about alike. Still, the results of one chief engineer are significantly better than those of the other. Why is this? The answer is that the one is simply a better manager, that he is able to supervise the functions of his department in a manner which allows him to get the job done with and through the people of his department. The difference between a good supervisor and a poor supervisor, assuming that their technical skill is alike, is the difference in their managerial ability.

Surprisingly enough, however, the managerial aspect of the supervisor's position has long been neglected. Rather, the emphasis has always been put on the technical and clinical competence for doing a particular job. Consider your own job, for example. It is very likely that you were appointed to this job from the ranks of one of the various professional services or crafts. As a result of your ingenuity, effort, and willingness to work hard, you were promoted to the supervisory level and were expected to assume the responsibilities of managing your particular department. But precious little was done to acquaint you with these responsibilities or to help you cope with the managerial aspects of your new job. More or less overnight you were made a part of administration without having been prepared to be an administrator. Ever since, you have done the best you could and your department is probably functioning reasonably well. But there are likely to be some problems and these may be eased by a better understanding of the managerial aspects of your job so that you will be the manager running the department instead of the department running you.

It is the aim of this text to show the supervisor how to become a better manager. Of course, this does not mean that he can neglect or underestimate the actual work involved in getting the job done. As you know, one of the requirements of a good supervisor is that he thoroughly understands the clinical, professional, and technical operations. Often the supervisor is actually the most skilled man of the department and he can do a more efficient and quicker job. But he must not be tempted to step in and take over the job, except for purposes of instruction or in case of an emergency. Rather, the supervisor's responsibility is to see to it that his employees can do the job, and do it properly. As a supervisor, he must plan, guide, and manage. Let us concentrate further on these managerial requirements of the supervisory position.

THE MEANING OF MANAGEMENT

First, let us consider what is meant by management. Simply stated, *management is the function of getting things done through and with people, and directing the efforts of individuals toward a common objective.* You have undoubtedly learned from your own experience that in most endeavors one person can accomplish relatively little by himself. For this reason, people have found it expedient and even necessary to join with others in order to attain the goals of an enterprise. In a business or service situation, it is the manager's function to achieve the goals of the enterprise with the help of his subordinates and fellow employees.

But achieving goals through and with people is only one aspect of the manager's job. He must also create a working atmosphere within which his subordinates can find as much satisfaction of their needs as possible. In other words, a supervisor must provide a climate which will make it conducive for his employees to fulfill such needs as the need for recognition, the need for achievement, the need for companionship, etc. If these needs can be met right on the job, employees are more likely to strive willingly and enthusiastically toward the achievement of departmental objectives as well as the over-all objectives of the institution. Thus, we must add to our earlier definition of management by saying that the manager's job *is getting things done through and with people by enabling them to find as much satisfaction of their needs as utterly possible while at the same time motivating them to achieve both their own objectives and the objectives of the institution.* The better the supervisor performs these duties the better will be the performance of his department.

You may have noticed by this time that we have been using the terms supervisory, managerial, and administrative interchangeably. Although the exact meaning of these titles varies with different institutions, the term *administrative* is usually used for top level management positions, whereas *managerial* and *supervisory* usually connote positions within the middle or lower rungs of the institutional hierarchy. But for our purposes these terms will be used interchangeably.

Our reason for doing this will become clearer when you understand the somewhat surprising fact that the managerial aspects of all supervisory jobs are the same. This is true regardless of the department or section in which the supervisor is engaged and regardless of the level within the administrative hierarchy on which he finds himself. Thus, the managerial content of your supervisory position is the same whether you are director of nursing services, head of the housekeeping division, chief engineer in the maintenance department, or chief therapeutic dietitian. And, by the same token, the managerial functions are the same whether you are the supervisor on the firing line (lowest level or first line supervisor), whether you are in the middle level of management, or in the top administrative group. And in addition to this, it does not matter in which kind of organization you are working. The managerial functions are the same whether the supervisor is working in an industrial enterprise, commercial enterprise, non-profit organization, fraternal organization, government, or in a hospital or other related health care facility. Regardless of his organization, his department, or his level, the manager's skills are the same.

These managerial skills, however, must be distinguished from the professional, clinical, and technical skills required of a supervisor. As stated above, all supervisors must also possess special technical skills and know-how in the particular field in which they do their daily work. Naturally, the technical skills will vary depending upon the department in which the supervisor works, but any supervisory position requires both the particular technical skills and the standard managerial skills.

It is very important to note, however, that as a supervisor advances upward in the administrative ladder, he will practice fewer professional and technical skills and more managerial skills. If you will observe your own institution, you will also find that the higher you go within the administrative hierarchy, the more administrative skills are required and the less technical know-how. Therefore, the top administrator generally uses far fewer technical skills than those who are employed under him. But in his rise to the top the administrator has had to acquire all the administrative skills necessary for the management of the entire enterprise. For example, a chief hospital administrator is concerned primarily with the over-all management of hospital activities; his functions are almost purely administrative. In this endeavor, of course, he depends upon the technical skills of his various subordinate administrators and managers, including all the first line supervisors, to get the job done. The chief administrator, in turn, uses his managerial skills in directing the efforts of all these subordinate managers toward the common objectives of the hospital. Therefore, throughout the organization the purpose of the managerial skills is the same.

MANAGERIAL SKILLS CAN BE LEARNED

At this point, you may be wondering how a supervisor acquires these very important managerial skills which we have been stressing. First of all, let us emphatically state that the standard managerial skills can be *learned*. They are not something with which you are necessarily born. Although it is often suggested that good managers, like good athletes, are born not made, this belief is patently false. It cannot be denied that men are born with different physiological and biological potential, and that they are endowed with an unequal amount of intelligence and many other characteristics. And it is true that a man who is not a natural athlete is not likely to run one hundred yards in record time. But many men who are natural athletes have not come close to that goal either.

A good athlete is made when a man with some natural endowment, by practice, learning, effort, sacrifice, and experience develops his natural endowment into a mature skill. The same holds true for a good manager; by practice, learning, and experience he develops his natural endowment of intelligence and leadership characteristics into mature management skills. The skills involved in managing are as learnable and trainable as the skills involved in playing tennis. If you currently hold a supervisory position, it is very likely that you have the necessary prerequisites of intelligence and leadership and that you are now ready to acquire the skills of a manager.

The benefits which you as a supervisor will derive from learning to be a better manager are obvious. First of all, you will have plenty of opportunity to apply managerial principles and knowledge to your daily work. Good management as a supervisor will make a great deal of difference in the performance of your department. It will function more smoothly, work will get done on time, you will probably find it easier to stay within your budget, and your workers will more willingly and enthusiastically contribute toward the ultimate objectives. The application of good management principles will put you as a supervisor on top of your job, instead of being completely swallowed up by it. You will also find that you will have more time to be concerned with the over-all aspects of your department, and in so doing you will become more valuable to those to whom you are responsible. For example, you will be more likely to contribute significant suggestions and advice to your superiors, perhaps in areas about which you have never before been consulted but which ultimately affect your department. You will also find it easier to see the complex interrelationships of the various departments throughout the health care center, and this in turn will help you to work in closer harmony with your colleagues who are supervising other departments. Briefly, you will be able to do a more effective supervisory job with much less effort.

In addition to the direct benefits of doing a better supervisory job for the hospital, there are other benefits for you personally. As a supervisor applying sound management principles, you will grow in stature. As time goes on you will be capable of handling larger and more complicated assignments. You will be able to fill better and higher paying jobs. You will move up within the managerial hierarchy and you will naturally want to improve your managerial skills as you advance.

As we noted above, an additional satisfying thought is that the principles of management are equally applicable in any organization and in any managerial or supervisory position. That is, the principles of management required to produce gyroscopes, to manage a retail department, to supervise office work, or to run a garage are all the same. Moreover, these principles are applicable not only in the United States, but also all over the world. Aside from local peculiarities and questions of personality, it would not matter whether you are a supervisor in a textile mill in India, a supervisor in a chemical plant in Italy, the foreman of a department in a steel mill in Gary, Indiana, or the supervisor of the medical records section in a hospital in St. Louis. By becoming a manager you will become more mobile in every direction and in every respect.

Obviously, then, there are great inducements for you to learn the principles of good management. However, you cannot expect to learn them overnight. You can only become a good manager by actually managing; that is, by applying the principles of management to your own work situation. As you go on, you will undoubtedly make mistakes here and there but you will, in turn, learn from your mistakes. The principles of management which we shall discuss in this book will be definite guidelines that you can apply in most situations. They will help you to avoid errors which often take a long time to correct. As we have seen, your efforts to become an outstanding manager will pay handsome dividends. As your managerial competence increases, you will be able to prevent many of the difficulties which make a supervisory job a burden instead of a challenging and satisfying task.

SUMMARY

The role of the supervisor is a most demanding one. To the employees in his department, the supervisor represents management. Toward his own boss, he is a subordinate. Toward the supervisors in other departments, he must be a good colleague, coordinating his efforts with theirs to bring about the achievement of the institution's objectives. The supervisor must possess technical competence for the functions to be performed in his department, and at the same time he must be the manager of that department. Management is the function of getting things done through people and with people. The way a supervisor handles the managerial aspects of his job will make the difference between running the department and being run by the department. The managerial aspects of any supervisory job are the same regardless of the particular kind of work involved and regardless of the position on the administrative ladder. As a supervisor climbs up this ladder, the managerial skills will increase in importance and the technical skills will gradually become less important. These managerial skills can be learned; a manager is not "born," he is made. A supervisor will benefit greatly both in a professional sense and in a personal sense if he takes the time to acquire the managerial skills.

CHAPTER 2

The Earmarks of a Manager

We have just spent considerable time discussing managerial skills, their importance to a supervisor, the fact that they can be learned, and the benefits of acquiring them. But we have not yet stated exactly what these all-important managerial skills are, and you must certainly be wondering by now. The managerial skills are the functions that a manager *must* perform in order to be considered a true manager. They are the functions necessary to carry out his managerial job.

THE MANAGERIAL FUNCTIONS

In this text, we shall consider five major managerial functions. They are planning, organizing, staffing, influencing, and controlling. The labels used to describe these functions vary from time to time, and also some textbooks list one more or one less managerial function. But regardless of the terms or number used, the managerial functions when taken together constitute one of the two major earmarks of a manager. If a person does not perform all of these functions to a certain extent, then he is not a manager in the true sense of the word, regardless of what his title may be. Of course, we must specify more precisely what we mean when we say that the managerial functions or skills are planning, organizing, staffing, influencing, and controlling. We will do so now only in a general way since most of the remainder of the book is devoted to the specifics involved in each of the functions.

Planning

Planning is the function that determines in advance what should be done. It consists of determining the goals, objectives, policies, procedures, and methods of the organization. In planning, the manager must think of the various alternative choices which are available to him. Thus, planning is mental work; it is intellectual in nature. It involves thinking ahead and preparing for the future. It is laying out in advance the road to be followed, the way the job should be done.

You may have observed supervisors who are constantly fighting one crisis after another. The probable reason for this is that they did not plan. They did not look ahead. It is every manager's duty to plan and this cannot be delegated to someone else. He may call on certain specialists to give him some assistance in laying out various plans, but by and large it is up to him, as the manager of the department, to make his own plans. Of course, these plans must coincide with the general over-all objectives of the hospital as laid down by the chief administrator. But within the over-all directives and general boundaries, the manager has considerable leeway as he maps out his own departmental course.

Planning must come before any of the other managerial functions. And even after the initial plans are laid out and the manager proceeds with the other managerial functions he continues to plan, revising his course and choosing different alternatives as the need arises. Therefore, although planning is the first function which a manager must tackle, it does not end when he goes on to the other functions. He continues to plan all the time he performs his organizing, staffing, influencing, and controlling duties.

Organizing

The organizing process determines how the work in a particular department will be divided and accomplished. It requires the manager to define, group, and assign job duties. More specifically, when the manager organizes he determines and enumerates the various activities which must be accomplished, he combines these activities into distinct groups (departments, divisions, sections, teams, or any other unit), he then further divides the group work into individual jobs, and defines the relationship between jobs.

In other words, to organize means to design a structural framework which sets up all the positions needed to perform the work of the department and to assign particular duties to these positions. Of course, the structural framework of any department must fit into the over-all structure of the institution. Furthermore, when the manager organizes his structural framework, he must also see to it that the authority relationships between his various subordinates are appropriately aligned. While organizing he will of necessity have to delegate a certain amount of his own authority to his subordinate managers so that they can carry out the duties for which they are responsible. Thus, it is through this organizing function that the manager clarifies problems of authority and responsibility within his department.

Staffing

By staffing, we mean the manager's responsibility to recruit new employees in order to make certain that there are enough qualified employees to fill the various positions needed in the department.

Staffing involves not only the selection but also the training of these employees. It involves the problem of promoting them, of appraising their performance from time to time, and of giving them opportunities for further development. In addition to this, staffing includes a wise and appropriate system of compensation.

Influencing

Influencing is concerned with motivating people at work to achieve the objectives of the job for which they are responsible. The influencing function of a manager includes directing, guiding, teaching, coaching, and supervising his subordinates. It is not sufficient for a manager to plan, organize, and staff. He must also stimulate action by giving directives and orders to his subordinates and by supervising and guiding them as they go about their work. Moreover, it is the manager's job to develop the abilities of his subordinates by leading, teaching, and coaching them effectively.

Thus, we can say that influencing is the process around which all performance revolves; it is the essence of all operations. This process has many dimensions such as morale, employee satisfaction and productivity, leadership, and communication. It is through the influencing function that the supervisor seeks to create a climate which is conducive to employee satisfaction and which, at the same time, gains the objectives of the institution. As you know from your own experience, much time is spent in influencing subordinates — as a matter of fact, most of your time is probably spent this way.

Controlling

The managerial function of control involves those activities that are necessary to see to it that events proceed as planned and that objectives are achieved as planned. In other words, to control means to determine whether or not the plans are being carried out, whether or not progress is being made toward objectives, and what actions to take to correct any deviations and shortcomings. Here again we can see the importance of planning as the primary function of the manager. It would not be possible for him to check on whether work was proceeding properly if there were no plans against which to check. Control can therefore include not only taking corrective action if objectives are not being met, but also revising the plans and the objectives themselves if circumstances require it.

The Interrelationships of Managerial Functions

It is helpful to think of the five managerial functions which we have just outlined as a management cycle. A cycle is a system of interdependent processes and activities. Each activity blends into the other and each affects the performance of the others. As a matter of fact, in your daily supervisory activities you may have often felt that your job looks like a vicious cycle without a beginning or an end. However, if you think of the managerial process as a cycle consisting of the five different functions, it will greatly simplify your job of supervising. As can be seen in Figure 2-1, the five functions flow into each other and at times there is no clear line of demarcation indicating where one function ends and the other begins. Because this is the case it is not possible for any manager to set aside a certain amount of time each day for one or another function. Rather, the effort spent on each function will vary as conditions and circumstances change. But there is little doubt that the planning function must come first. Without plans the manager cannot organize, staff, influence, or control. Therefore, in our later discussions we shall follow this sequence of planning first, then organizing, staffing, influencing, and controlling.

FIGURE 2-1

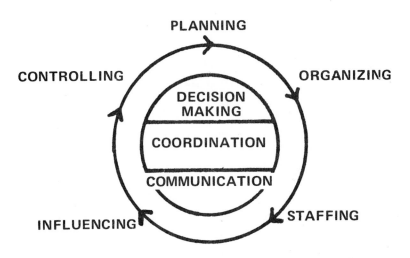

It is worthwhile to repeat that although we can separate the five managerial functions in our minds, in the daily job of the manager these activities are inseparable. Each function blends into the other and each affects the performance of the others. The output of one provides the input for another. That is why we are able to think of these functions as elements of a system such as is shown in Figure 2-2.

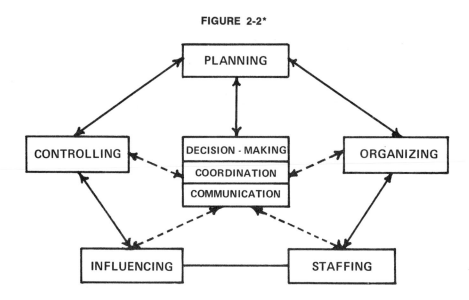

FIGURE 2-2*

*Adapted from Theo Haimann and William G. Scott, *Management in the Modern Organization* (Boston: Houghton Mifflin Company, 1970), p. 2. Reprinted with permission of the publisher.

The Universality of the Managerial Functions

As stated earlier, the managerial functions are universal. They are the responsibility of all managers regardless of whether they are the chairman of the board, the administrator, or the supervisor on the firing line. All of them perform all five functions. However, the time and effort that each manager devotes to each of these five functions will vary, depending upon the level within the administrative hierarchy on which he finds himself. For example, a chief administrator will spend more time in the planning and organizing functions and less time staffing, influencing, and controlling. A supervisor of a department, on the other hand will probably spend less of his time in planning and organizing and more of his time in staffing, and particularly in influencing and controlling. But the supervisor must still do some planning. The administrator will plan, let us say, for one year ahead, for five years ahead, or for even ten or twenty years ahead. You, as a supervisor, will make plans of much shorter duration. There are times when you may have to make plans for six months or so, but more frequently you will just make plans for the next four weeks, for this week, or even for this day or this shift. In other words, the span and the magnitude of your plans will be smaller. Nevertheless, you, as a supervisor, will plan just as the administrator plans.

The same is true of the influencing function. The administrator, if he is a capable administrator, will spend a minimum of time in direct supervision. You, as a supervisor, however, are concerned with getting the job done each and every day, and you will have to spend a large part of your time in this influencing or directing function. Therefore, we may repeat that all managers perform the same managerial functions regardless of their level in the hierarchy, but that the time and effort involved in each of these functions will depend on the rung of the administrative ladder. This is illustrated in Figure 2-3. Let us not forget, however, that unless a manager performs all five functions, he is not fulfilling his managerial duties.

FIGURE 2-3

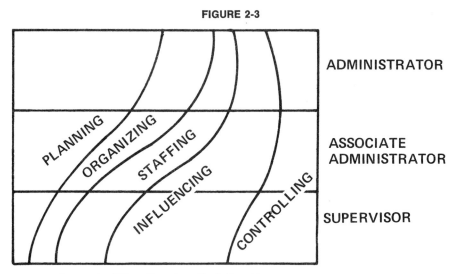

Amount of Time Spent on Each Function.

AUTHORITY

The second factor which earmarks a manager is the possession of authority. As with the managerial functions, the absence of authority means that you are not dealing with a true manager. But what is this authority without which the supervisor cannot be considered a manager? What is this authority which makes the managerial position real? Briefly speaking, authority can be defined as legal or rightful power, the right to act. It is the power by which a manager can ask his subordinates to do or not to do a certain thing which he, as the possessor of authority, deems appropriate and necessary in order to realize the objectives of the department. It is important to note that authority is not actually delegated to people but to positions within the enterprise. Unless these positions are manned by people, however, the delegation of authority would be meaningless. That is why one commonly speaks of the manager's authority rather than of the authority of the managerial position.

Our concept of authority must also include the possession of power to impose sanctions and to coerce. In case a subordinate refuses to carry out the manager's directive, his authority must include the right to take disciplinary action and, in the last instance, to discharge the employee. Without such power to enforce an order, the enterprise could become disorganized and chaos could result. Of course, this negative type of authority has many restrictions and limitations. These may be in the form of legal restrictions, union contracts, or considerations of morals, ethics, and human behavior. In the latter category, for example, every successful manager knows that in order to induce his subordinates to perform required duties it is best not to coerce them, but to utilize other ways and means to get the job done. In other words, it is far better not to depend on the negative aspects of power and authority. As a matter of fact, in practice most managers do not speak of authority at all. They prefer to speak of the "responsibility" or the "tasks" or "duties" which they have. Such managers rightfully consider it better human relations to say that they have the responsibility for certain activities instead of saying that they possess the authority within that area. Using the words responsibility, tasks, and duties in a loose sense allows the manager to avoid the big stick.

But as a supervisor you should not be misled by the loose use of these terms. You should know that having authority delegated to you means that you have the power and right to issue directives. You should know that tasks and duties have been assigned to you and that you have accepted the responsibility for getting them done. This responsibility has been exacted from you by your superior. It is important to understand that the concept of responsibility is always connected with authority. They go hand in hand and one cannot exist without the other.

In Chapter 9 we shall discuss the concepts of authority and responsibility in far greater detail. At that time we shall also examine how subordinates and workers react to authority, and how authority is delegated. This latter means the process by which a supervisor receives authority from his superior manager, as well as the process by which he delegates some of the authority which has been delegated to him to his own subordinate managers. Just as the possession of authority is the lifeblood of any managerial position, this process of delegating authority to the lower ranks within the managerial hierarchy makes it possible to build an organizational structure with effective managers on every level. These points will become clearer in our later discussions. At this time, it will suffice to remember that authority is one of the basic earmarks of the managerial job. Without authority the other earmark of management, the managerial functions, would be meaningless and management itself would cease to exist.

SUMMARY

The five managerial functions of planning, organizing, staffing, influencing and controlling are the first earmark of the manager's job. Each of these functions blends into the other, and each affects the performance of the others. The output of one provides the input for another. These five functions are universal for all managers regardless of where he stands in the managerial hierarchy. The time and effort involved in each of these functions will vary depending on the rung of the administrative ladder the manager occupies.

A second earmark of the managerial job is the possession of authority; it makes the managerial position real. This organizational authority is delegated to positions within the organization. Since these positions must of necessity be staffed by people, one commonly speaks of the manager's authority rather than of the authority of the managerial position.

PART TWO

The Connecting Processes

CHAPTER 3

Decision-Making

We have just seen that the earmarks of a manager are his authority and his performance of the five managerial functions. We have also seen that these five functions are interrelated and interconnected. This is the case partly because we find that binding the five managerial functions together are three connecting processes, namely decision-making, coordination, and communication. These connecting processes are not functions in and of themselves; rather they link the functions together into a continuous management system and make it possible for the manager to run his department as a smoothly working unit which is an integral part of a larger institution and of a total health care system.

Decision-making, coordination, and communication are essential to the performance of each of the managerial functions. For example, when the manager plans he most certainly must make decisions, he must also coordinate these decisions so that they will not contradict one another or result in duplication of effort, and finally, he must communicate his decisions to those who are to carry them out. Similarly, when the manager performs his organizing function he must make decisions as to the kind of organizational structure to set up, he must coordinate this structure with that of the rest of the institution, and he must communicate and explain it to his subordinates so that they will understand their place and their duties in relation to each other and to the whole. The same pattern of deciding, coordinating, and communicating holds true for the other functions of staffing, influencing, and controlling.

Thus, we can see that the three connecting processes are a vital force for all the managerial functions and must be developed in order to hold the managerial system together. Since they overlay the functions, so to speak, these three processes will be discussed in separate chapters before we go into the detailed analysis of each of the functions.

DECISION-MAKING

If you were to ask practicing managers to define in one or two words the essence of their jobs, they would very likely reply that what permeates their jobs more than anything else is "making decisions." This process of decision-making is in reality at the heart of all five managerial functions. As a matter of fact, to make decisions is a substantial part of everybody's activities. All of us have to solve problems in many areas of endeavor. Therefore, decision-making or problem-solving should not be foreign to us. However, for many of the problems with which we are confronted in our daily lives we have found a pat answer. Solving these problems does not usually cause us much difficulty because we are quite familiar with them. But when new problems confront us, problems which are of considerable significance and which cover unfamiliar situations, then we find it increasingly difficult to make decisions.

THE IMPORTANCE OF DECISION-MAKING SKILLS

In your experience as a supervisor you are constantly called upon to find practical solutions to problems which are caused by changing situations or unusual circumstances. Normally, you are able to arrive at a satisfactory decision. As a matter of fact, one reason why you are in a supervisory position is that you have made many more correct decisions than wrong decisions as problems presented themselves. It is true that many of the decisions you have made cover problems which arise out of the daily working situation; nevertheless, they are real problems which required you to come to a conclusion as to what should be done.

All managers go through — or should go through — the very same process of problem-solving or decision-making that you go through as a supervisor. The only difference is that the decisions made at the top of the administrative hierarchy are usually more far-reaching and affect more people and areas than those which you have to make within your own department. Thus, decision-making, like the five managerial functions, is an essential process which permeates the entire administrative hierarchy.

Of course, it must be kept in mind that once a decision has been made, effective action is necessary. Every decision made should be put into practice and should be carried out. Obviously, there is nothing as useless as a good decision about which nobody does anything. But getting effective action is not the problem with which we are concerned in this chapter. Our other chapters will deal mainly with ways in which the manager can achieve effective action. At the present time, however, we will discuss the process which should come *before* the action, the process which you as a manager should go through in order to decide what action to take.

Let us be a little bit more specific about the timing of this decision-making process. When we think of a man as a decision-maker, a picture often comes to our mind of an executive with horn-rimmed glasses bent over some papers, his pen in his hand ready to sign on the dotted line. Or we picture a gentleman in a smoke-filled board of directors meeting raising his arm to vote a certain way. Such images have one point in common: they portray the decision-maker at the very moment of choice when he is ready to select one alternative which leads him from the crossroads down a particular path of action. We do not want to emphasize this moment of decision-making here because it cannot describe the long, difficult process which must come before the final moment of selecting one alternative over the other.

But although it is long and difficult, the decision-making process is worthwhile knowing for, like the managerial skills, the skills involved in decision-making can be learned and once they are learned they provide great benefits for the manager. These benefits will, of course, accrue to the manager no matter what position he is in because the decision-making process is used throughout the entire administrative organization. Moreover, it is important to note that your managerial job involves not only making decisions yourself, but also seeing to it that those who work under you make decisions effectively. Obviously, a supervisor cannot make all the decisions necessary for running his department himself. Many of the daily decision-making activities for which you as a supervisor are responsible will be delegated by you to your subordinates. It is therefore necessary that you train your subordinates in this process of making decisions as well as develop better decision-making skills for yourself.

THE DECISION-MAKING PROCESS

As we have said, a decision is something that takes place prior to the actual performance of the action that has been decided upon. It is a conclusion that the manager has reached as to what he or others should do at some later time. Thus, to make a decision means to cut off deliberation and come to a conclusion. However, it is this deliberation which is the essence of the decision-making *process*. That process requires the manager to follow certain steps, arranged in a certain sequence:

1) Define the problem.
2) Analyze the problem.
3) Develop alternative solutions.
4) Decide upon the best solution.

A detailed discussion of each of these steps follows.

Definition of the Problem

You have often heard supervisors say, " I wish I had the answer," or "I wish I had the solution to this," or "I wish I knew what to do about this." All of these "wishes" indicate that the supervisor is overly concerned with having an *answer*. Instead of seeking an answer, however, he should be looking for the problem. His first task is always to find out what the problem is in the particular case in question; only then can he work toward the solution, the answer. As someone has put it, "There really is nothing as useless as having the right answer to the wrong question."

To define the problem, in most cases, is not an easy task. What often appears to be the problem might be merely a symptom of it which shows up prominently on the surface. It is therefore necessary to dig deeper in order to locate the real problem and to define it. For example, it might appear that a supervisor is confronted with a problem of conflicting personalities within his department. Two of his employees are continually quarrelling and cannot get along together. Upon checking into this situation, however, the supervisor may find that in reality it is not a problem of personalities. Rather, the problem is that he, as manager, has never really defined the functions and duties of each employee. He has not specified where the functions begin and where they end; he has never clarified where the other employee takes over.

Thus, what appeared on the surface to be a problem of personal conflict was actually a problem of an organizational and structural nature. Only after he realizes the true nature of the problem, can the supervisor do something about it, and the chances are good that once he clarifies the activities and duties of the two employees, the friction will stop.

There is little doubt that defining a problem like this may be a time-consuming chore, but it is time well spent. There is no need to go any further in the process of decision-making until you as a supervisor have clearly defined your own problems.

Analysis of the Problem

After the problem — and not just the symptoms — has been defined, the manager can set out to analyze it. The first step in the analysis of any problem is to assemble the facts, to gather all pertinent information. Only after a clear definition of the problem can the supervisor decide how important certain data are and what additional information he may need. He will then gather as many facts as he possibly can.

Many supervisors complain, however, that they never have enough facts. Although it is normal for a supervisor to feel that he does not have all the facts he would like to have, this complaint is often just an excuse to delay making a decision. As a manager, you will never have *all* the facts available. Therefore, it is necessary to make decisions on those facts which you do have available and also on those additional facts which you can gather without too much delay and expense.

At the same time, it is wise to remember that what is considered a fact is to a certain extent colored by subjectivity. You should bear in mind that one cannot completely free oneself of the subjective elements involved. As much as we may want to exclude prejudice and bias, we are only human and subjectivity will creep in somehow. Of course, we should make an effort to be as objective as possible in gathering and examining facts. However, the process of analysis requires the supervisor to think not only of objective considerations but also of intangible factors which may be involved. These are very difficult to assess and to analyze, but they do play a significant role especially in health care institutions. These intangibles may be factors of reputation, quality of patient care, morale, discipline, etc. It is hard to be specific about such factors, but you should nevertheless take them into consideration in the analysis of the problem on which you have to come to a decision.

Development of Alternatives

After having defined and analyzed the problem, the manager's next step is to search for and develop various alternative solutions. As a manager, you must make it an absolute rule that all possible alternatives will be taken into consideration. Always bear in mind that the decision you finally make can only be as good as the best of the alternatives which you considered. It can never be better than the best alternative you thought of. Therefore, the more alternatives you have, the greater the likelihood that the best is among them.

It is almost unthinkable that a situation should not offer at least several alternatives. These choices, however, might not always be obvious, yet it is the duty of the manager to search for them. Also, some of the alternatives may not be desirable, but the manager should not decide this until he has carefully considered all of them. If he does not do this, he is likely to fall into the "either-or" kind of thinking. You have often heard it said after one minute's deliberation: "There is only one of two things that we can do, namely, ... or ...." The type of manager who says this is too easily inclined to see only one of these two alternatives as the right one to follow.

Nor is it enough for you as a supervisor to decide between the various alternatives with which you have been presented by your subordinates. The routine alternatives normally suggested by them may not include all the possible choices. It is your job as a manager to conceive of more and possibly better alternatives. Even in the most discouraging situations there are several choices and although none of them may be desirable, the manager still has a choice to make. Let us suppose that a business concern is in financial difficulties. The creditors have the choices of driving the enterprise into bankruptcy, agreeing to a moratorium to extend the payment of the bills for approximately a year, or compromising on a small percentage of the outstanding debts and thus clearing out the indebtedness. Here in a most unpleasant situation the creditors have three alternatives, none of which of course is desirable; but alternatives do exist and there is a choice.

Evaluation and Selection From Among Alternatives (Choice)

As stated above, the purpose of decision-making is to select or choose from among the various alternatives that specific one which will provide the greatest amount of wanted consequences and the smallest amount of unwanted consequences. After developing the alternatives, the manager should test each of them by imagining that he had already put each into effect. He should try to foresee the probable desirable and undesirable consequences of each. Once he has thought them through and appraised their consequences, he will be in a position to compare the desirability of the various alternatives.

In making this comparison, the supervisor should bear in mind the degree of risk which is involved in each course of action. He must remain aware of the fact that there is no such thing as a riskless decision, and that one alternative will simply have more or less risk than another. It is also possible that the question of timing will make one alternative preferable to another. There is usually a difference in the amount of time required to carry out each alternative and this should be considered by the supervisor. Moreover, in this process of evaluating the different alternatives, the supervisor should also bear in mind the resources, facilities, know-how, equipment, records, and so on which are available to him. Finally, he should not forget to judge the different alternatives along the lines of economy of effort; in other words, which action will give the greatest result for the least amount of effort and expenditure.

Using the above criteria of risk, timing, resources, and economy, it is often possible for the manager to see that one alternative clearly provides a greater number of desirable consequences and fewer unwanted consequences than any other alternative. In such cases, his decision is a relatively easy one. However, the choice of the best alternative is not always so obvious. It is conceivable that at certain times two or more alternatives may seem equally desirable. In such a case, the choice is simply a matter of the manager's personal preference. On the other hand, it is also possible for the manager to feel that no single alternative far outweighs any of the others or is sufficiently stronger. In this case, it might be advisable for him to combine two of the better alternatives and come up with a compromise solution.

But what about a situation where the manager finds that none of the alternatives is satisfactory and that all of them have too many undesirable effects? As a supervisor, you might have been in a situation where the undesirable consequences of all the alternatives were so overwhelmingly bad that they paralyzed any action. At such a time, you might have thought that there was only one available solution to the problem, namely, to take no action at all. However, in so thinking you were deceiving yourself. A supervisor is wrong to believe that taking no action will get him "off the hook." In practice, taking no action is as much a decision as deciding to take a specific action, although few people are aware of this. Most people feel that taking no action relieves them of making an unpleasant decision. The only way for the manager to avoid this pitfall is to try to visualize the consequences of his inaction. The manager need only think through what would happen if no action were taken, and he will probably see that in so doing, he is in reality choosing an undesirable alternative.

Having ruled out inaction in most cases, you may still be in a position where all alternatives that you have considered seem undesirable. In such a case, you would do well to force yourself to search for more and different alternatives. Be a bit creative and try to develop at least a couple of new solutions. Also check to see that all the steps of the decision-making process have been followed. Has the problem been clearly defined, have all the pertinent facts been gathered and analyzed, and finally, have you really thought of all possible alternatives? Chances are that some new solutions will be thought of and that a good decision can then be made. In making this decision, however, you might have to employ some additional factors such as experience, intuition, and actual testing.

Experience

The manager's final selection from among the various alternatives is frequently influenced and guided by past experience. History often repeats itself, and the old saying that "experience is the best teacher" still holds true. There is no denying that the manager can often decide wisely on the basis of his own experience or that of other managers. Knowledge gained by past experience can frequently be applied to new situations and no manager should ever underestimate the importance of such knowledge. On the other hand, it is dangerous to follow past experience blindly.

Therefore, whenever the manager calls upon experience as a basis for his choice among alternatives, he should examine the situation and conditions which prevailed at the time of the past decision. It may be that current conditions are still very much the same, and thus the present decision should be the same as the one made on that previous occasion. More often than not, however, you will find that conditions have changed considerably and that the underlying circumstances and assumptions are no longer valid. In these cases, of course, the decision should not be the same.

Previous experience can also be very helpful in the event the manager is called upon to substantiate his reasons for making a particular decision. Experience is a good defense tactic and many superiors use it as valid evidence. But there is still no excuse for following experience blindly. Past experience must always be viewed with the future in mind. The underlying circumstances of the past, the present, and the future must be considered. Only within this framework is experience a helpful approach to the selection of the best alternative.

Hunch and Intuition

Managers will at times admit that they have based their decisions on hunch and intuition. At first glance, it might seem that certain managers have an unusual ability for solving problems satisfactorily by intuitive means. However, a deeper search will disclose that the "intuition" on which the manager thought he had based his decision was actually past experience or knowledge. In reality, the manager is recalling similar situations in which he had been involved previously and which are now stored in his memory; but he labels this type of recall "having a hunch." No superior would look favorably upon a subordinate who continually justified his decisions on the basis of intuition or hunch alone. These factors might come into play once in a while but they must always be supplemented by more concrete considerations.

Experimentation

The avenue of experimentation or testing is another approach to decision-making. In the scientific world where conclusions are reached through laboratory tests, experimentation is essential. But in the field of management it is often too costly and too time consuming to experiment to see what happens. Moreover, it is difficult to maintain controlled conditions and to test various alternatives fairly in a normal workday environment. There may be certain instances, however, where a limited amount of testing and experimenting is advisable, as long as the consequences are not too disruptive. For example, a supervisor might decide to test out different work schedules or different assignments of duties. In this small, restricted sense, experimentation may be valid. But, normally, in a supervisory situation experimentation is at best a most expensive way of reaching a decision.

SCIENTIFIC DECISION-MAKING

During the last twenty-five to thirty years a new group of highly sophisticated tools has become available to aid the manager in decision-making. These tools are of a quantitative nature, involving complicated mathematical techniques which can only be applied by mathematicians, statisticians, programmers, systems analysts, or other types of scientists with the help of a computer. The overall process is known as scientific decision-making or operations research.

Of course, only certain kinds of management problems lend themselves to this type of quantitative solution. In a hospital situation, for example, it could be applicable to problems involving scheduling, inventory, arranging the best possible use of facilities and employees during various shifts, planning for the most effective use of existing equipment, etc. However, such scientific problem-solving is often a very complicated and costly way of reaching decisions and it should only be used by the administration when the magnitude of a particular problem warrants considerable effort and expenditure. Normally, the problems with which a single supervisor is confronted are not of this magnitude. But if similar problems are found in several departments, in a whole unit, or a section, it may be advisable for management to employ the quantitative approach. And since many health care centers today have easy access to a computer, it should not be too difficult to contact someone within the computer center to see if they could lend some quantitative assistance in the solution of the problem. The programmers and systems analysts may produce not only an optimum solution, but their research may also lead to other findings which are welcome by-products. However, management should not forget that it could be a long and tedious as well as an expensive process to arrive at a solution through quantitative, scientific decision-making.

ACTION AND FOLLOW-UP

No matter what method has been used to arrive at the solution, it must be kept in mind that effective action is necessary once the decision has been made. There is no use going through the lengthy and tedious decision-making process unless the manager goes all the way and sees to it that his decision is carried out effectively. As stated before, there is nothing so useless as a good decision about which nobody does anything. In other words, decision-making is only one aspect of the manager's job; achieving effective execution of the decision is at least as important. And such execution is impossible without two other essential processes — those of communication and coordination. Unless a decision is clearly communicated to the people who must carry it out and unless it is coordinated with other decisions and other departments, it will be quite meaningless. Thus, we must look more closely at the two additional connecting processes which are vital to management's over-all task of "getting things done through and with people."

SUMMARY

To select the best alternative by facts, study, and analysis of various proposals is still the most generally approved avenue of making a managerial decision. If an objective, rational, systematic method is used in the selection, the manager is likely to make better decisions. The first step in such a method is to define the problem. After you have defined it, you must analyze the problem. Then you must develop all the alternatives you possibly can, think them through as if you had already put them into action, and consider the consequences of each and every one of them. You may also evaluate each alternative on the basis of past experience which you or some other manager have had. By following this method, you will most likely be able to select the best alternative, the one with the greatest amount of wanted and the least amount of unwanted consequences.

Not only can this sound method of decision-making be learned by you, but as a supervisor you can also teach the same systematic step approach to your subordinates. In so doing, you have the assurance that whenever they are confronted with a situation where they have to make a decision they will do it in a systematic manner also. Although this is not always a guarantee for arriving at the best decisions, it is certainly apt to produce more good decisions than would otherwise be the case.

CHAPTER 4

Coordination

THE MEANING OF COORDINATION

We defined management as the process of getting things done through and with people. We also defined it as directing the efforts of individuals toward a common objective. In the final analysis, this means that management involves the coordination of the efforts of all members of an organization. As a matter of fact, some writers have even defined management as the task of achieving coordination or more specifically, of achieving the orderly synchronization of the efforts of employees to provide the proper amount, timing, and quality of execution so that their unified efforts lead to the stated objective namely, the common purpose of the enterprise. Other writers have preferred to look at coordination as a separate managerial function. However, we prefer to look at it not as a separate activity of the manager and not as *the* defining characteristic of management, but as *a process* by which the manager achieves orderly group effort and unity of action in pursuit of the common purpose. The manager engages in this process *while* he performs the five basic managerial functions of planning, organizing, staffing, influencing, and controlling. The resulting coordination, the resulting synchronization of efforts, should be one of the goals that the manager keeps in mind when he performs each of the five managerial functions.

You can probably see that the task of achieving coordination is a much more difficult one on the administrative level than on your supervisory level. The administrator has to achieve the synchronization of efforts throughout the entire organization, throughout all of its many departments. As a supervisor of a single department, you have to carry out this task only within your own division. Nevertheless, the achievement of coordination is necessary regardless of the scope of your division. We have suggested that you look at coordination as something which comes about as you perform your five managerial functions appropriately. Coordination should result as a by-product of performing these functions, and it should not be looked upon as a separate managerial function. As a supervisor, you should

31

bear coordination in mind in everything you do. Thus, synchronizing the efforts of your subordinates should be a prominent consideration whenever you plan, organize, staff, influence, and control.

Coordination and Cooperation

The term *coordination,* however, must not be confused with *cooperation* for there is a considerable difference between them. Cooperation merely indicates the willingness of individuals to help each other. It is the result of a voluntary attitude of a group of people. Coordination is much more inclusive, requiring more than the mere desire and willingness of the participants. For example, consider a group of men attempting to move a heavy object. They are sufficient in number, willing and eager to cooperate with each other, and trying to do their best to move the object. They are also fully aware of their common purpose. However, in all likelihood their efforts will be of little avail until one of them — the manager — gives the proper orders to apply the right amount of force at the right place and the right time. Only then will their efforts be sufficiently coordinated to actually move the object. It is possible that by coincidence mere cooperation could have brought about the desired result. But no manager can afford to rely upon such coincidental occurrence. Although cooperation is always helpful and its absence could prevent all possibility of coordination, its mere presence will not necessarily assure that process. Coordination is therefore superior in order of importance to cooperation.

COORDINATION AND THE FIVE MANAGERIAL FUNCTIONS

We have already stated that as a manager performs his managerial functions he must remember that coordination is one of the desired by-products. Let us look more carefully at how this important by-product is related to each of the five functions as well as to the other connecting processes.

When the manager plans he must strive for coordination immediately. As a matter of fact, the planning stage is the ideal time to bring about coordination. As a supervisor, you must see to it that the various plans within your department are properly interrelated. You should discuss these plans and alternatives with the employees who are to carry them out so that they have an opportunity to express any doubts about synchronization or any objections. If employees are involved in departmental planning at the initial stages, then the supervisor's chances for coordination are good. His employees will get a clear picture of the purpose and direction of their department and will be better able to help achieve departmental and institutional goals.

The same concern for coordination should exist when the manager organizes his department. Indeed, the prime purpose for setting up a structural framework outlining who is to do what, when, where, and how, is to assure coordination. This is the only way to obtain stated objectives in a synchronized fashion. Thus, whenever a manager groups activities and assigns them to various subordinates, the task of coordination should be in his mind. By placing related activities which need to be closely synchronized within the same administrative area, coordination will of course be facilitated.

Moreover, in the process of organizing management defines authority relationships among departments and among employees. It should define them in such a way that coordination will result. Often poor coordination is caused by a lack of understanding of who is to perform what or by the failure of a manager to delegate authority and exact responsibility clearly. Such fuzziness can easily lead to duplication of efforts instead of to synchronization. This is most likely to happen when two subordinates or two departments both feel they are responsible for the same activity.

Coordination should also be in the manager's mind when he performs his staffing function. He must make certain that he has the right number of employees in the various positions to assure the proper performance of their functions. He should see to it that they are of such quality that they will be able to coordinate their efforts willingly.

When a manager influences and directs he is also involved in coordination. As a matter of fact, the very essence of giving instructions, coaching, teaching, and generally supervising subordinates is to coordinate their activities in such a manner that the over-all objectives of the institution will be reached in the most efficient way. Or as some writers have put it in more sophisticated terms, coordination is that phase of supervision which is devoted to obtaining the harmonious and reciprocal performance of responsibilities of two or more subordinates. As a supervisor, you must continuously watch the performance of the different jobs under your direction in order to be sure that they are proceeding harmoniously.

Last but not least, when the manager performs his controlling function he is concerned with coordination. In controlling, he checks to see whether or not the activities of his department conform with the pre-established goals and standards. If he finds any discrepancy, he should take immediate remedial action so goals will be achieved and coordination will be assured at least from then on. Frequent evaluation and correction of departmental operations in this manner helps to synchronize not only the efforts of employees, but also the activities of the entire organization. Thus, by its very nature the controlling process is the one that brings about the overall coordination necessary to lead the organization to its desired objectives.

COORDINATION AND DECISION-MAKING

Since the process of decision-making is at the heart of all managerial functions, achieving coordination must be an overriding thought in every manager's mind whenever he makes decisions. When he chooses from the various alternatives, he must never forget the importance of achieving synchronization of all efforts. Thus, he will select that alternative which is most likely to bring about the best coordination within his department. There may be times when a certain alternative *taken by itself* would seem to constitute the best choice. However, a second choice might result in better coordination throughout the department. In such a case, the supervisor would be far better off to follow the second solution since achieving coordination is an important objective. In other words, each decision a manager makes is an exercise in the synchronization and integration of his department's activities.

COORDINATION AND COMMUNICATION

In all coordination efforts, good communication will be of immeasurable help. It is not enough for a manager to make decisions which will bring about coordination. It is at least as important to have them carried out effectively. In order to achieve successful execution, the supervisor must first be able to communicate his decisions to his subordinates in such fashion that they understand them correctly. Therefore, good communication is actually essential for achieving coordination. Personal oral face-to-face contact is probably the most effective means of communicating to obtain coordination. However, there are other means such as written communications, reports, procedures, rules, bulletins, as well as numerous modern mechanical devices which insure the speedy dissemination of information to employees. Recent developments in electronic data processing can also be of considerable help in communicating and coordinating. The importance of good communication for achieving coordination will become even more obvious as we discuss this final connecting process in the next chapter.

INTERNAL AND EXTERNAL COORDINATION IN HEALTH CARE CENTERS

Due to the proliferation and specialization of medical sciences and technologies, health care centers have become very large and complex organizational structures. More and more positions have had to be created and this increasing division of labor has generated a need for more and better coordination. Of course, the division of labor arises from the recognition that work divided into smaller specialized tasks permits a group of people, performing together, to accomplish more than one individual attempting the whole task by himself. As a result of such specialization, however, the synchronization of daily activities has become extremely complicated and coordination has become increasingly difficult to attain. You yourself know that as the number of positions in your department increases and as more specialized tasks are to be performed, the greater is your need for coordination and synchronization to secure a unified result — namely, the best possible patient care.

As a supervisor, you also know that you must be concerned with more than just coordination inside your own department. You also have to coordinate the efforts of your department with those of many other departments. Of course, the process of bringing about the total coordination of *all* the divisions and levels within a health care facility is primarily the concern of the chief administrator. It is he who must deal with the fact that each special departmental interest in the health care center is likely to stress its own opinion of how the best possible patient care should be accomplished and each is likely to favor one route or another depending upon its particular functions and experience. This problem of different viewpoints also holds true among the numerous levels of the administrative hierarchy. It takes considerable thoughtfulness and understanding on the part of the chief administrator to coordinate the working relationships of the groups above, below, and alongside of each department. Even with cooperative attitudes, self-coordination, and self-adjustment by most members of the health care center, there can still be duplication of actions and conflicts of efforts unless the administration very carefully synchronizes all activities. Only through such coordination can management bring about a total accomplishment which is far in excess of the sum of the individual parts. Although each part is significant, the result can be of greater significance if management achieves success in coordination.

It is very important to emphasize that the task of securing harmonious action and internal coordination within a health care center belongs solely to its regular management. This task cannot be delegated to a specialist, often called a "coordinator". The regular management is in a far better position than any special "coordinator" to view the various functions and to determine how they should be coordinated in order to bring about the desired objective. Although some hospitals do have special positions labeled "coordinator," there are usually regular managerial and supervisory jobs and they should be named as such and not as "coordinators." The important point is that *all* managers must coordinate as they perform their five managerial functions and therefore it is wrong to think that the task of securing internal coordination can be shifted or assigned to a special department or individual.

In addition to this need for internal coordination, however, there exists a need for coordination with factors external to the institution. There are a number of these factors such as changes in the general economy, governmental activities, medical and technological advances, and the interests of the general public in health care facilities. There should also be a certain amount of external coordination between each hospital and other health care institutions and the health care system at large. And in those situations where a hospital is trying to coordinate many of its activities with other health care institutions or with any other external factors, a special coordinator or liaison person may be utilized. Such a person should be thoroughly familiar with the conditions and thinking of his institution, he must be able to explain these to the others with which he is dealing, and he must report the findings and intentions back to his own institution. Normally, however, an external coordinator does not have any authority to commit his institution. In most instances, he will have to check back with the administrator or executive director as to how far his own institution will go to support whatever action has been decided upon. In this sort of a situation, then, we are not dealing with a manager in the same sense that the term is being used in our text.

Nevertheless, the importance of such external coordination should not be underestimated. Obviously, the more external coordination among medical centers and related institutions, the better will be our over-all health care system. Thus, a great deal is being said today about interface relationships, that is, analyzing behavior among health care centers at the point where they are tangent to one another.

But, in the final analysis, management's ever increasing problems of coordination, both internal and external, can only be offset by an ever increasing knowledge of how to perform the managerial skills. Fortunately, this knowledge is becoming broader due not only to the emergence of new tools and devices, but also to a more thorough understanding of the over-all dependence and relationships among health care systems within the community, state, and country.

SUMMARY

Coordination is the orderly synchronization of all efforts of the members of the organization to achieve the stated objectives. It is not a separate managerial function but a by-product which comes about when the manager performs his five managerial functions. There is a significant difference, however, between cooperation and coordination. Although cooperation is always helpful in achieving coordination, the latter is superior in importance to the former.

As a supervisor plans, organizes, staffs, influences, and controls he must remember that he needs to achieve coordination or the synchronization of all efforts. The same overriding thought permeates his mind whenever he makes decisions and communicates these to his employees. Achieving coordination is a valid consideration for all managers regardless of their particular positions, their level within the administrative hierarchy, or the kind of enterprise in which they work. Due to the proliferation and specialization of medical sciences and technologies, the task of obtaining coordination in a health care center has become increasingly difficult. However, coordination is clearly a part of the regular managerial positions in a hospital and cannot be shifted or assigned to a special position labeled "coordinator."

In addition to the need for internal coordination in a hospital, there exists a need for coordination with factors external to the institution such as government agencies, local health councils, and so forth. For this external coordination, a liaison person or special coordinator can be utilized in order to provide the necessary contacts between the hospital and outside factors.

CHAPTER 5

Communication

Communication is the third process which serves to link the managerial functions in an organization. Employees look for and expect communication since it is a means of motivating and influencing people. Communication is vital to them not only for purposes of social satisfaction but also to carry out their jobs effectively. Thus, the communication process fulfills both human needs and institutional needs.

You already know that as a supervisor your job is to plan, organize, staff, influence, and control the work of the employees of your department and to coordinate their efforts for the purpose of achieving departmental objectives. But in order to do this you must explain and discuss the arrangement of the work. You must give directives. You must describe to each subordinate what is expected of him. You will very likely need to speak to your employees regarding their performance. All of this is communication.

As you go on supervising your employees, you probably will come to realize that your skill in communication determines your success. Communication is the most effective tool you have for building and keeping a well-functioning team. Just consider your own job and you will quickly see why communication is essential to successful supervision. Is there any area of responsibility within your job as a supervisor that you could fulfill without communicating? Certainly not.

You probably know some supervisors who are competent, technically knowledgeable, and good mannered. Nevertheless, they do not seem to get anywhere. Deep down you probably know the reason: they cannot use words to sell themselves or to sell their plans; they cannot communicate. And in your career you may also have observed supervisors who have lost their skill in communicating or who think that communication is no longer worth the effort. Before they knew it they lost touch with their employees because they failed to communicate. This ability to communicate is absolutely essential to leadership. It is the only means you as a supervisor have to take charge of and train a group of employees, to direct them, motivate them, and to coordinate their activities so that the goal which you have pointed out can be reached. The problem of communication is vital for any organization. Without effective communication the organizational structure cannot survive.

THE MEANING OF COMMUNICATION

Plainly stated, *communication is the process of passing information and understanding from one person to another*. Communication — fundamental and vital to all managerial functions — is a means of imparting ideas and of making oneself understood by others. The exchange is successful only when mutual understanding results. Since managing is getting things done through others, it is an obvious requirement that the manager communicate with the members of his group.

If you were to estimate it, you would find that as a supervisor you spend approximately ninety percent of your time in either sending or receiving information. Of course, it would be incorrect to assume that real communication is actually taking place all of this time. The mere fact that a supervisor is constantly engaged in sending and receiving messages is most certainly not any assurance that he is an expert in communicating. There is no need to point out to you the many instances where communication has not taken place: where the result has been utter confusion and errors.

We defined communication as the process of passing information and understanding from one person to another. The significant point here is that communication always involves two people: a sender and a receiver. It is wrong to think of communication as merely a matter of sending. There must be a receiver. One person alone cannot communicate; communication is not a one-way street. For example, a man who is stranded on a deserted island and who is shouting at the top of his voice does not communicate because he has no receiver. In such a case, this is obvious. But it may not be so obvious to a manager who sends out a letter. Once he has mailed his letter he is inclined to believe that he has communicated. However, he has not communicated until and unless information and understanding have passed *between himself and the receiver*.

This understanding aspect of communication is another very important part of our definition. Effective communication requires not only two people but also the two ingredients of information and understanding. A receiver may hear a sender because he has ears but still not understand what the sender means. Understanding is a personal matter between people. If the idea received by the listener or reader is the one which was intended, then we can say that communication has taken place. If the idea received by him is not the one which was intended, then communication has not taken place; the sender has not communicated, he has merely spoken or written. "Simply telling" somebody something is not enough to guarantee successful communication. As long as there is no reception or imperfect reception of the idea intended, we cannot speak of having communicated.

However, communication does not require the receiver to agree with the statement of the sender. Communication occurs whenever the receiver at least understands what the sender means to convey. Agreement is therefore not necessary for communication to be successful. Two people can fully understand each other and still not agree. Thus, as a supervisor your subordinates do not have to agree with everything that you communicate to them. But they must understand it. No subordinate can be expected to comply with a directive unless there is understanding on his part. Similarly, the supervisor must know how to receive knowledge and understanding in the messages which are sent to him by his subordinates, by his fellow supervisors, and also by his boss.

Only through such communication can policies, procedures, and rules be formulated and carried out. Only with such communication can misunderstandings be ironed out, long-term and short-term plans achieved, and the various activities within a department coordinated and controlled. The success of all managerial functions depends upon effective communication. Communication is a skill which can be acquired. All of us can improve our natural endowments to a great degree and become more effective communicators; in other words, better managers.

FORMAL CHANNELS OF COMMUNICATION

In every organization, the communication network has two distinct but equally important channels: the formal channel of communication and the informal channel, usually called the grapevine.* Both channels carry messages from one person or group to another in downward, upward, sideward, and diagonal directions.

The formal communication channels are established mainly by the organizational structure. They follow the lines of authority from the chief administrator all the way down. You are probably familiar with the expression that messages and information "must go through channels." This, of course, refers to the formal flow of communication through the organizational hierarchy.

Downward Communication

When it moves in a downward direction, this formal flow of communication begins with someone at the top issuing a directive and the next person in the hierarchy passing it along to the men who

*The grapevine is discussed at the end of this chapter.

report to him, and so on further down the line. The downward direction is the one which management relies upon most heavily for its communication. It is used to convey not only directives but also information, objectives, policies, procedures, and so forth to subordinates. The downward flow thus helps to tie the different levels of the organizational structure together.

Upward Communication

Upward communication is a second but equally important direction in which messages flow through the official network. Any person who is charged with supervisory authority accepts an obligation to keep his own superior informed. Moreover, his subordinates must feel free to convey to him their opinions and attitudes and to report on activities and actions regarding their work. Management should encourage a free flow of upward communication, as this is the only means by which it can determine whether or not its messages have been transmitted and received properly and whether or not appropriate action is taking place.

Generally speaking, downward communication starts action by subordinates. Its content is mostly of a directive nature, whereas upward communication is of an informative and reporting nature. As a supervisor, you should encourage and maintain upward communication channels and pay proper attention to the information transmitted through them. You must show that you want the facts and want them promptly. Unfortunately, the reaction of many managers to upward communication is still very much like that of ancient tyrants who executed the "bearer of bad news." In your supervisory capacity, therefore, you must make a deliberate effort to encourage upward communication by showing a genuine desire to obtain and use the ideas and reports of your subordinates, by being approachable, and by recognizing the importance of upward communication. Lack of an effective upward flow will throttle the natural desire of your employees to communicate, will lead to frustration, and will ultimately cause your employees to seek different outlets such as the grapevine.

In addition to encouraging your employees to communicate upward to you, you must likewise communicate upward to your own superior. Every person who has been put into a supervisory position accepts an obligation to keep his own boss informed. As we stated at the outset, the supervisor is the man in the middle. He is not only responsible for providing good communication downward *to* his workers, but he is also responsible for stimulating good communication upward *from* his workers and then for passing this and other information further up to the next higher level in the administrative hierarchy. However, most supervisors will agree with the statement that it is much easier for them to "talk down" to their subordinates than to "speak up" to their superior, especially if they have ever had to tell their boss that they did not meet a certain schedule due to bad planning, or that they forgot to carry out an order, or that something else went wrong.

Nevertheless, it is the supervisor's job to keep his boss advised of up-to-date facts concerning the department. The supervisor should inform his superior of any significant developments as soon as possible after they occur. It would be most unfortunate if the boss were to learn such news elsewhere, because this would indicate that he was not allowing proper upward communication or that you were not providing it. You as a supervisor have the duty to keep him up-to-date even if the information reveals errors that have occurred. It is his right to have complete information, and it is your duty to provide complete information about the functioning of your department. After all, he is still responsible if anything goes wrong.

Moreover, your superior may have to act on what you tell him. Therefore, the information must get to him in time and in a form which will enable him to take the necessary action. As a supervisor, you must assemble all facts that are needed and check them carefully before you pass them on to your boss. Try to be as objective as possible. This, of course, will be quite difficult at times since all subordinates want to appear favorably in the eyes of their boss. Thus, there is a danger that you may want to soften the information a bit so that things will not look quite so bad in his eyes as they actually are. However, it is likely that sooner or later the full extent of the malfunctioning will be discovered. So when difficulties arise it is best to tell your superior what the complete score is even if this means admitting mistakes on your part. Always keep in mind that your boss depends upon his supervisors for upward communication just as you depend upon your employees to pass along their bits of information to you.

Sideward Communication

In addition to downward and upward communication, there is a third direction of communication which is essential for the efficient functioning of an enterprise. This is sideward or lateral communication. It is concerned mainly with communication between departments or people on the same level but in charge of different functions. For example, lateral communication will often take place between the operating room supervisor and the head nurse on the floor.

Diagonal Communication

Diagonal communication, on the other hand, is the flow of messages between positions which are not on the same lateral plane of the organization structure. Communication between line groups such as nursing personnel and staff groups* such as the laundry is an example of diagonal communication. In order to achieve coordination

*See Chapter 8.

among the various functions in any organization, a free flow of both lateral and diagonal communication is absolutely essential.

Once all the formal channels of communication are set up and understood by the employees of an organization, it is necessary that they be used properly. Therefore, the following section will be concerned mainly with the essential media which make the communication process possible, with the many barriers which prevent communication, and with the ways and means which you have available to overcome such barriers. Remember that it is not sufficient merely to have good channels of communication; it is even more important that they be used for real communication in the sense that we have defined it.

THE COMMUNICATION MEDIA

The media for communication can be words, pictures, and actions. Words are, of course, the most important symbols used in the communication process. But it would be wrong to ignore the power of pictures and actions in conveying meaning and understanding to other people.

Pictures

Pictures are visual aids and it is wise for a manager to resort to them from time to time. They are particularly effective if he uses them in connection with well-chosen words to complete a message. Most enterprises make extensive use of pictures in the form of blueprints, charts, drafts, models, posters, and so on. Motion pictures and the comic strips also offer clear proof of the power of pictures to communicate understanding.

Action

Action is another medium used in communication. The manager must not forget that what he does is interpreted as a symbol by his subordinates and that his actions often speak louder than words. Due to his managerial status, all observable acts communicate something to the employee whether he intended it to be so or not. Purposeful silence, gestures, a handshake, a shrug of the shoulder, a smile, all have meaning. For instance, a frown on someone's face may at times mean more than ten minutes of oral discussion or a printed page. By the same token, a manager's inaction is also a way of communication. Moreover, an unexplained action on his part can often communicate a meaning which was not intended. Suppose, for example, that some piece of equipment has been removed from the department without telling employees the reason why. To subordinates apprehensive of a reduction in activities, such unexplained action could be interpreted to carry a message which the supervisor probably had no intention whatsoever of sending.

Spoken and Written Words

Of course, words are the communication medium most widely used in today's "verbal environment." We all know that words can be tricky and that instructions which mean one thing to one employee can have a completely different meaning to someone else. You may have heard the often told story about the maintenance foreman who asked the new worker to go out and paint the canopy in front of the building green. When the foreman checked on the job an hour later he found that the wastecan had been painted bright green. The new employee did not know what a canopy was. Perhaps he should have known, but no one had ever told him. Thus, a supervisor must be extremely careful to define his words clearly in both oral and written communications.

Written Communication

A well balanced communication system, of course, must pay due attention to both the oral and the written media. Although oral communication is the most frequently used, written messages are indispensable in certain activities of the health care field. They provide a permanent record to which the receiver can refer as often as necessary in order to make sure that he understands what has been said. The spoken word, in contrast, generally exists only for an instant. But detailed and specific instructions may be so lengthy and cumbersome that they must be put into writing so that they can be studied for a longer period of time. Also, it is advisable to use the written medium for widespread dissemination of information which may concern many people. Furthermore, there is a degree of formality connected with written communications which orally delivered messages usually do not carry. However, while there are many occasions in the health care field where written messages are necessary, most of the supervisor's communication will take place by word of mouth. Therefore, in the following paragraphs we are primarily referring to spoken or oral communication.

Oral Communication

In most instances, oral communication is superior to the written medium since it normally achieves better understanding and saves time. This is true of both oral telephone and oral face-to-face communication. As a matter of fact, in the supervisor's daily performance man-to-man personal discussions between him and his subordinates are the principal means of two-way communication. Such daily contacts are at the heart of an effective communication system. They provide the most frequently used channels for the exchange of information, points of view, instructions, and motivation. There is no form of written communication that can equal oral, especially the face-to-face oral, communication between a supervisor and his employees. Therefore, the effective supervisor will utilize this medium more than any other. He knows that his subordinates like to see and hear their boss in person, and that oral communication is usually well-received because most people can express themselves more easily and more completely by voice than by writing.

Aside from these features, the greatest single advantage of oral communication is that it provides an immediate *feedback*, although such feedback may only be an expression on the listener's face. By merely looking at the receiver the sender can judge how he is reacting to what is being said. Oral communication thus enables the sender to find out immediately what the receiver is hearing and what he is not hearing. Oral communication also enables the recipient to ask questions right then and there if the meaning is not clear, and the sender can explain his message more thoroughly and clarify unexpected problems raised by the communication. Moreover, the manner and tone of the human voice can endow the message with meaning and shading which even long pages of written words simply could not convey. The manner and tone create the atmosphere of communication and the response is influenced accordingly.

Inasmuch as this is the case, the good communicator must be concerned with the total impact of his message. He must be aware of the listener and of his responses, both verbal and non-verbal. These responses will provide him with the feedback which will indicate whether or not his message is getting across. If not, the communicator must search for the reason why. He must be familiar with the many barriers to effective communication which may plug the communication lines. In other words, the effective communicator must realize that the speaker and the listener are two separate individuals who live in different worlds and that there are many factors which can interfere and play havoc with the messages that pass between them. Always remember that there is no communication until and unless the meaning which is received by the listener is the same as that which the sender intended to send. Therefore, we must now turn to those factors which may create a roadblock to the intended meaning of a communication. Afterwards, we shall discuss ways and means of successfully overcoming these roadblocks.

ROADBLOCKS TO COMMUNICATION

All of you are familiar with the confusions, frictions, and inconveniences that arise when communications break down. These breakdowns are not only costly in terms of money, but they also create misunderstandings which may hurt your teamwork and morale. Indeed, many of a supervisor's problems are due to faulty communication. That is, the way you as a supervisor communicate with your subordinates is the essence of your relationship, and most problems of human relations grow out of poor communications or even lack of communication. Although the number of communication barriers is large, the more important ones can be grouped into three general categories. These are language barriers, status and position barriers, and barriers due to general resistance to change.

Language Barrier

Normally, words serve us well and we generally understand each other. But it sometimes happens that the same words may suggest different meanings to different people. In such a case, the words themselves create a barrier to communication. You have often heard it said that people on different levels "speak a different language." There are many instances where a frustrating conversation ends with the admission that "we are just not speaking the same language," yet both participants have been conversing in English. In order to avoid such a breakdown in communication the communicator should use the language of the receiver and not his own language. He should speak a language which the receiver is used to and which he understands. It is not a question of whether the receiver *ought* to understand it; the question is, simply, does he? The supervisor must therefore use plain, simple words — direct, uncomplicated language.

Of course, this is difficult at times because the English language assigns several meanings to one word. For example, the word "round" has many meanings. We speak of round as a ball — he walks round and round — a round dozen of eggs — a round trip — a round of beef — round as a cylinder, etc., etc. When using words which have such different meanings, the communicator must be certain that he clarifies the exact meaning he intends. He should not just assume that the receiver will interpret the word in the same way he does. Always bear in mind that the listener tends to listen and to interpret the language based on *his own* experience and frame of reference, not yours.

Barriers Due to Status and Position

It cannot be denied that an organizational structure and the resulting administrative hierarchy creates a number of different status levels among the members of an enterprise. Status refers to the regard and attitude which is displayed and held toward a particular position and its occupant by the other members of the organization. There is certainly a difference in status between the level of the administrator and that of the supervisor, and between the level of the supervisor and that of his employees. This difference in status and position becomes more apparent as one level communicates with the other.

For example, when an employee listens to a message from his supervisor several factors become operative. First of all, the employee evaluates what he hears in relation to his own position, background, and experience; he also takes the sender into account. It is difficult for a receiver to separate what he hears from the feelings he has about the person who sends the message. It often happens therefore that the receiver adds nonexistent motives to the sender. Union members are frequently inclined to interpret a management statement in a negative manner due to the fact that they are often convinced that management is trying to weaken and undermine the union. Such a mental block obviously does not make for good understanding.

The supervisor who is trying to be an effective communicator must realize that these status and position differences influence the feelings and prejudices of his employees and thus create barriers to his efforts to communicate with them. He can overcome these barriers by putting himself in the employee's place and by trying to analyze and anticipate the employee's reaction before he sends his message. Moreover, not only might the employee evaluate his boss's words differently, but he might also place undue importance upon a superior's gesture, silence, smile, or other facial expression. Simply speaking, the boss's words are not just words; they are words that come from a boss.

Similar obstacles due to status and position also arise in the upward flow of communication since every subordinate is eager to appear favorably in his boss's eyes. Therefore, he conveniently and protectively screens the information which he passes up the line. A subordinate, for example, is likely to tell his superior what the latter likes to hear and will omit or soften what is unpleasant. And by the same token, the subordinate is anxious to cover up his own weaknesses when talking to a person in a higher position. Thus, a supervisor often fails to pass on important information because he believes that such information would reflect unfavorably upon his own supervisory abilities. You can imagine how after two or three protective screenings of this sort by different levels of the administrative hierarchy the message is likely to be considerably distorted or even totally obliterated.

Barriers Due to Resistance to Change

Most people prefer things as they are and do not welcome changes in their working situation. This natural resistance to change can constitute a serious barrier to communication because very often a message intends to convey a new idea to the employee, something which will change either his work assignment, his position, or his daily routine. Many employees resist such a change, feeling that it is safer to leave the existing environment in its present state. Ultimately each and every one of us lives in his own little world; although it may not be a perfect world, we sooner or later learn to make peace with it and to live within it more or less happily.

Consequently, a message which will change this world is greeted with suspicion and the listener's receiving apparatus works just like a filter, rejecting new ideas if they conflict with what he already believes. He is likely therefore to receive only that portion which confirms his present beliefs, and to ignore anything that conflicts. Sometime his filters work so efficiently that in reality he does not hear at all. Even if he does hear, he will either reject that part of the message as false or he will find some convenient way of twisting its meaning to fit his preconceived ideas. Ultimately, the receiver hears only what he wishes to hear. If he is insecure, worried, and fearful in his position this barrier to receiving communication becomes even more powerful.

As a supervisor, you may have been confronted with situations where it appeared that a subordinate only half listened to what you had to say. Your employee was so busy and preoccupied with his own thoughts that he paid attention exclusively to the ideas he had hoped to hear. He simply selected those parts of the total communication which he could readily use. The information which he did not care for or which he considered irreconcilable was just conveniently brushed aside, not heard at all, or easily explained away. The selective perception of information constitutes a serious barrier to a supervisor's communications, particularly when the message he intends to convey contains a change, a new directive, or anything which could conceivably interfere with the employee's routine or working environment. But only if a supervisor is aware of such reactions can he anticipate the difficulties and attempt to word his messages in a way which will not seem so threatening to the employee. This is why it is important for you as a supervisor to be familiar with the usual manner in which your subordinates react toward any change.

Additional Barriers to Communication

In addition to the above-mentioned barriers, there are many other road-blocks to communication which arise in specific situations. For example, there are obstacles due to emotional reactions such as deep-rooted feelings and prejudice, as well as obstacles due to physical conditions such as inadequate telephone lines or lack of a private place in which to talk. Or it may be indifference, the "don't care" attitude, which stands in the way of communication. In such a case, the message may get through all right, but it is acted upon only half-heartedly or not at all. Or there may be complacency on the subordinate's part which prevents the message from getting across.

All of these and many other barriers form serious roadblocks to clear communication. Unless the supervisor is familiar with such road-blocks, he is in no position to overcome them. He should not just assume that the messages which he sends will be received as intended. Since the effectiveness of the supervisory job depends largely on the accurate transmission of messages and orders, the manager must do everything within his power to overcome these barriers and to improve communication.

MEANS FOR PREVENTING AND OVERCOMING BARRIERS TO COMMUNICATION

There are numerous ways and means of preventing and overcoming the major communication barriers. These can be expressed in terms of a few essential rules which we shall now discuss.

Prepare Adequately

The first step toward preventing communication barriers from arising is to know exactly what you want to communicate. You must think the idea through until it becomes hard and solid in your mind — do not just proceed with imprecise thoughts and desires that you have not bothered to put into final form. Only if you understand your ideas can you be sure that another person will understand your instructions. Therefore, know what you want to communicate and plan the sequence of steps necessary to attain it. Study the subject until it is so clear in your own mind that you have no difficulty explaining it. In other words, do not start talking or writing before you know what you are going to say.

For example, if you want to make a job assignment, be sure that you have analyzed the job thoroughly so that you can explain it properly. If you are searching for facts, decide in advance what information you will need so that you can ask intelligent, pertinent, and precise questions. If your discussion will entail a disciplinary problem, be certain that you have sufficiently investigated the case and have enough information before you reprimand or even penalize. Briefly speaking, take care that you do not start to communicate before you know what you are going to say and what you intend to achieve by your communication.

Obtain Feedback

Once you are in the process of communicating, feedback is probably the most effective tool you have to prevent roadblocks. The sender must always be on the alert for some signal or clue indicating that he is being understood. Merely asking the receiver and getting a simple "yes, sir" answer is not usually enough. Most of the time more than this is required to make sure that the message is received as intended and that understanding is actually taking place.

The simplest way to obtain such reassurance is to observe the receiver and judge his responses by non-verbal clues such as a facial expression of bewilderment or understanding, the raising of an eyebrow, or a frown. This kind of feedback is, of course, only possible in face-to-face communication, and it is one of the outstanding advantages of using the oral face-to-face channels. Another way of obtaining feedback is for the sender to ask the receiver to repeat in his own words the information that has just been transmitted. This is much more satisfactory than merely asking the receiver whether or not he understands or if the instruction is clear, both of which require only a yes answer.

If the receiver can state in his own words the content of the message, then the sender will really know exactly what the receiver has heard and what he did or did not understand. At the same time, the receiver may ask additional questions which the sender can answer right there and then. This direct feedback is probably the most useful way to make certain that a message has gotten across. Without being aware of it, you as a supervisor have probably already been using the principle of feedback in your daily communications with subordinates.

Use Direct and Simple Language

Another helpful way to overcome roadblocks in communication is for the manager to use words which are as understandable and simple as possible. Long, technical, and complicated words should be avoided. As we said before, the sender should use language which the receiver will actually understand and not language which he ought to understand. The single most important question is not whether he should have understood it, but, rather, did he understand it?

Listen Effectively

An additional means for overcoming barriers to communication is for the sender to take more time to listening effectively. Due to different backgrounds, education, etc. the world of the subordinate is often significantly different from that of the superior. Yet some common ground is necessary for understanding. Therefore, you must give the other party a chance to tell what is on his mind. The only way you can convince the other party of your interest in him and your respect for his opinions is to listen to him carefully and completely.

The supervisor who pays attention and listens to what his subordinate is saying learns more about him and more about his job. In other words, he learns more about the employee's values and relationships to his working environment. There is no need to agree, but there is a great need for the supervisor to try to understand the other person. It may even be advisable for him to state from time to time what has been expressed by asking the common question, "Is this what you mean?" The listener must be patiently listening to what the other person has to say even though he may believe it to be unimportant. Such listening will greatly improve communication since it will reduce misunderstandings. By careful listening, moreover, a speaker can adjust his message to fit the responses and the world of his receiver. This again is the great advantage which oral communication has over written messages.

However, it should be noted that careful listening is not as easy as it might seem. Much of the difficulty in listening is caused by the fact that the speed of thought moves several times faster than the speed of speech. It is too easy for the listener to let his mind wander and daydream. Instead, he should make an effort to use the idle time for thinking, to use the lag between speech and thought to concentrate on what is being said. The listener can do this by summarizing in his mind what the speaker has said, by trying to read the thoughts behind the words, by analyzing their implications. The fact that the mind is actively working on what the other party is saying improves listening skill. One of the worst things a listener can do is to sit with faked attention while his mind is on a mental daydreaming excursion. Only by actually tuning in to the world and thinking of the other party can mutual understanding take place. Thus, in order to communicate successfully, the sender must also be a good receiver; in other words, an effective listener.

Remember That Actions Speak Louder Than Words

The manager who fails to bolster his talk with action fails in his job as a communicator no matter how capable he is with words. A supervisor must realize that he communicates by his actions as much as by his words. As a matter of fact, actions usually speak even louder than words. Therefore, one of the best ways to give meaning to a message is to behave accordingly. Whether he likes it or not, the supervisor's superior position makes him the center of attention for his employees, and he communicates through all observable actions regardless of whether or not he intended to do so. If his verbal announcements are backed up by appropriate action, it will help the supervisor overcome barriers to communication. However, if the supervisor says one thing but does another, sooner or later his employees will "listen" primarily to what he "does." For example, a statement by the Director of Nursing Services that she is always available to see a subordinate with a problem will have no meaning whatsoever if she keeps her door closed all the time.

Be Redundant

Another means of preventing barriers to communication is for a supervisor to repeat his message several times, preferably using different words and means of explanation. A certain amount of redundancy is especially advisable when each word is important or when the directives are complicated. The degree of redundancy will, of course, depend both upon the content of the message and the experience and background of the employee. But the sender must caution himself not to be so repetitious that his message may be ignored because it sounds overly familiar. However, in case of doubt a degree of repetition is safer than none.

THE GRAPEVINE: THE INFORMAL CHANNEL OF COMMUNICATION

At the beginning of this chapter we stated that in addition to the formal communication channels, there is an informal network of communication commonly referred to as the grapevine. Although the management tries its best to develop sound formal channels, informal systems will also emerge within an organization. Every organization has its grapevine. It is a logical outgrowth of the informal groupings of people, their social interaction, and their natural desire to communicate with each other. The grapevine must be looked upon as a perfectly natural activity. It fulfills the subordinate's desire to be "in the know" and to be kept posted on the latest information. The grapevine also gives the members of the organization an outlet for their imagination and an opportunity to relieve their apprehensions in the form of rumors. At the same time, it offers the supervisor excellent insight into what his subordinates think and feel. An efficient manager will acknowledge the grapevine's presence and will put it to good use if possible.

The Workings of the Grapevine

Sometimes the grapevine carries factual information and news, but most of the time it carries inaccurate information, half-truths, rumors, private interpretations, suspicions, and other various bits of distorted information. The grapevine is active all day long and it spreads information with amazing speed, often faster than most official channels could. The grapevine has no definite pattern or stable membership. Its path and behavior cannot be predicted, and the path followed yesterday is not necessarily the same as today or tomorrow.

Most of the time only a small number of employees will be active participants in the grapevine. The vast majority of employees hear information through the grapevine but do not pass it along. Any person within an organization is likely to become active in the grapevine on one occasion or another. However, there are some individuals who tend to be active more regularly than others. They feel that their prestige is enhanced by providing the latest news, and hence they do not hesitate to spread the news or even change it so as to augment its "completeness" and "accuracy." These active participants in the grapevine know that they cannot be held accountable, so it is understandable that they exercise a considerable degree of imagination whenever they pass information along. The resulting "rumors" give them as well as other members of the organization an outlet for getting rid of their apprehensions. In general, the grapevine serves as a safety valve for the emotions of all subordinates, providing them with the means to freely say what they please without the danger of being held accountable. Since everyone knows that it is nearly impossible to trace the origins of a rumor, employees can feel quite safe in their obscurity as they participate in the grapevine.

Uses of the Grapevine

Because the grapevine often carries a considerable amount of useful information in addition to distortions, rumors, and half-truths, it can help to clarify and disseminate formal communication. It often spreads information which could not be disseminated through the official channels of communication.

The manager should accept the fact that he can no more eliminate the grapevine than he can abolish the informal organization that develops among employees. It is unrealistic to expect that rumors can be stamped out; the grapevine is bound to flourish in every organization. In order to deal with it the supervisor must tune in on the grapevine and learn what it is saying. He must look for the meaning of the grapevine's communication, not merely for its words. He must learn who the leaders are and who is likely to spread the information. He must also learn that by feeding the grapevine facts, he can counter rumors and half-truths. This is one way to utilize the grapevine's energy in the interest of management.

The wise supervisor will, of course, have to tailor his use of the grapevine to suit the particular needs of the situation. He will realize that rumors can be caused by several different factors such as wishful thinking and anticipation, uncertainty and fear, or even by malice and dislike. For example, it is quite common for an employee who wants something badly enough to suddenly start passing the word. If he wants a raise, he may start a rumor that management will give everybody an across-the-board pay increase. No one knows for certain where or how it started, but this story spreads like wildfire. Everyone wants to believe it. Of course, it is bad for the morale of a group to build up their hopes in anticipation of something that will not happen. If such a story is getting around which the supervisor realizes will lead to disappointment, he ought to move quickly to debunk it by presenting the facts. A straight answer is almost always the best answer. In other words, the best prescription for curing this type of rumor is factual medicine.

The same prescription applies to rumors caused by fear or uncertainty. If, for example, the activities of an enterprise decline and management is forced to lay off some employees, stories and rumors will quickly multiply. In such periods of insecurity and anxiety the grapevine will become more active than at other times. Usually the rumors are far worse than what actually happens. Here again, it is better to give the facts than to conceal them. If the supervisor does not disclose the facts, the employees will make up their own "facts" which are usually a distortion of reality. In many instances, much of the fear and anxiety can be eliminated if the facts of what will happen are disclosed. Continuing rumors and uncertainty are likely to be more demoralizing than even the most unpleasant facts. Thus, it is usually best to explain immediately why employees are being laid off, why orders are being given, and so on. When emergencies occur, when new procedures are introduced, when policies are changed, explain why. Otherwise your subordinates will make up their own explanations and often they will be incorrect.

There may be situations, however, where you as a supervisor do not have the correct facts either. In such instances, let your superior know what is bothering your employees. Ask your superior for specific instructions as to what information you may give, how much you may tell, and when. Next meet with your chief assistants and lead employees. Give them the story and guide their thinking. Then they can spread the facts before anyone else can spread the rumors.

Although this procedure may work with rumors caused by fear or uncertainty, it might not be appropriate for rumors which arise out of dislike, anger, or malice. Once again, the best prescription is to try to be objective and impersonal and to come out with the facts if this is possible. Sometimes, however, a supervisor will find that the only way to stop a malicious rumor peddler is to expose him personally and then reveal the untruthfulness of his statement. A superior should always bear in mind that the receptiveness of any group to rumors of this type is directly related to the strength of the supervisor's leadership and the respect his subordinates have for him. If your employees believe in your fairness and good supervision they will quickly debunk any malicious rumor once you have exposed the person who started it or given your answer to it. Thus, you can see that although there is no way to eliminate the grapevine, even its most threatening rumors can be counteracted to management's advantage. Every supervisor, therefore, will do well to listen to the informal channels of communication and to develop his skill in dealing with them.

SUMMARY

In order to perform his managerial functions effectively, a supervisor must realize the importance of good communication. Without it, objectives cannot be achieved. Communication means the process of passing information and understanding from one person to another, from the sender to the receiver. As long as two people understand each other, they have communicated although they may not agree. Agreement is not necessary for communication to be successful.

Throughout every organization there are formal and informal channels of communication. They carry messages downward, upward, sideward, and in diagonal directions. The formal channels are established mainly by the organizational structure and the authority relationships. The position of the supervisor plays a strategic role in the communication process in all of these directions. He is a vital link in every dimension.

Although words are the most significant medium of communication in our "verbal environment," we must not overlook the importance of pictorial language as another meaningful medium in which to communicate. In addition to these two, action is a communication medium which often speaks louder than words. In the health care field, the written word is a major medium of communication. But of all media, oral face-to-face communication is still the most effective one since it provides some sort of immediate feedback.

There are many reasons why messages frequently become distorted or do not come across. There are roadblocks to communication due to language, due to status and position, due to normal resistance to change, and so forth. The supervisor must be aware of these potential barriers and must make an effort to either prevent or overcome them. Feedback is the most effective remedy. The use of direct and simple language will also help. Furthermore, the supervisor must make himself an effective listener by tuning in on the world of the receiver. Since a supervisor communicates not only by what he says but also by what he does, he must make certain that his actions bolster his words and do not contradict them. Often a certain degree of redundancy will also help in preventing and overcoming various roadblocks to communication.

In addition to the formal communication channels, there is an informal network usually referred to as the grapevine. It is a natural outgrowth of the informal organization and the social interactions of people. It serves a useful purpose in every organization. The grapevine spreads information with great speed but without a definite pattern or a stable membership. The supervisor should accept the grapevine as a natural outlet of his employees, he should tune in on it, and even at times feed it and cultivate it.

PART THREE

Planning

CHAPTER 6

The Managerial Planning Function

Planning, the first of the five managerial functions, is the primary task of every manager. Planning is deciding in advance what is to be done in the future. Logically, planning must come first. It must come before any of the other functions because it determines the framework in which the other functions are carried out. Planning vitally influences each of the managerial functions. Every organization must plan ahead because it dare not face the future unprepared. In planning, management is concerned with establishing the objectives to be achieved and determining how to achieve them. Planning information is assembled, planning premises are set out, and decisions are made in order to reach organizational goals. These decisions made in planning provide the other functions with their objectives and standards of performance.

Thus, when the manager plans a course of action for the future, he attempts to achieve a consistent and coordinated structure of operations aimed at the desired results. Of course, plans alone do not bring about these results; in order to achieve them the operation of the enterprise is necessary. But without plans it is likely that only random activities will prevail, producing confusion and possibly chaos.

THE NATURE OF PLANNING

Planning as a Continuous Mental Process and a Primary Function

Planning is mental work, and for many managers it is therefore quite difficult to perform. But there is no substitute for the hard thinking which planning demands. It is necessary to think before acting and to act in the light of facts rather than guesses. For this reason planning is the primary function which must come before the manager can intelligently perform any of the other managerial functions. Only after having made his plans can he organize, staff, influence, and control. How could a supervisor properly and effectively organize the workings of his department without having a plan in mind? How could he effectively staff and supervise his employees without knowing which avenues to follow and without knowing what the objectives are? And how could he possibly control the activities of his employees? He could not perform any of these functions without having planned first.

However, planning does not end abruptly when the supervisor begins to perform the other functions. It is not a process used only at occasional intervals when he is not too engrossed in his daily chores. Rather, planning is a continuous process which must be used consistently every day. By his day-to-day planning, the supervisor realistically anticipates future problems, analyzes them, determines their probable effect on the activities of the enterprise, and decides on the plan of action which will lead to the desired results. In other words, he decides in advance which of the alternative courses are to be followed, which policies, procedures, methods, and so on will be used as the basis of operations.

Planning as a Task of Every Manager

The question often has been raised as to who does the planning. It is the managers who do the planning and it is the job of every manager whether he is the chairman of the board, the chief administrator of a hospital, or the supervisor of a small department. By definition all of them are managers, and therefore all of them must do the planning. However, as we noted in an earlier chapter, the importance and the magnitude of plans will depend upon the level on which they are determined. Naturally, planning on the top level of management is more fundamental and more far-reaching. As we descend toward the supervisory levels of management, the scope and extent of planning becomes narrower and more detailed. Thus, the chief administrator is concerned with the overall aspects of planning for the entire health care center, whereas the supervisor is concerned with plans for getting the job in his department done promptly and effectively each and every day.

Although planning is the manager's function, this does not mean that he cannot call upon others to advise him. A supervisor may feel that certain areas of his planning require special knowledge, for example, those areas dealing with personnel policies, accounting procedures, or technical aspects. In such instances, he must feel free to call upon specialists within the organization to help him with his planning responsibilities. In other words, a manager should avail himself of all the possible help he can get to effectively do his planning. But in the final analysis it is still his responsibility to plan.

Planning as a Cost-Saver

Planning is important because it makes for purposeful organization and activities which in turn minimize costs. Deciding in advance what is to be done, how and by whom, where it is to be done, and when, promotes efficient and orderly operations. All efforts are directed toward a desired result, haphazard approaches are minimized, activities are coordinated, and duplications are avoided. A minimum amount of time is needed for the completion of each planned activity because only the necessary amount of work is done. Facilities are used to their best advantage and guesswork is also eliminated. Thus, we can see that planning by its very nature is a cost-saving activity which no manager can afford to neglect.

As a supervisor you are entrusted with the management of both a group of employees and a set of physical resources. You have to work with people and factors such as space, equipment, tools, materials, and so on. Only by planning will you be able to make the best possible use of these resources. Only by planning will you as a supervisor be able to bring out the best in your employees, the most valuable resource you have. Plans for the proper utilization of your physical resources are also essential because of the capital investment that the hospital has made in them. Even in the smallest department the total investment in working space, equipment, tools, materials, and supplies is substantial. Only by planning can all of these resources be utilized most effectively.

THE MAJOR PLANNING CONSIDERATIONS

The Planning Period

For how long a period in the future should the manager plan? Usually a distinction is made between long-range and short-range planning. The exact definition of long-range and short-range planning depends upon the manager's level in the organizational hierarchy, upon the type of enterprise, and the kind of activity in which it is engaged. For all practical purposes, however, short-term planning can be defined as planning which covers a period of up to one year. Long-term planning usually involves a considerably longer interval of time. In recent years, there has been an increasing trend for many health care facilities to plan for five, ten, or even twenty years ahead. The board and the administrator must plan along these lines in addition to making short-term plans.

It is likely that the supervisor's planning period will be short-range, that is, planning for one year at the most, or maybe for six months, one month, one week, or perhaps even just for one day. There are activities in certain departments for which a supervisor can definitely plan three, six, nine, or twelve months in advance; for instance, the planning of preventive maintenance by the engineering department. On the other hand, there are those activities in a hospital or related health facility where most supervisory planning will be for a shorter time, namely a week, a day, or only a shift. Such short-range planning is frequently needed in nursing services. For example, it is more desirable if the supervisor is able to make longer-range plans, but for all practical purposes he must give most of his attention to seeing to it that the work of each day gets accomplished. Such short-range planning for the day is always necessary. It requires the supervisor to take the time to think through the nature and the amount of work that is to be done each day by his department, who is to do it, and when. Furthermore, this daily planning must be done ahead of time; many supervisors like to do it at the end of the day when they can size up what has been accomplished that day in order to formulate plans for the following day.

There are occasions when a supervisor will be also involved in long-range plans. For example, his boss may want to discuss with him the part he is to play in the planning of broader future objectives for the institution. Or a supervisor may be informed of a contemplated expansion or the addition of new facilities, and he will be asked to estimate what his department can contribute, what he will need in order to achieve the new objectives, and questions of that type. From time to time the supervisor might also be requested by the administrator to project the long-run trend of his particular activity, especially if it seems apparent that such activity will be affected by changes in medical science and technology or by increasing mechanization and automation. Much time and effort will be spent by the supervisor in making these long-range plans, and even more time will be needed to carry them out once they are made and approved.

Nevertheless, it is important for the supervisor to participate in such long-range planning because the plans may require him to reassign some of his employees or to give them an opportunity to acquire additional education. Or the long-range plans may indicate that subordinates with completely new skills are needed and that a search must be made for them. Or training in new procedures and new techniques might be necessary as a result of new equipment which will be introduced. In these types of situations, therefore, there is need for the supervisor to participate in long-range planning, but generally this will not be the case and his primary planning period will be that of a shorter duration.

The Integration and Communication of Plans

It is always necessary that the short-range plans made by the supervisor be integrated and coordinated with the long-range plans of the top administration. It is wrong to look at long-range planning as an activity separate from and independent of short-range planning. Rather, it is essential for the top administration to keep all its managers well informed of the new and existing long-range plans and objectives of the institution, and to make certain that the short-range plans of lower level management are in accordance with them. The better informed a supervisor or lower level manager is, the better will he be able to integrate his short-range plans into the over-all plans of the enterprise.

All too often, however, there is a gap between the knowledge of top management and lower level management as far as planning is concerned. This gap is often justified by the claim that many of the plans are confidential and cannot be divulged for security reasons. Of course, most employees know that very little can be kept secret in any organization. Therefore, internal security cannot always be used as an excuse. On the other hand, supervisors should realize that there are some limitations and that the top administration does not have to disclose all of its plans as long as lower level managers are made aware of those plans that will directly affect their particular activities.

To this extent, then, plans should be communicated and fully explained to subordinate managers so that they are in a better position to formulate derivative plans for their departments. And by the same token each supervisor should always bear in mind that his own employees will be affected by the plans that he makes. Since the work of the employees is needed to execute whatever he has planned, the supervisor will do well to take them into his confidence and to explain to them in advance what is being planned for the department. The employees may even be in a position to make contributions, and their ideas may be very helpful. The supervisor should also bear in mind that a well-informed employee is a better employee for the department.

THE PLANNING PROCESS AND THE DIFFERENT TYPES OF PLANS INVOLVED
Objectives

Effective management is always management by objectives. This holds true for the executive director of a hospital as well as for the supervisor on the firing line and for all managers on the levels in between. Formulating objectives should therefore be foremost in every manager's mind. Policies, procedures, methods, rules, and performance standards are then derived from the objectives. Moreover, the objectives will largely determine how the managers go about their organizing, staffing, and influencing functions. And, of course, controlling would be meaningless without objectives as guidelines.

Primary Objectives

The very first step in planning is therefore a statement of the over-all or primary objectives to be achieved by the enterprise. Every member of the organization should be familiar with this statement of objectives because it outlines the goals and end result toward which all plans and activities are directed. The objectives constitute the purpose of the enterprise, and without them no intelligent planning can take place. To set these over-all objectives is a function of the top administration: the board together with the chief administrator. In other words, the top administration must clearly define the primary purpose for which the undertaking is organized.

Of course, in any organization there is a multitude of objectives and the real difficulty lies in ranking and balancing them. This is especially true for health care facilities. Broadly speaking, in most hospitals and related institutions we find such primary objectives as care of the sick and injured, research and advancement of medical knowledge, help in the prevention of sickness, and education and training in all the professional and non-professional activities customarily associated with a hospital. A home for the aged might state as its primary objective the total care of elderly people in a home-like atmosphere.

In adition to these, there are many other over-all objectives which a health care facility can have. Maintaining a fine reputation among hospitals, practicing the best possible medicine, discharging numerous social and charitable responsibilities are just a few examples. Moreover, another primary objective of even not-for-profit health care facilities is to operate without a loss or to have an occasional operating surplus. There are also other less tangible objectives toward which a health care facility can strive. In relation to those who work there, for instance, there is the goal of being a good employer, a good place to work. Although it would go beyond the confines of this book to discuss all of the objectives of all types of health care facilities, the above examples show sufficiently well the multiplicity of objectives and why top administrators have a continuous challenge in balancing and achieving them.

Secondary Objectives

While the goals established for an institution as a whole are called the primary objectives, those set up for each of the institution's various departments are called the secondary objectives. Since each department or division has a specific task to perform, it follows that each must have its own clearly defined objectives as a guide for its functioning. Of course, these secondary goals and objectives of the departments must stay within the overall framework set by the primary objectives of the total organization; they must contribute to the achievement of the over-all institutional objectives.

However, because they are concerned with only one department, the secondary objectives are necessarily narrower in scope. Whereas the over-all objectives are broad and general, the objectives of a department have to be much more specific and detailed. Such departmental objectives are purposely designed to serve as specific guides for subordinate units. They enable departmental managers to operate at their own discretion although always within the limits of the over-all hospital goals.

This may become clearer if we look at an example. Suppose, for instance, that the stated objective of a hospital's medical records department is as follows: To provide a central file of the medical records compiled during the treatment of each patient to be used as a permanent record in case of future illness, as an aid in clinical and statistical research, as an administrative tool for planning and evaluating the hospital's program, and as a potential legal protection for the patient, hospital, and physician. Obviously, these departmental objectives are quite narrow, but their fulfillment contributes significantly to the achievement of over-all hospital goals. As a matter of fact, the primary hospital objectives could not be achieved at all if the subsidiary departmental ones were not fulfilled.

This is why it is essential for all supervisors and their employees to clearly understand not only the objectives of their own department but also those of the entire institution. The two sets of objectives must be carefully defined and stated, so that they can be integrated, coordinated, and explained on the departmental level. The supervisor must bear in mind that the successful completion of a task depends upon the full understanding of its purpose by those who have to carry it out. It is therefore good management to make certain that all employees at all levels are thoroughly informed and indoctrinated about the objectives to be achieved.

Once the objectives of the enterprise have been determined, the managers can set about to make the rest of the plans which are necessary to implement them. There are a number of different types of plans devised in order to implement objectives: namely, policies, procedures, methods, rules, budgets, and so on. All of these types of plans must be designed to reinforce one another, in other words, they must be integrated and coordinated. Since every manager will probably have to make or at least use each type of plan at some time in his career, he should be familiar with all of them. Of course, the major plans are formulated by the top administrator, but each department supervisor will have to formulate his own departmental plans in accordance therewith. The purpose of all the plans is to insure that the thinking and the actions taken on different levels and in different departments of the institution are consistent with its over-all objectives.

Policies

Among the various plans which a manager must devise, policies are probably the most frequently used. Policies are broad guides to thinking. They are general statements which channel the thinking of all personnel charged with decision-making. Although they are broad, policies do have definite limitations at either end. As long as a subordinate stays within these limitations, he will make an appropriate decision, one which conforms to the policy. Thus, policies serve to keep decision-makers on the right track, and in this way they facilitate the job of both managers and subordinates.

The Flexibility of Policies

Defining a policy as a broad guide to thinking implies a certain amount of flexibility. Some policies even have flexibility explicitly stated by such words as "whenever possible," "whenever feasible," etc. If these clauses are not built in, then the manner in which the supervisor applies the policy will determine its degree of flexibility. He must intelligently adapt the policy to the existing set of circumstances. Such flexibility, however, mut not lead to inconsistency; policies must be administered by supervisors in a consistent manner. Anything else would defeat the basic purpose of a policy, namely, its effort to provide subordinate managers with a uniform guide for thinking.

Policies as an Aid in Delegation

By issuing policies, the top administration sanctions in advance the decisions made by subordinate managers as long as they stay within the broad policy guidelines. After having set policies, a superior manager should feel reasonably confident that whatever decisions his subordinate managers make will fall within the limits of the policies. In fact, the subordinates will probably come up with just about the same decisions that the superior manager would have made himself. Hence, policies make it easier for the superior to delegate authority to his subordinates. By the same token, policies are a great help to the subordinate manager also. They provide specific guidelines for his thinking which facilitate his decision-making and at the same time insure uniformity of decisions throughout the entire enterprise. Therefore, the clearer and the more comprehensive the policy guides are, the easier and better will it be for the superior manager to delegate authority and for the subordinate manager to exercise authority.

The Origin of Policies

Obviously, policies do not come about by chance. They are determined by management, particularly by the higher administrative levels. Indeed, to formulate policies is one of the most important functions of top management. The top manager is in the best position to establish the various types of over-all policies which will enable the enterprise's objectives to be achieved. Once the broad policies have been set by the top administrator, they in turn will become the guides for narrower policies covering smaller areas of departmental scope. Such departmental policies are originated by the various managers lower down in the managerial hierarchy. Of course, all of these departmental policies will implement and coincide with the broader policies of the enterprise as set by top management. This type of policy formulation, originated by the top administrative level and pursued by the lower levels, is the most important source of policies.

However, there are occasions when a supervisor may find himself in a situation for which no policies appear to exist. In such a dilemma, the supervisor has only one choice; that is, to go to his boss and simply ask him whether or not any of the existing policies are applicable. If there are none, then the supervisor will appeal to his boss to issue a policy to cover such situations. Suppose, for instance, that one of your employees asks you for a leave of absence. In order to make the appropriate decision, you would like to be guided by a broad policy so that whatever decision you arrive at would be in accord with all other decisions regarding leaves of absence. However, you may find that the administrator never issued any policies on the granting or denial of a leave of absence. Instead of making an individual decision, you ask your boss to issue a policy, a broad guide for thinking to be applied whenever leaves of absence are requested. It is not likely that you will have to make such a request very often for a good administrator usually foresees most of the areas where policies are needed. On occasion, however, you may have to appeal to your own boss, stimulating the formulation of what is known as *appealed* policy.

In addition to appealed and originated policies, there are a number of policies which are *imposed* upon an organization by external factors such as the government, accrediting agencies, trade unions, trade associations, and so on. The word "imposed" indicates compliance with a force which cannot be avoided. For instance, in order to be accredited hospitals and other health care facilities must comply with certain regulations issued by the accrediting agency. These regulations must be translated into hospital policy and all employees must abide by them. Any policy originating outside the enterprise in this manner is known as an externally imposed policy.

Clarity of Policy Statements

Because policies are such a vital guide for thinking and thus for decision-making, it is essential that they be explicitly stated and communicated so that those in the organization who are to apply them will fully understand their meaning. This is no easy task. It is difficult to find words which will be understood by all people in the same way since different meanings can be attached to the same word. Although there is no guarantee that even the written word will be properly understood, it still seems desirable that all policies be communicated in a written statement. However, many enterprises simply never get around to writing their policies down and others purposely do not write them down.

Nevertheless, the benefits derived from written policies are well worth the time and effort spent in doing so. The mere process of putting the policies into writing requires the top administrator to think them out clearly and consistently ahead of time. The subordinate managers can then read them as often as they care to. Moreover, the meaning of a written policy cannot be changed by word of mouth because if there is any doubt the written policy can always be referred to. Furthermore, written policies are especially helpful for new employees who want to speedily acquaint themselves with how the organization runs.

Although the advantages are far more significant, there is one disadvantage connected with written policies. Once they are written down management may become reluctant to change them. Thus, many enterprises prefer to have their policies communicated by word of mouth because they feel that this is more flexible, allowing the verbal policies to be adjusted to different circumstances with greater ease than written policies. But the exact meaning of a verbal policy might become scrambled, making it difficult to apply the policy properly. Thus, written policy statements are generally considered more desirable.

The Supervisor and Policies

If a manager heads a major department which has many employees and several subdivisions within it, he may sometimes find it necessary to issue and write policies himself. However, for the most part supervisors do not actually have to issue policies. Instead, they are called upon primarily to apply existing policies in making their daily decisions. It is also the supervisor's job to interpret and explain the meaning of policies to the employees of his department. Thus, although he will seldom have to issue policies, the supervisor must continuously use them. Therefore, it is essential that he clearly understands the policies and that he learns how to apply them appropriately.

Periodic Review of Policies

Regardless of how well thought out the policies were when originated, the dynamic nature of activities in today's health care centers makes it probable that some policies will sooner or later become outmoded. It is therefore necessary to periodically review and appraise policies in order to see whether they ought to be changed, modified, or completely abandoned. Such an investigation may uncover practices which are a complete contradiction to current written policies. Or it may uncover policies which have become so outdated that no one follows them. In such cases, the top administration must either rewrite or abandon the questionable policies, for an institution certainly cannot afford to let its various subordinate managers decide whether policies are still current or whether they should be observed any longer. Hence, it is absolutely essential for policies to be periodically reviewed by top management.

Procedures

Like policies, procedures are also plans for achieving the institution's objectives. But procedures are much more specific than policies. While the supervisor will not have much opportunity to issue policy, there will be many occasions for him to issue procedures. Procedures are a guide to *action*, not a guide to thinking. Procedures show the sequence of definite acts. They define a chronological order for the acts which are to be performed. (See Figure 6-1) Procedures specify a route which will take subordinates between the guideposts of the policies and lead them to the final objectives. In brief, procedures pick a path toward the objectives.

FIGURE 6-1*

The Relationship of Policies, Procedures, and Methods

*Adapted from Theo Haimann and William G. Scott, *Management in the Modern Organization* (Boston: Houghton Mifflin Company, 1970), p. 105. Reprinted with permission of the publisher.

If a supervisor were fortunate enough to have only highly skilled employees under his direction, he could depend upon them to a great extent to select an efficient path of procedure. But this is very unlikely, and most employees look to their supervisor for instructions on how to proceed. Since the supervisor is the manager of the department, he is the one to determine how the work is to be done. And, of course, effective work procedures designed by the supervisor will result in definite advantages.

One of these advantages lies in the fact that the mere process of preparing a procedure necessitates analysis and study of the work to be done. The supervisor is more likely therefore to assign work fairly and to distribute it evenly among his employees. Moreover, once a procedure has been established it assures uniformity of performance. In addition to these benefits, procedures give the supervisor a standard for appraising the work of his employees. And since a procedure specifies the chronological sequence of how the work is to be done, it decreases the need for further decision-making. This makes the supervisor's job as well as that of his employees easier. Naturally, therefore, a good supervisor will spend considerable time and effort in devising efficient procedures to be applied throughout his department. From time to time, of course, it will be necessary for him to review all departmental procedures for they are likely to become outdated just as policies do.

Methods

A method is also a plan for action, but a plan which is even more detailed than a procedure. Whereas a procedure shows a series of steps to be taken, a method is concerned only with a single operation, with one particular step. The method tells exactly how this particular step is to be performed. (See Figure 6-1) For the majority of work done by the employees of a department there exists a "best method," a best way for doing the job. Again, if the supervisor had only highly skilled subordinates, they would probably know the best method without having to be told. But, in most cases, it is necessary for the supervisor to specify for his employees exactly what he considers the best method under existing circumstances. Indeed, a large amount of the supervisor's time is spent in devising methods. But once a method has been devised, it carries with it all the advantages of a procedure, as cited above. In determining the best method, a supervisor may occasionally need to call on the help of a methods engineer or a time and motion study man, if such a person is available in the organization. Most of the time, however, the supervisor's own experience is probably broad enough to allow him to design the "best" work methods by himself.

Standard Procedures and Practices

In some activities of the hospital there will be no need for the supervisor to be overly concerned with devising procedures and methods because his employees will already have been thoroughly trained in standard practices and procedures. For instance, nurses, technicians, and medical specialists are exposed to many years of schooling and training during which great emphasis is placed on the proper procedures and methods for performing certain tasks. In managing a department where such highly skilled employees are at work, the supervisor's job is greatly simplified. One of his main concerns is to see to it that good, generally approved procedures and methods are carried out in a professionally accepted way. However, in addition to these highly trained professionals, the supervisor will probably have other employees in his department who are not highly skilled and for whom procedures and methods must definitely be devised by him.

Rules

A rule is somewhat different from a policy, procedure, or method, although it is still a plan which has been devised in order to bring about the attainment of the enterprise's objectives. A rule is not like a policy because it does not provide a guide to thinking and it does not leave any discretion to the party involved. It is, however, related to a procedure insofar as it is a guide to action and states what must or must not be done. But a rule is not the same as a procedure because it does not specify a time sequence for the particular action. No smoking, for instance, is a rule which could be made by management, probably just one of a long list of safety rules. This rule is a guide to action, or more precisely to inaction. But there is no order of steps involved, it is simply no smoking wherever and whenever it is in effect. There will be many occasions when a supervisor has to set up such rules on his own or see to it that the rules set up by the administration are obeyed.

Repeat-Use and Single-Use Plans

The different kinds of plans mentioned above — objectives, policies, procedures, methods, and rules — are commonly known as repeat-use or standing plans because they are plans which are followed each time a given situation is encountered. In other words, they are used again and again. They are applicable whenever a situation presents itself which is similar to that for which the standing plan was originally devised.

The opposite of repeat-use plans are those plans which are no longer needed once their objective is accomplished. They are known as single-use plans. Once the goal is reached, the plan is used up. Within this single-use plan category, we find programs, projects, and budgets. Programs and projects are a complex set of plans designed to reach a major goal, for instance, a hospital building program. However, since programs and projects are mainly the concern of the top administrator, it will suffice in this discussion to concentrate on budgets.

Budgets

Budgets are usually thought of only in connection with the function of controlling; but this is incorrect. Budgets are also plans, plans which express the anticipated results in numerical terms, be this in dollars and cents, nursing hours, man hours, kilowatt hours, or units to be produced. Indeed, a budget may be stated in time, material, money, or any other unit which is used to perform work or to measure specific results. However, since most values are ultimately convertible to monetary terms, money budgets are the most frequently used. Although budgets are an important tool for controlling, the preparing and making of a budget is part of the planning function, and planning as we know is the duty of every manager.

Since a budget is a plan expressed in numerical units, it has the distinct advantage that the goal is stated in exact and specific terms instead of in generalities. The figures which a supervisor puts into a budget represent actual plans which will become the standards to be achieved. These plans are not mere projections or general forecasts, but will be considered as a basis for daily operations. They will be looked upon as goals to live up to.

Because budgets are so important for the daily operations of every department, it is essential for the supervisors who have to function under them to participate in their preparation. It is only natural that people resent arbitrary orders, and this applies to budgets. Thus, it is necessary that all budget objectives and allowances be determined with the full cooperation of those who are responsible for executing them. Every supervisor should actively participate in the budget-making process and this should not be mere pseudo-participation. In order to assure the true type of participation, these subordinate managers should be allowed to submit their own budgets; that is, they should participate in what is commonly known as grass roots budgeting. Of course, each supervisor will have to substantiate his budget proposals in a discussion with his boss and possibly with the top administrator who sets and adjusts the final budgets. Indeed, this is what is meant by active, real participation in budget-making, and this is what insures the effectiveness of the process. Such participation, however, should not be construed to mean that the suggestion of the supervisor will always prevail. The supervisor's budget should not be accepted by his boss if he feels that it is based on plans which are inadequate or incorrect. Differences between budget estimates should be carefully discussed by them, but the final decision rests with the superior manager. Nevertheless, if a budget is arrived at with the participation of the supervisor, then the likelihood that he will live up to it is better than if the budget had been handed down to him by his boss.

In conclusion, it is important to remember that the budget is an example of a single-use plan. It will serve as a guideline only for the period for which it is drawn up. When this particular period is over, this plan — this budget — will not be called upon again. It has served its usefulness and is no longer valid. A new budget will have to be drawn up and a new planning period will be established.

SUMMARY

Planning is the managerial function which determines in advance what is to be done in the future. It is the function of every manager ranging from the top administrator to the supervisor of each department. Planning is important because it assures the best utilization of resources and economy of performance. The planning period on the supervisory level is usually of a much shorter duration than is on the top administrator's level. Nevertheless, even the short-range plans of the supervisor must coincide with the long-range plans of the enterprise. Setting objectives is the first step in planning. Although the over-all objectives are determined by the top administration, there are many secondary objectives which must be clarified by the supervisor and which must be in accordance with the primary objectives of the over-all undertaking. In order to reach all the objectives, different kinds of plans must be devised. Policies are one kind of plan. They are guides to thinking and the majority of them originate with the chief administrator. In most cases, the supervisor's concern with policies is primarily one of interpreting them, applying them, and staying within them whenever he makes decisions for his department. There may be occasions, however, when the supervisor has to appeal to his boss for the issuance or clarification of certain policies. Although the supervisor does not usually originate policies, he will often be called upon to design procedures and methods. These types of plans are guides for action, not guides for thinking. The supervisor also will participate in the establishment of budgets, which are plans expressed in numerical terms.

CHAPTER 7

Planning on the Supervisory Level

Planning, as we have said, is deciding in advance what is to be done in the future. Although the future is fraught with uncertainties, the manager must make certain assumptions about it in order to plan. These assumptions are based on forecasts of what the future will hold. Since the appraisal of future prospects is inherent in all planning, the success of an enterprise depends in large measure upon the skill of management first in forecasting and then in preparing for the future conditions.

FORECASTS AS THE BASIS OF PLANNING

Administrative Forecasts

All managers must make some assumptions about the future. However, the chief administrator must make an effort to forecast the future in a much more far-reaching manner than a supervisor would do. But since both are managers, both must make forecasts. Such forecasts are possible in widely diverse areas. Normally, of course, management confines its forecasting efforts to those factors which experience suggests are important to its own planning. Thus, the chief administrator of a hospital or related facility would select and use only those forecasts which have a direct material bearing on the health care field.

In his endeavor to predict the outlook of things to come, one of the factors that the administrator will be concerned with is the general economic and political climate in which his institution must operate during the next few years. This includes government attitudes, government spending policies, and possible future laws which would ultimately affect the activities of hospitals and related health facilities. The administrator will try to predict the general trends for the delivery of health care. He will be concerned with the outlook of monetary policy and with the over-all volume of economic activities within the country. He will be vitally interested in forecasts of changes in our population. He will pay serious attention to forecasts for, say, the year 2000 when the U.S. population is expected to considerably exceed 300 million people. The breakdown of population figures according to age patterns will be even more meaningful for him, depending upon whether he is the administrator of a general short-term hospital, of an extended health care facility, or of a nursing home.

All of these types of economic and political conditions will affect the operations of a health care facility. Since the administrator's job is to take the broad and long-run outlook, he will have to make forecasts in these far-reaching fields.* Although lower level managers are not directly concerned with making such overall assumptions, they will ultimately be affected by them since they affect the institution in general.

Departmental Forecasts

Technological Developments

When it comes to departmental forecasts, the supervisor will also have to make certain assumptions as to what the future will hold. But his assumptions will cover a much narrower field. A supervisor must try to forecast only those factors which may have some bearing on the future of his particular department. For example, he should try to determine whether there is a growing trend for simplification of the function which he oversees or whether his particular function seems to be on the increase or decrease. He must keep a keen eye on developments in the area of technology and automation. Based on what has happened in the past, he should venture some kind of assumption as to what the future will hold in this respect. In making such an assumption, he can look for assistance to the sources of supplies and equipment which he uses. He can learn much by attending their meetings, exhibitions, and so on. He could discover that technology is progressing so rapidly that in a number of years his department's functions may be significantly different from what they had been. Consider, for instance, the impact of further mechanization in laboratories or the impact of disposables on the laundry department. Such a projection of the future would be essential for a laboratory supervisor and the laundry manager to have in order to plan properly.

Employees and Skills

A supervisor will also have to make forecasts in relation to the kind of employees who will be working for him. He may foresee the need for employees who are better educated and more skilled and whose increasing demands the department must be ready to meet. This

---

*Hospital administrators do not, of course, have to actually do the research and the statistical analysis for all forecasts themselves. They frequently use already published statistics and forecasts made available by experts in various fields. For example, population forecasts would generally come from studies of the U.S. Bureau of the Census.

refers both to monetary demands, and also to demands that the positions offer enough of a challenge. For example, the supervisor may find that the current pattern of wages and fringe benefits cannot be maintained in the future, and he would do well to start planning accordingly at an early time. Similarly, he should be aware of the noneconomic demands which young people coming out of school, whether it is a university, junior college, vocational training program, or high school, expect to fulfill on their jobs. Meeting both types of demands will be particularly important if the supervisor has to look for people who possess skills which up to now have never been required in his department or perhaps anywhere in the hospital.

A supervisor may also discover a trend toward the upgrading of certain duties. For instance, the supervisor of the operating room suite might foresee an increasing number of operating room technicians. He will have to plan for the impact that this will have on the position of the graduate operating room nurses. Or, the director of the nursing services might have to view the future in terms of more nurse specialists, more physicians' assistants, and so forth.

On the other hand, it may very well be that due to increased mechanization, less and less people will be necessary to perform the functions currently performed. Indeed, a supervisor might find that the department which he is supervising will lose its function altogether. It is conceivable that due to new discoveries or new means of doing the work an entire department may become obsolete. Although this is not a very pleasant thought, it is better for the supervisor to realize it early instead of being confronted with such an event without having prepared for it. If obsolescence is threatened, the far-sighted supervisor should inform the administrator accordingly. Sooner or later the administrator should make it his business to carve out a new supervisory position for the particular supervisor who has been so far-sighted. He is too valuable an employee to lose and he can probably be just as good in the supervision of another department, perhaps a department which heretofore has never existed. In such a case, the supervisor will probably have to acquire special skills with which he has not been familiar up to this time. If so, he should get busy and learn these particular skills, taking advantage of appropriate technical assistance when he can. Only in this way will he be able to plan competently for his own future as well as for that of his department. Only in this way will he be ready with a plan if and when the forecasted technological events occur.

It should always be remembered that at the base of all forecasts lie certain assumptions, approximations, and average conditions. It must be emphasized that forecasting is an art and not a science and as yet there is no infallible way of predicting the future. However, forecasting accuracy increases with experience. As time goes on, making assumptions about the future should become a normal activity for all managers from the administrator down to the supervisor. The managers should exchange ideas, help each other, and supply information whenever available. In all likelihood, they will act as a check upon each other and their final analysis of what the future holds will probably be quite reliable.

But even if some of the events which have been anticipated do not materialize or do not materialize exactly as forecast, it is better to have foreseen them than to be suddenly confronted with them. Having foreseen these events, the supervisor has readied his mind and his state of affairs so as to be able to incorporate changes whenever they are needed. Although this may sound like a formidable task for a supervisor, all that is asked of him is to be alert to all possible changes and trends. This is the only way he can prevent his own and his employees' obsolescence, so that with the help of hindsight he won't have to recall the time when certain trends were already visible and wish he had taken them seriously at that time.

PLANNING THE UTILIZATION OF RESOURCES

As we already know, every supervisor is entrusted with a large number of valuable resources to be used to accomplish the job of his department. It is the supervisor's duty to plan specifically how to utilize the resources available to him so that the work of his unit can be carried out most effectively. This means that he must make detailed plans for the utilization of his equipment and tools, of the space available to him, of his materials and supplies, and last but not least of his own and his employees' time.

Plan Utilization of Equipment and Tools

The supervisor must plan the full utilization of the equipment and tools provided for his department. These tools frequently represent a substantial investment that the institution has made for him. Therefore, he must plan for their efficient use so that the institution will get a good return on their investment. It is the supervisor's job to see to it that his employees respect the equipment and tools and treat them carefully. It is his job to ascertain whether or not the equipment serves its purpose and whether or not there are better facilities available for doing the work. This does not mean that a supervisor must always have the very latest model of each tool available; but, on the other hand, he should plan to get rid of inefficient tools and equipment if he can replace them with better ones.

Of course, the supervisor must plan such replacements very carefully. He must look at professional journals, listen to what salesmen of equipment and tools have to show him about their products, read the literature which is circulated by hospitals and related associations, and keep himself aware of the general development within his field. Only with this type of background can the supervisor submit intelligent plans for the replacement of tools and equipment to his superior or to the administrator. He should be able to support his recommended changes with all the possible reasons he can think of, but he will have to leave the final decision to those above him. Even if his request should be turned down at the moment, the supervisor has demonstrated that he is on top of the job, planning for the future. In the long run, he will probably find that his plans for the replacement of equipment will be accepted and the administrator will have to admit that the supervisor did plan for the proper utilization of his department's equipment.

Plan Work Methods and Procedures

In our discussion of the planning process, it was pointed out that the supervisor is deeply involved in the design and development of procedures and methods. Indeed, the supervisor should continually make plans concerning improved work methods and processes in his department. The difficulty is that many supervisors work under considerable pressure and find little time for this type of planning. Moreover, the supervisor is often so close to the jobs performed in his department that he believes that the prevailing work methods are satisfactory and that not much can be done about them. Nevertheless, in order to maintain high efficiency in the department it is necessary from time to time to study the operations performed so that improvements can be planned in the work methods being used.

The supervisor would do well to try to look at his department's operations from the point of view of a stranger coming into the department for the first time. In other words, he should look at his operations with a detached point of view, observing all methods and processes objectively. He should ask himself if each operation is really necessary, what the reason for it is, and whether or not it could be combined with something else. Are the various steps performed in the best possible sequence, are there any avoidable delays, and so on? In his efforts to devise more efficient work methods, it may be possible for the supervisor to call on the help of a staff specialist, such as a systems analyst or a methods engineer, who may be available within the hospital. Even if a specialist is not available, however, it is likely that the supervisor can plan better methods and processes on his own.

Plan Use of Space

A supervisor must also plan for the best utilization of space. He will first have to determine whether or not the space assigned to his department is now being used effectively. In making this determination, he may again call on some industrial engineering help if it is available. If not, he should make a layout chart for himself, showing the number of square feet he has to work with, the location of equipment and supplies, and the work paths of his employees as they carry out their tasks. Such a chart can then be studied to determine whether the allocated space has been laid out appropriately or whether things need to be rearranged so that the department's work can be done more efficiently.

This type of layout planning could also show the need for additional space. If such a request is placed before the administrator, based upon thorough planning of the space currently allotted, then the likelihood that it will be granted is better than otherwise. The supervisor must realize, however, that he has to compete with many other managers who probably also request more space. Even if the request is denied, these space allocation plans will not have been drawn up in vain. In all probability, they will have made the supervisor more aware of some of the conditions under which his employees are working, and perhaps he will be able to use that information to plan more efficient work methods considering the existing conditions.

Plan Use of Materials and Supplies

The supervisor must plan for the appropriate use and conservation of the materials and supplies entrusted and charged to his department. These would include such things as cotton balls, tongue blades, alcohol, sponges, medicine cups, paper supplies and so forth at a nursing station. In most departments, the quantity of materials and supplies used is substantial. Even if each single item represents only a small value, the aggregate of these items adds up to sizeable amounts in the budget of a hospital or related health care facility. Proper planning will insure that materials and supplies are used as conservatively as possible, thus bringing about good performance within the department. The supervisor must teach his employees proper use because many of them are careless and do not realize the significance of the amount of money involved. By careful explanation the supervisor can call his workers' attention to this fact, pointing out to them that the economic utilization of supplies is to their own advantage because whatever is wasted cannot be used to raise their wages or improve their working conditions. Although proper planning for the utilization of materials and supplies will help significantly in performance, it will not prevent all waste.

Plan the Use of Time

Last but not least, the supervisor must plan the use of time. The old saying "time is money" applies with equal force to the supervisor's own time and to his employees' time. Thus, the supervisor must not only plan his employees' time, but he must also consider at least as carefully the use of his own time.

The Supervisor's Time

The supervisor's own time is one of the human resources for which he is responsible. Every supervisor has probably experienced days that were so full of pressures and demands that he began to feel as though he could never take care of all the matters that needed attention. The days and the weeks just were too short. The only way to keep such days at a minimum is for the supervisor to plan his time for the most effective use.

Unfortunately, the supervisor's problems come up on a continual basis but without any order of importance. Thus, the first thing the supervisor must do is sort and grade them; that is, he has to decide between those matters which he must attend to personally and those which he can delegate to someone else. There are some matters which the supervisor actually cannot delegate; but the majority can be assigned to his employees. Every time the supervisor dispenses with one of his duties by assigning it to an employee he is gaining time for more important matters. This is worthwhile even if he has to spend some valuable time training one of his employees in a particular task. In case of doubt, therefore, the supervisor should be inclined to delegate. Then he should plan his available time so that it is divided among those matters to which he alone can attend. He will again have to classify them according to their urgency.

Unless the supervisor does distinguish between those matters which *must* be done and those which *ought* to be done he is inclined to pay equal attention to all matters before him, and the more important ones may not get the attention they truly deserve. But by distinguishing he will be giving priority to those matters which need immediate attention. He shoud therefore plan his time so that the most important things he has to attend to will appear at the top of his schedule. The supervisor must make certain, however, that he leaves some flexibility in his time schedule because not every contingency can be anticipated. There will be some emergencies to which he must turn his attention when they arise. The flexibility will permit him to take care of these situations without significantly disrupting the other activities planned on his time schedule.

Many techniques have been devised to help supervisors control their time schedules. One of the simplest methods is to use a desk calendar to schedule those things which need attention such as appointments, meetings, reports, discussions, etc. The supervisor should schedule these events far in advance and in so doing they will automatically come up for his attention when they are due.

Another effective way of planning each week's work in advance and also of knowing what is being accomplished as the week goes on, is to keep a planning sheet. Such a planning sheet is prepared at the end of one week for the week to follow. It shows the days of the week divided into morning and afternoon columns and a list of all things to be accomplished. Then, a time for accomplishment is assigned to each task by placing it in the morning or the afternoon blocks of the assigned day. Thus, at a glance the supervisor knows what is planned for each morning and afternoon of the week. As a task is accomplished its box is circled. Those tasks that have been delayed during the day must be rescheduled for another time by placing them in an appropriate block on a subsequent day. Those tasks which are planned but have not been accomplished during the week (they are still uncircled) must be rescheduled for the following week. Such a record will show how much of the original plan has been carried out at the end of the week and will provide a good answer to the question of where the supervisor's time went. Based on this record he will then be able to plan his next week, and so on. Regardless of whether he uses this particular system or another, the supervisor must make it his duty to schedule his own time each week and to have some method of reporting the tasks that are planned and those which have been accomplished. (See Figure 7-1)

FIGURE   7 -1

MONDAY 10/23	TUESDAY 10/24	WEDNESDAY 10/25	THURSDAY 10/26	FRIDAY 10/27
AM	AM *work on job descriptions*	AM *See Personnel Director about Helen* / *Talk to Maintenance about new el. outlets*	AM *Arrange dates for evaluation interviews*	AM *Work on dress code revisions*
PM *Check leave of absence Policy*	PM	PM *Read minutes last meeting of infection Com.*	PM *Start work on new budget*	PM *Attend Management Seminar*

The Employee's Time

When planning for the effective use of his subordinates' time much will depend on the supervisor's basic managerial strategy and his assumptions about human nature. According to Douglas MacGregor, a well known author and professor of management, most managers base their thinking on one of two sets of assumptions about human nature which he calls Theory X and Theory Y. The Theory X manager believes that the average employee dislikes work, will avoid work, and tries to get by with as little as utterly possible. He has little ambition and has to be forced and closely controlled in each and every job. The Theory Y manager operates with a drastically different set of assumptions regarding human nature. He believes that most employees consider work natural, that most are eager to do the right thing, that they will seek responsibility under the proper conditions, and that they will exercise self-control and do not need to be continually urged. Theory Y further states that external controls and threats are not a good means for producing results. Rather, since work is as natural to man as play or rest, it will not be avoided. Although there may be some situations where a manager has no choice but to follow Theory X, in all likelihood he would much prefer to practice and believe in Theory Y. A great deal more will be said about MacGregor's theories in Chapter 17, but it is appropriate to bring them up now because they are important when planning for the effective utilization of employees' time.

For example, if a supervisor is a Theory Y manager he will expect his employees to do the right thing and to turn in a fair day's work. Of course, he will not expect his employees to work indefinitely at top speed. Thus, his plans for their time will be based on a fair output instead of a maximum output. Allowances will be made for fatigue, unavoidable delays, and for a certain amount of unproductive time during the work day.

In planning employees' time, as in other aspects of planning, the supervisor may be able to get assistance from a staff specialist employed by the hospital, preferably a motion and time specialist. But, normally, most supervisors can use work methods studies and the like to come up with a pretty fair idea themselves as to what can be expected of their employees timewise. Such reasonable estimates of employees' time are necessary because the supervisor must depend upon the completion of certain tasks at certain times. The supervisor himself may have been given deadlines, and in order to meet them he must have a fairly good estimate or idea of how fast the job can be done. Most supervisors are capable of planning reasonable performance requirements which their employees accept as fair. Such requirements are, of course, based on average conditions and not on emergencies.

There are also situations in hospitals where due to the peculiarity of the activity performed, the subordinate's time is paced and set by someone other than the supervisor. For instance, the time an operating room technician spends on a case is in reality determined by the speed and skill of the particular surgeon doing the operation. Furthermore, unexpected complications may add to the time normally necessary to complete the job. In cases of this sort, average time estimates can still be made; but the time allotted must allow for the various contingencies which can arise.

In addition to planning for the normal employee time, there may occasionally be the necessity to plan for overtime. Overtime should be considered only as an emergency matter. If the supervisor finds that overtime is regularly required, then he should change his plans by altering work methods, obtaining better equipment, or hiring more employees. The supervisor must also plan for employee absences. Of course, he cannot plan for those instances when employees are absent without notice. But he can plan for holidays, vacations, layoffs for overhaul, etc. Plans for this kind of absence should be worked out as far in advance as feasible so that the functioning of the department will suffer as little as possible.

Plan Utilization of Work Force

Although a supervisor must plan for the utilization of equipment and tools, for improved work methods and processes, for the utilization of space, for the conservation of materials and supplies, and for the proper use of his own and his employees' time, the most important planning of all is that connected with the utilization of his work force. Alter all, the employees that a manager has available in his department are his most valuable resource. Therefore, to plan for their full utilization must be uppermost in every manager's mind.

This, of course, does not mean planning to squeeze an excessive amount of work out of each employee. Rather, utilization means giving employees as much *satisfaction* as possible in their jobs. To plan for the best utilization of the work force also means to develop methods for recruiting good employees, to search for all available sources of employees. Furthermore, it means to search continually for the best ways to group their activities. It includes the problems and plans of training, supervising, and motivating employees. Finally, the question of effective utilization of workers means the continual appraisal of their performance, appropriate promotions, adequate plans for compensation and rewards; and at the same time, fair disciplinary measures.

All of these considerations play an important role when the supervisor plans for the best utilization of his employees. Only by such human resource planning can he create a situation wherein his workers willingly contribute their utmost in order to achieve both personal satisfaction on the job as well as the attainment of the department's objectives. The supervisor may rest assured that the efforts he makes in this connection will be rewarded amply by his employees. Actually, the matter of planning for the best utilization of employees is at the heart of expert supervision. It is discussed here only briefly, but in reality this entire book is concerned with bringing about the best possible utilization of employees.

TACTICAL CONSIDERATIONS IN PLANNING

While doing all this planning, the supervisor must keep in mind the impact of his plans on those around him. He must be aware that the success or failure of planning will depend largely upon the reaction of those involved in the plans, be they his employees, the supervisors of other departments, or his own boss. There are a number of tactical or political strategies at the supervisor's disposal to help minimize negative reactions and facilitate the success of his plans. He may choose to use one or a combination of these, depending upon the situation at hand.

Since timing is a critical and essential factor in all planning, the manager may choose the strategy which tells him to *strike while the iron is hot*. This strategy obviously advocates prompt action when the situation and time for action are propitious. On the other hand, he may want to invoke the old saying that *time is a great healer*. This is not an endorsement of procrastination, but it is often advisable to create an opportunity for cooling off because many things take care of themselves after a short while.

When significant changes are involved in his planning, the supervisor may do well to use the strategy known as *concentrated mass offensive*. This strategy advocates a quick radical change made all at once. On the other hand, the supervisor may prefer to just *get a foot in the door*. This tactic implies that it may be better to propose merely a portion of the plan in the beginning, especially if the program is of such magnitude that its total acceptance would be doubtful.

Sometimes one supervisor's plan may involve changes which could come about more easily if supervisors of other departments would join in the action. It may therefore be advisable to seek allies in order to promote the change; that is, to adopt the strategy which states that *there is strength in unity*. For example, if a supervisor plans to increase the salaries of his employees it may be expedient to try to get the other supervisors to join with him in presenting a general request for higher remuneration to the administrator. Of course, this may involve another strategy which is well known in politics: *You scratch my back and I'll scratch yours*. This tactic of reciprocity is practiced not only in political circles and in the activity of purchasing agents, but also among colleagues who wish to present joint action on a particular issue.

There are, of course, many other strategies which can frequently be of help in initiating and carrying out plans. Mentioning of these tactics, however, should not be construed to mean that they are always recommended. The choice and the application of political tactics will depend upon the people involved, the situation, the urgency of the objective, the timing, the means available, and a number of other factors. Properly applied, they can minimize difficulties and increase the effectiveness of the manager's planning.

SUMMARY

All planning must be done with forecasts of the future in mind. Since the future is uncertain, it is necessary to make various assumptions as to what it holds. Over-all forecasts or assumptions are made by the top administrator, and the supervisor narrows these down to forecasts for his particular activity. Based on such forecasts, the supervisor will then make plans for his department. He must plan for the full utilization of all the resources he has at his disposal. More specifically, he must plan for proper utilization of equipment and tools, and of work methods and processes; he must make plans to effectively utilize the space available to him and the materials and supplies under his supervision; and he must plan the efficient use of his own and his employees' time. And even more important, he must plan for the best over-all utilization of the employees in his unit. This means, among other things, seeing to it that his employees are able to find satisfaction in their work. Throughout all such planning, the supervisor should be concerned with the effects of his plans on other members of the organization. At times he may need to resort to various tactical considerations which will be helpful in getting his plans accepted and effectively carried out.

PART FOUR

Organizing

CHAPTER 8

Establishing the Formal Organizational Structure

Organizing is closely related to planning. It is based on the goals and objectives of the institution which are formulated in the planning process. Organizing enables an enterprise to accomplish its planned objectives. Organizing plots the activities needed and establishes the relationships among various functions. These activities and functions form subsystems which are synchronized and harmonized into a larger system, called the formal organization.

Formal organization theory rests on several major principles or premises: namely, that the *division of work* is essential for efficiency; that *coordination* is a primary responsibility of management, fulfilled by performing the managerial functions properly; that the *formal structure* is the main network for organizing and managing the various activities of the enterprise; that the *span of supervision* sets outside limits on the number of subordinates a manager can effectively supervise; that *unity of command* must prevail; and that the lifeblood of the organization is the process of *delegation of authority*.

These major principles of organization are a primary concern of the chief administrator. He is the one who must translate them into a formal organizational structure for his institution. He is the one who must establish this structure in such a way that it enables the institution to operate smoothly and to accomplish its objectives. However, since the application of these formal organizational principles involves all levels of management, it is also necessary for you as a supervisor to understand them and to know how they are used. This knowledge will help you in organizing your own department and in coordinating its activities with those of the rest of the institution. In your supervisory capacity, you will certainly be asked to carry out, and may be even asked to help make, decisions involving departmentalization or the division of work, the span of supervision, the delegation of authority, etc. And as you move up in the managerial hierarchy, you will probably be called upon to participate in more and more such organizational decisions. Thus, although it is the chief administrator who initially applies the formal principles in order to establish the organization's over-all structure and activities, it is the supervisors and other lower and middle level managers who must make these principles and the resulting structure work. This is why it is essential for us to discuss the organizing process on an over-all or institutional basis before we can discuss it on the departmental or supervisory level.

DEPARTMENTALIZATION

The first step in the process of establishing the formal organizational structure for the over-all institution is to departmentalize. Departmentalization arises from the division of work and the resulting need for coordination. The division of work, as you can probably guess, simply means to break down a whole job into smaller, more specialized tasks. Man has been dividing his work in this manner for thousands and thousands of years, the reason being that he could see that a group of people, each performing a small, specialized part of the over-all job, could accomplish more than the same size group where each individual was trying to do the whole job alone. In other words, the division of work results in greater efficiency and higher production. To take a rather exaggerated example, a group of doctors would probably find it impossible to run a hospital, even a small one, all by themselves. The hospital is likely to be a much better institution if the doctors hire managers, nurses, dietitians, maintenance men, etc., each to do a specialized and necessary task, while they themselves concentrate on those special medical tasks for which only they are trained.

It is because the division of work into such specialized tasks produces a much more efficient operation that nearly every organization must departmentalize. By departmentalization, we understand the process of grouping various activities into natural units. A department is such a unit; it is a distinct area of activities over which a manager or supervisor has been given authority and for which he has accepted responsibility. Of course, the terminology may vary and a department may be called a division, a service, a unit, or some similar term, but it still represents a closely related set of activities.

For all practical purposes, the major departments in an organization are established by the top administrator. He is the one who groups the various activities and assigns them to be a distinct department. Some of the departments which he establishes will be small and will require no further subdivision. But in a hospital many of the departments will be of sufficient magnitude that their managers will have to further subdivide; that is, set up subdepartments or smaller units within the overall department. For this reason, it is necessary that every manager become acquainted with the various alternatives available for grouping activities. The grouping can be done on the basis of functions, product, territory, customer, process and equipment, or time. We shall now explore each of these alternatives more fully.

By Functions

The most widely accepted practice of departmentalizing is to group activities according to function — the job to be done. This is the guiding thought in the establishment of most departments within hospitals and related health care facilities. All those activities that are alike and that involve a particular function are placed together into one department, under a single chain of command. For instance, a director of nursing services would be put in charge of all nursing activities throughout the center, a director of dietary services is put in charge of all kinds of food-related activities, and so forth, as can be seen in Figures 8-1 and 8-2. As the institution grows and undertakes additional work, these new duties are added to the already existing departments. Such increased activities, however, necessitate the addition of more levels of supervision within the functional departments, a topic which we shall discuss further in the next section.

To departmentalize by function in this manner is a natural and logical way of arranging the various activities of any enterprise. It takes advantage of specialization by putting together the functions which belong together and which are performed by the same specialists with the same kind of education, background, equipment, and facilities. Each supervisor is concerned with only one type of work and all of his energy is concentrated on it. Functional departmentalization also facilitates coordination since one supervisor is in charge of all of one type of activity. It is easier to achieve coordination in this way than it would be in an organization where the same function is performed in several different divisions. Another advantage of functional departmentalization is that it makes the outstanding abilities of one or a few individuals available to the enterprise as a whole. Functional departmentalization, moreover, is a simple method and one which has been successful over the years. In short, it makes good sense. Hence, it is the most widely used method of setting up departments.

By Product

Industry very frequently invokes the principle of product departmentalization. To departmentalize on a product basis in industry means to establish each product or groups of closely related products as a product line, as a relatively independent unit within the over-all framework of the enterprise. In product departmentalization, the emphasis is shifted from the function to the product. For example, a

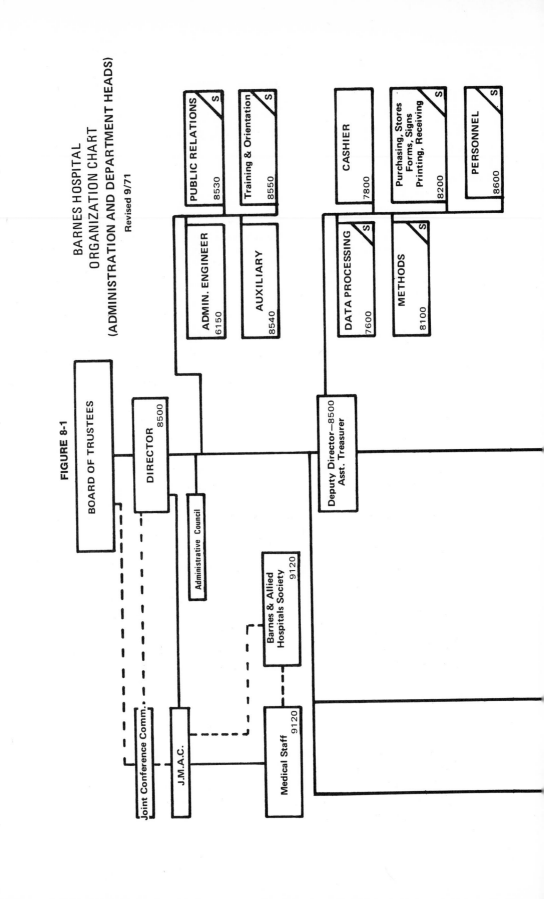

FIGURE 8-1

BARNES HOSPITAL
ORGANIZATION CHART
(ADMINISTRATION AND DEPARTMENT HEADS)

Revised 9/71

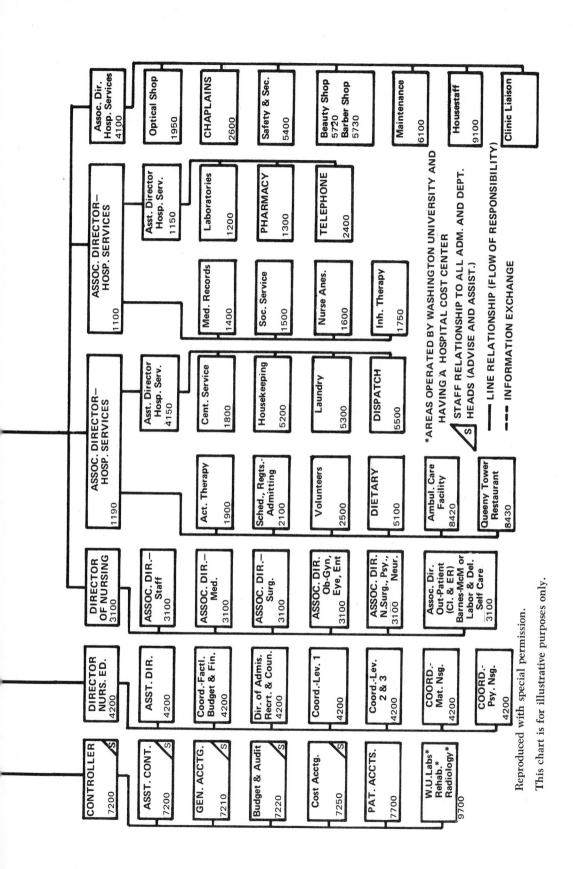

*AREAS OPERATED BY WASHINGTON UNIVERSITY AND HAVING A HOSPITAL COST CENTER

STAFF RELATIONSHIP TO ALL ADM. AND DEPT. HEADS (ADVISE AND ASSIST.)

—— LINE RELATIONSHIP (FLOW OF RESPONSIBILITY)

– – – INFORMATION EXCHANGE

Reproduced with special permission.

This chart is for illustrative purposes only.

FIGURE 8-2

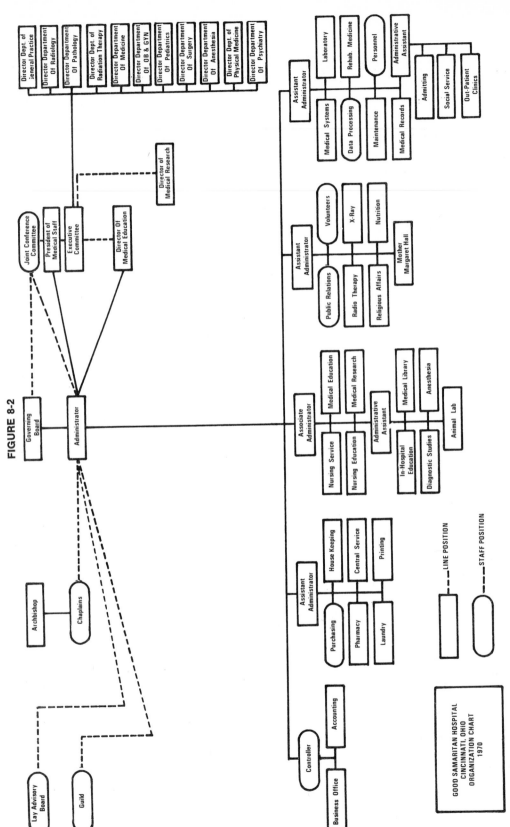

Reproduced with special permission.

hospital supply company may have a separate division for furniture, another one for surgical supplies and a third one for uniforms.

Product departmentalization in a health care facility would involve dividing a hospital into departments based on the "product" turned out; for example, maternity, surgery, intensive care, etc. Each such department would have its own supervisor of nursing, its own dietary supervisor, its own maintenance staff, etc. And each such "product" department would have its own boss, the director of surgery, the director of intensive care, the director of maternity, etc. These directors would be in charge of all functions within their "product" departments, including nursing activities, food services, laundry, maintenance, etc.

As you can see, such product departmentalization will result in duplication of effort. Instead of a single director of nursing there are many — as many as there are departments. Moreover, coordination among all nursing services would be difficult since each supervisor reports to a different boss. And the same difficulties would, of course, be found in every department. Thus, product departmentalization is not applicable in a health care institution.

By Territory

Another way to departmentalize is by geographical considerations. Again, this kind of departmentalization is more important in industrial enterprises, but applications of it can be made within a hospital. For instance, a hospital may be confronted with a setup where there are numerous physically dispersed units. That is, if the same functions are performed in different locations — different buildings — then geographic departments may be feasible. The same considerations may be applicable even if all activities are performed in one building, but on different floors and wings, e.g. the medical-surgical nursing unit, third floor, west wing.

By Customer

At times, a manager may find it advisable to group activities based on customer considerations. This is commonly known as customer departmentalization and it means that the paramount interest of the enterprise lies in the peculiarities of its customers. Two examples of non-industrial organizations which have departmentalized along customer lines are: a university where night programs and day programs comply with the requests and special needs of the various "customers", namely, part-time and full-time students; and a hospital where certain activities are grouped for outpatients and inpatients. This is "customer" departmentalization.

By Process and Equipment

Activities can also be grouped according to the process involved or the equipment used. This way of departmentalizing is often found in hospitals because they usually handle certain processes and operate certain equipment which requires special training and expertise. Everything involving the use of the particular equipment would be referred to its special department. It is important to note that this kind of organizational structure may come close to functional departmentalization. For instance, in an X-ray department specific equipment is used, but also only certain functions are performed. Therefore, in such a situation departmentalization by function and equipment become closely allied.

By Time

An additional way to departmentalize is to group activities according to time. An enterprise such as a hospital or related health care facility, which of necessity is engaged in a continuous process, must departmentalize activities on the basis of time at least to a certain extent. In other words, it must set up different time shifts, usually day, afternoon, and night shifts. Of course, the activities which have to be performed on the later shifts are largely the same as those performed during the regular day shift. Thus, such groupings often create serious organizational questions of how self-contained each shift should be and what relationship should exist between the regular day shift supervisors and the off-shift supervisors.

Composite Structure

Departmentalization is not an end in itself. In grouping activities, management should not attempt to merely draw a pretty picture. Its prime concern should be to set up departments that will facilitate the realization of the institution's objectives and the coordination of its functions. In so doing, management will probably have to use more than one of the guides for grouping activities and they may end up with mixed departmentalization, i.e. a nursing supervisor (functional) on the surgical unit (sub-function), west wing third floor (geographical), of the night shift (time). In practice, most enterprises do have this composite type of departmental structure invoking functional, geographical, time and many other considerations. All of these choices are also available to the supervisor who has to subdepartmentalize and any kind of mixture is acceptable within his own department as long as it is consistent with the over-all structure and objectives of the institution.

MANAGERIAL LEVELS AND THE SPAN OF SUPERVISION

The establishment of departments in an organization is not an end in itself. It is not desirable *per se* because departments are expensive; they must be headed by various supervisors and staffed by additional employees, all of which runs into large sums of money. Furthermore, departments are not desirable *per se* because the more there are, the more difficulties will be encountered in communication and coordination. However, as we discussed earlier, departments do make possible the division of work. And what is equally important, they allow an organization to incorporate what is commonly known as the principle of the span of management or the span of supervision. This principle states that there is an upper limit to the number of subordinates a manager can effectively supervise. Sometimes the same principle is referred to as the span of managerial responsibility, the span of authority, or the span of control. Regardless of the phrase used, however, span is a very important concept in organizational theory and practice.

Almost every manager knows himself that there is a limit to the number of employees he can effectively supervise. He knows that there is a limit to the number of superior-subordinate relationships and cross relationships that he can handle. Since no one can manage an infinite number of subordinates, there is the necessity for the administrator to create departments, distinct areas of activities over which he places a manager in charge. To this manager, the administrator delegates authority. The manager, in turn, will redelegate authority to some of his lower subordinates who, in turn, will supervise only a limited number of employees. In this manner, not only are departments and subdepartments created, but also the *span of supervision,* or the number of employees under each manager, is established *and* the number of managerial *levels* in the organization is determined.

The Relationship of Span to Levels

In order to examine this relationship between the span of supervision and the levels of an organization, imagine a situation where 256 subordinates report to one executive, thus representing one organizational level. Then let us assume that it is concluded that 256 subordinates are way too many and that only four should report to the top administrator. Under each of these four associate administrators there would now be 64 employees reporting. By creating associate administrators, however, we have established two levels of organization and a total of five executives. Now, assuming that 64 subordinates are still too many and this number is reduced to 16, the organization will require three executive levels totaling 21 executives. Each of the five executives on the upper two levels will have four subordinates reporting to him, and each of the sixteen supervisors on the lowest level will have sixteen subordinates reporting to him. The span of supervision has thus been reduced drastically from the original 256 to a maximum of 16.

This obviously extreme example is illustrated in Figure 8-3. The figure shows very clearly what occurs when one begins to narrow the span of supervision. It shows that the narrower the span becomes, the more levels of management have to be introduced into the organizational setup. As with departments, this is not desirable *per se* again because levels cost money and because they complicate communications and control. Therefore, there is a constant conflict between the width of the span and the number of levels. The problem is whether to have a broader span of supervision or more levels, or vice versa. This problem is one with which every manager is faced throughout his entire career.

Moreover, the problem of span vs. levels is as old as mankind. And we have still not found a pat answer to it. It is simply not possible to state a definite figure as to how many subordinates a manager can have reporting to him. It is correct to say only that there is an upper limit to this figure. Although we do not know exactly what the upper limit should be, it is interesting to note that in many enterprises the top administrator has only from five to eight subordinate managers reporting directly to him. As we descend down the managerial hierarchy, we find that the span of supervision generally increases. It is not unusual to have anywhere from fifteen to twenty people reporting to the supervisor's level. Upon closer inspection, we find that the number of subordinates who can be effectively supervised by one manager actually depends upon numerous different factors. These factors determine not only the actual number of relationships but also their frequency and intensity. Therefore, before deciding the proper span of supervision in a particular organization it is necessary to examine the more important factors that influence the magnitude of the span.

Factors Determining the Span of Supervision

One of the factors that influences the magnitude of the span is the *supervisor's qualifications* — his training, experience, and know-how. Obviously, there are some supervisors who are capable of handling more subordinates than others. Some are better acquainted with good management practices; some have had more experience and are simply better all around managers. If a man is a "good manager," he probably can supervise more employees. But he is still limited by his human capacity and by the amount of time he has available during the working day.

What the manager does with his time is of utmost importance in determining his span. For example, it takes more time for a supervisor to make an individual decision for every problem that comes up, than it does for him to take the time initially to make policy decisions which anticipate problems that might arise later. Clear and complete policy statements reduce the volume of, or at least simplify, the per-

FIGURE 8-3

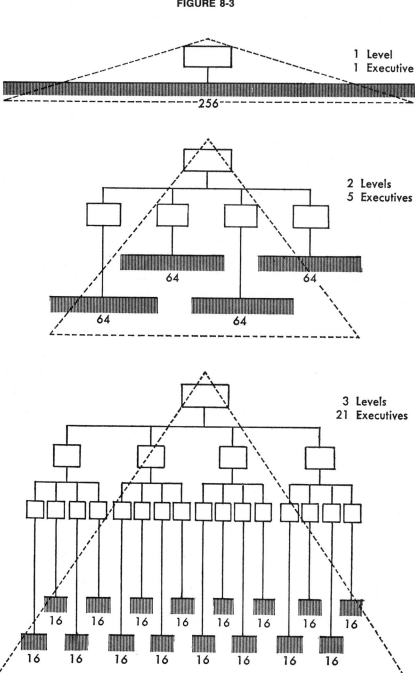

sonal decision-making required of a manager, and hence can increase his span of supervision. The same applies to other managerial processes that determine in advance definitions of responsibility and authority, performance standards, programs, procedures, and methods. Predeterminations such as these also reduce the number of decisions the manager has to make, and likewise increase his potential span of management. Thus, we can see that one of the important factors in determinig the quantity of employees a manager can effectively supervise is the quality of his managerial ability, and more specifically how he spends his managerial time.

Another factor which will determine how broad a span a manager can handle is the *capacities and the makeup of the employees* in his department. The greater the capacities and self-direction of the employees, the broader the manager's span can be. The training possessed by the subordinates is also of importance. The better their training, the less they will need their supervisor; hence, the more subordinates he can manage.

Another factor on which the manager's span depends is the amount and nature of the work he must do, and more particularly whether he can count on *help from specialists* within the organization. If a hospital has a range of experts who provide various kinds of advice and service, then the manager's span can be wider. For instance, if the personnel department does a good job in servicing and assisting the supervisor in the procurement of employees, then he will have more time and energy available to increase the number of subordinates he can manage. But if the supervisor has to do all the recruiting, preinterviewing, and testing himself, then obviously he cannot devote that portion of his time to the management of his department. Therefore, the amount of additional help available within the institution will influence the width of the span of supervision.

The number of subordinates which can be supervised will also depend on the *variety and importance of the activities* performed by them. If these activities are highly important and/or frequently changing, it follows that the span of supervision will of necessity have to be small. But the simpler and more uniform the work, the greater can be the number of persons supervised by one supervisor. If the task to be performed is repetitious, the span may even be as broad as twenty-five to thirty employees. If the activities are varied and demanding, the span might have to be as small as three to five employees.

Closely related factors that have a bearing on the span of supervision are the *dynamics and complexity of a particular activity*. Some aspects of the hospital routine are most certainly of a dynamic nature whereas others are of a more stable character. In those departments which are engaged in dynamic and unpredictable activities, like the coronary intensive care unit, the span will have to be narrow. In those departments which are concerned with more or less stable activities, for example, the dietary department, the span of supervision can be broader.

Another factor which will determine the span of supervision is the degree to which *objective standards* are or can be applied. If there are enough objective standards available for a subordinate to check whether or not he is on the right track, he will not need to constantly report to and contact his boss. Good objective standards will result in less frequent relationships and therefore make for a broader span of supervision.

Although we have now discussed most of the major factors which influence the span of supervision, we still cannot state a definite number of subordinates that a supervisor can effectively manage in each and every instance. It will always depend upon the particular circumstances and the factors which are operative. The principle of span of supervision tells us only that an upper limit exists for this number.

LINE AND STAFF

In hospitals and related health facilities, it is common to speak of the medical staff, the nursing staff, the maintenance staff, the administrative staff, etc. In this context, the word "staff" applies to a group of people who are engaged primarily in one activity to the exclusion of others. That is, the word "staff" is used to define all those people who do about the same thing, e.g. nurses, doctors, dietitians, and so on. However, in the general field of management and administration the meaning of the word "staff" is very different — "staff" is spoken of in connection with "line," and both of these terms refer to authority relationships which we shall discuss below. In this book, any reference to "staff" will be in the line/staff sense, not in the sense to which most people working in health care centers are usually accustomed.

Much has been written and said about the concepts of line and staff, and there probably is no other area in the field of management which has evoked as much discussion as these concepts. It is probably also true that many of the difficulties and frictions encountered in the daily life of an organization are due to line and staff problems. Misconceptions and lack of understanding as to what line and staff really are can cause bitter feelings and conflicts of personalities, much disunity, duplication of effort, waste, lost motion, and so on.

As a supervisor of a department, you should know whether you are attached to your organization in a line capacity or a staff capacity. You might be able to find this out by reading the job description and if that does not clarify it, by asking your superior manager. Line and staff are not characteristics of certain functions, rather they are characteristics of authority relationships. Therefore, the ultimate way to determine whether a department is related to the organization structure as line or as staff is to examine the intentions of the administrator. It is he who confers line authority upon certain departments and places others into the organization structure as staff. Staff is not inferior to line authority or vice versa; they are just of a completely different nature. As we discuss these differences, it is well to keep in mind, however, that the objectives of the staff elements, are ultimately the same as those of the line organization, namely, the achievement of the institution's over-all goals.

Line

The simplest of all organizational structures is the line organization. The line organization depicts the primary chain of command and is inseparable from the concept of authority. Thus, when we refer to line authority we mean a superior and a subordinate with a direct line of command running between them. In every organization, there is this straight, direct line of superior-subordinate relationships which runs from the top of the organization down to the lowest level of supervision. Figure 8-4 depicts an example of one direct line of authority running from the board of trustees to the administrator of the institution, to the director of nursing services, to a nursing supervisor, from her to a head nurse, then on to a team leader, and finally to the rest of the nursing employees.

Unity of Command

The uninterrupted line of authority from the administrator to the team leader assures that each superior exercises direct command over his subordinate and that each subordinate has only one superior to obey. This is known as the principle of *unity of command*. It is a principle which every administrator should follow while arranging line authority relationships. Unity of command means that there is one person in each organizational unit who has the authority to make the decisions appropriate to his position. It means that each employee has a single immediate supervisor who is in turn responsible to his immediate supervisor, and so on up and down the chain of command. Thus, everyone in the line organization knows precisely who his boss is and who his subordinates are. He knows exactly where he stands, to whom he can give orders and whose orders he has to obey.

From what we have said thus far, it is easy to see that line authority can be defined as the authority to give orders, to command. It is the authority to direct others, and to require them to conform to decisions, plans, policies, and objectives. The primary purpose of this line authority is, of course, to make the organization work by evoking appropriate action from subordinates. Directness and unity of command have the great advantage of assuring that results can be achieved precisely and quickly.

However, this kind of direct line structure does not answer all of the needs of the modern organization. It was adequate at a time when organizations were not as complex as they are today. In most enterprises now, activities have become so specialized and complicated

FIGURE 8-4

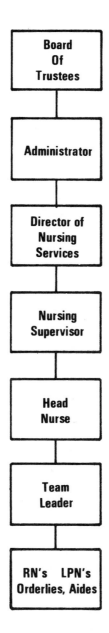

that an executive cannot be expected to properly and expertly direct all of his subordinates in all phases of their activities without some additional assistance. Line management today definitely needs the help of others to carry out its job. That is, in order to perform his managerial functions well, almost every line executive needs someone to lean on, someone who can give him counsel, advice, and service. In short, he needs a staff.

Staff

Staff is auxiliary in nature, but it helps the line executive in many ways. It provides counsel, advice, and guidance in any number of specialized areas. However, staff cannot issue orders or command line executives to take their advice. Staff can only make recommendations to the line. Within each staff division, of course there exists a line of command with superior-subordinate relationships just like in any other department. But staff's own chain of command does not extend over to the line organization. Rather, it exists alongside of the line organization as shown in Figure 8-5. The function of staff is to provide guidance, advice, counsel, and service to all members of the organization whenever and wherever there may be a need. Obviously, staff is not inferior to line and line is not inferior to staff. They are just different and both are needed to complement each other in order to achieve over-all objectives.

You can probably now see more clearly why every supervisor must know whether he is attached to the organization in a line or a staff capacity. He must know this so that he will understand his function and his relation to the other members of the organization. If he is staff, then his function is to provide guidance, counsel, advice, and service in his specialized area to whomever may ask him for it. But as far as his own department is concerned it will not matter whether he is line or staff. Within every department, the supervisor is the line manager. He is the only boss regardless of whether the department is attached to the organization in a staff or in a line capacity.

At this point, we must distinguish between *personal* staff and *specialized* staff. When an executive finds himself in a position where he needs a personal aid who will help him in the performance of duties that he cannot delegate, he may create a personal staff position. The person in this position is a staff aid to the particular executive, rather than to the organization at large, for example, the Assistant to the Administrator as shown in Figure 8-5. Eventually, however, a personal staff will usually become inadequate because many other managers in the organization also need expert advice and guidance. At this juncture, specialized staffs are introduced into the institution to provide counsel and advice in various special fields to any member of the organization who needs it.

Relations of Staff and Line

It is common practice for certain activities in each organization to be undertaken as staff. But this does not mean that one can assume that these activities are always staff. Line and staff, as stated before, are characteristics of authority relationships and not of functions. Thus, even a title will not offer any clue in recognizing line or staff. In industrial enterprises, it is common to find a vice-president of

FIGURE 8-5

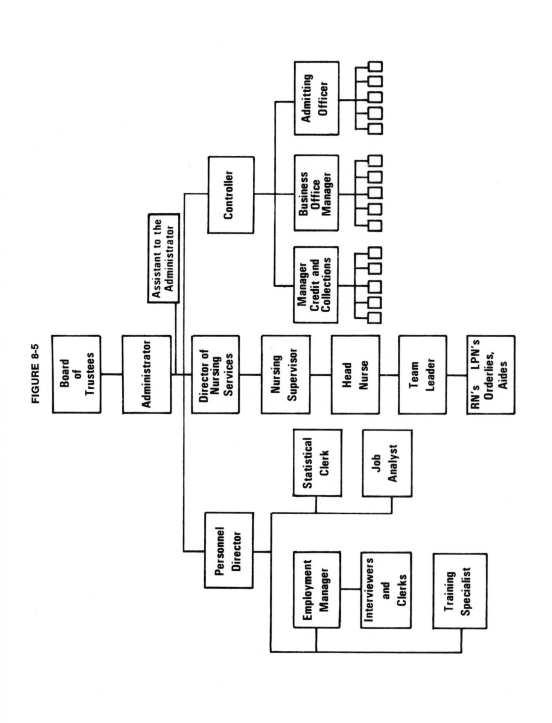

engineering, a vice-president of industrial relations, a vice-president of production. None of these titles, however, indicates whether the position is line or staff.

The same situation applies in hospitals and related health care facilities. For example, most hospital personnel managers and their departments operate in a staff capacity, although you could not tell this from their titles. The function of a staff personnel department is to provide advice and service on personnel matters to all the other departments of the institution. The personnel department is there to recruit, screen, and test applicants, to keep personnel records, to help provide reasonable wage and salary administration, to advise line managers when difficult problems of discipline arise, and so on. Whenever a line manager has a personnel problem, therefore, he should call upon the specialized services of this staff department. Certainly, the personnel manager is the one who is best qualified to supply the current advice and information since this is his background and his only duty.

But all the personnel manager can do is submit suggestions to the line manager, who in turn can accept, alter, or reject them. If the line manager should feel that the suggestions of the personnel department are not feasible, he is at liberty to make his own decision. But inasmuch as the reason for establishing a staff in most instances is to obtain the best advice, it is usually in the interest of the line manager to follow staff suggestions. After all, staff people are the ones who really ought to know best. So, for all practical purposes, the "authority" of the staff lies in their thorough knowledge of and expertise in dealing with the problems in their specialized field. They will sell their ideas based on their authority of knowledge, not on their power to command. Thus, if any of the suggestions of staff are to be carried out, they are carried out under the name and the authority of the line officer and not that of the staff man. A person who acts in a staff relationship must know that his task is to advise, counsel, and guide, and not to give orders except within his own department. He must understand that if his ideas are accepted by the line executive, the orders to carry them out must be issued by that same executive following the regular chain of command.

Functional Authority

It is correct in most instances, then, to say that staff provides advice and counsel to line managers, but that it lacks the right to command them. However, there is one exception to this concept of staff which should be pointed out here. A staff man may have been given *functional authority*. Functional authority is authority restricted to a very narrow area; it is a special right given to someone who normally would not have authority and therefore could not command. This right is based on expertise in the person's specialized field.

For example, let us assume that an administrator decided that his personnel director should have the final word in cases of discharge.* In this instance, the administrator has conferred upon staff (assuming that the personnel department was a staff activity) functional authority in the special area of firing. Now the personnel director has this authority and it no longer adheres to the line supervisor who would normally have had the authority to do his own firing. This would be an example of functional staff authority.

There is no doubt that functional authority violates the principle of unity of command. This principle, as the reader will recall, states that the subordinate is subject to orders from only one superior regarding all his functions. Functional authority, however, introduces a second superior for one particular function, such as the discharging of employees in our example.

Nevertheless, functional authority is advantageous because it allows for the maximum effective use of a staff specialist. It makes it possible for staff to intervene in line operations in questions which top management designates. The price for this, as stated above, is violation of unity of command which may cause real frictions in some organizations. It is up to the administrator to weigh the advantages versus the disadvantages before he assigns functional authority.

THE AUTHORITY OF OUTSIDE PHYSICIANS AND SURGEONS

At this point, it becomes necessary to discuss another source of authority which is found only in a hospital setting, namely, the authority exercised by physicians and surgeons. Here we are not referring to those medical men who are full-time chiefs of the medical staff group, or full-time chiefs of a medical specialty, or members of the resident house physicians group. Let us assume that all the latter are regular employees of the hospital, who do not have a private practice, and who receive their salary from the hospital. We are not speaking of these types of doctors now. Rather, our reference is to those physicians and surgeons who are in the private, fee-for-service practice of medicine and who have been admitted to practice at the hospital. There is little doubt that such outside doctors are in charge of their patients whom they bring into the hospital. In this connection, they exercise substantial influence throughout the hospital structure at many organizational levels and in many functions.

However, these outside physicians admitted to practice at the hospital (usually referred to as the medical staff) are not shown on the hospital organization chart in any direct line or staff relationship. They practice medicine at the hospital, but they are outside of the

---

*This type of situation and the difficulties it can cause will be discussed further in Chapter 13 in connection with the supervisor's staffing function and the activities of the personnel director.

administrative line of authority. They are "guests" who are granted practice privileges. Yet, as the physician or surgeon on the case, they have a great deal of authority over various people in the hospital.* Their authority is exercised over the patient, and especially over the nursing staff when it comes to the medical aspects of the case. But they also give orders to and expect compliance from many other employees of the hospital, for instance from personnel in the x-ray section, in the laboratories, from the dietary supervisor and so forth.

As a second line of "authority," such orders from a physician or a surgeon clearly violate the principle of unity of command. They may lead to a situation where nursing personnel in particular are accountable to two "bosses" — i.e. they must take orders from and are responsible not only to their supervisor but also to the physician on the case. This, of course, can cause great difficulties when the administrative source of authority and the medical professional source of authority are not consistent. Nevertheless, in a hospital the physician on the case can give orders to an employee without being his line supervisor. In other words, the physician constitutes an outside source of authority who can marshal the resources of the hospital without being in the chain of command and without being responsible to the administrator, except for his professional responsibility owed to the medical world. Of course, it is assumed that the physician's medical competence warrants the right and the authority to remain in practice at the hospital.

This dual command obviously creates administrative and operational problems as well as human problems. It causes difficulties in communication, difficulties in the area of discipline, and it can make organizational coordination an extremely difficult task. Moreover, it can cause considerable confusion in cases in which it is not clear where authority and responsibility truly reside. This can lead to frequent efforts on the physician's part to circumvent administrative channels. And by the same token, the administration may think that the physician through his power and authority is interfering with administrative responsibilities. In all likelihood, there will be some changes in this situation as hospitals' over-all legal responsibilities are defined more clearly in the future. However, regardless of all the complications inherent in this duality of command, it is for the time being an integral part of every general community hospital and it exists in most other health care facilities as well. Hospital supervisors and personnel just have to learn to live and cope with the problem of dual authority when it applies to the medical or surgical aspects of the case.

*These remarks of necessity have to be general. They apply primarily to *general, private, community hospitals.* There are many ramifications in teaching hospitals or in hospitals operated by government agencies and so forth where our statements would not apply or would have to be modified.

SUMMARY

Management's over-all organizing function is to design a formal structural framework which will enable the institution to achieve its objectives. The chief administrator establishes this framework initially, using the basic principles of formal organization theory as guidelines. He begins by applying the principle that the division of work is necessary for efficiency. Thus, he knows that he must group the various activities of the institution into distinct departments or divisions and assign specific duties to each. There are several ways in which the administrator can approach this departmentalizing task. The most widely used concept of departmentalization is grouping activities according to functions, that is, placing all those who perform the same functions into the same department. Besides departmentalization by functions, it is possible to departmentalize along geographic lines, or by product, by customer (patients), by process and equipment, or by time (shifts). A composite structure made up of several of these alternatives is also used quite frequently.

A second step in the over-all organizing process is for the administrator to determine the number of managerial levels in the organizational hierarchy and the span of supervision at each level. The span of supervision is another of the basic principles of organization which states that there is an upper limit to the number of employees that a manager can effectively manage. The actual width of this span is determined by such factors as the capability of the supervisor, the previous training and experience of the subordinates, the amount and nature of the work to be performed, and the availability of special staff assistance. No definite figure can be quoted as the ideal number of subordinates to be supervised by one manager, but the administrator knows that whenever the span of supervision is decreased, meaning that the number of employees to be supervised is reduced, an additional manager has to be introduced for the excess employees. In other words, the smaller the span of supervision, the more levels of supervisory personnel are needed. This will shape the organization into either a tall, narrow pyramid or in the case of a broad span of supervision into a shallow, wide pyramid.

As a third step in establishing the formal organizational structure, the administrator will have to decide whether each department is attached to the organization in a line or in a staff capacity. Since line and staff are quite different, it is essential for every supervisor to know in which capacity he serves. If he finds himself in the straight, direct chain of command which can be traced all the way up from his position to that of the top administrator, then he is part of the line organization. The line organization generally follows the principle of unity of command which means that each member of the organization has a single immediate superior who in turn is responsible to his immediate superior and so on up and down the line of command. If the supervisor does not find himself within this line of command, then he is attached to the organization as a staff man to provide expert counsel, service, and advice in his own specialized field to whomever in the organization needs it. Staff people are not inferior to line or vice versa, rather they represent different types of authority relationships. The line manager has the authority to give orders whereas the staff manager usually only has the authority to make recommendations which the line manager does not have to accept. Sometimes, however, the administrator may confer functional authority upon a staff manager; that is, the right to command in a very narrow area based upon the staff manager's expertise in that specific area. Such functional authority violates the principle of unity of command, as does the authority of the private outside physician who is admitted to practice at the hospital. Nevertheless, these additional channels of command have to be coped with in almost every health care center.

Formal Organizational
Charts and Manuals

Once the administrator has established the formal structure of the organization by setting up departments and levels, determining the span of supervision, and deciding which functions are to be line and which are to be staff, he can depict this entire structure graphically by using organization charts and manuals including position descriptions. These are very important organizational tools for they provide a clearcut picture of the over-all institution which can be used by all levels of management. For the supervisor, organization charts and manuals can be particularly helpful in understanding the formal organizing process and the goals and intent of the administration. By familiarizing himself with them, the supervisor can see the position and relations of his own department within the over-all structure and he will learn about the functioning and relationships of all other departments as well. Although the administrator is responsible for preparing charts and manuals for the institution as a whole, it may be necessary for the supervisor to devise some of these organizational tools himself on a departmental level if they are not available or not up-to-date or if he needs to use them for planning purposes. Thus, we must look more carefully at how such tools are prepared and at the information which they supply.

ORGANIZATION CHARTS

Organization charts are a means of graphically portraying the organization structure at a given time. The chart shows the skeleton of the structure, depicting the basic relationships and groupings of positions and functions. Most of the time the chart starts out with the individual position as the basic unit shown as a rectangular box. Each box represents one job. The various boxes are then interconnected to show the groupings of activities which make up a department, division, or whatever other part of the organization is under consideration. It can readily be determined who reports to whom merely by studying the position of the boxes in their scalar relationships. For example, we saw in the organization charts on pages 88-90 some of the scalar relationships which can be found in a typical hospital.

Although different types of charts are available, those on pages 88 and 90, like the vast majority of organizational charts, are of the vertical type. They show the different levels of the organization in a step arrangement in the form of a pyramid. The chief administrator is placed at the top of the chart and the successive levels of administration are depicted vertically in the pyramid shape. One of the main advantages of this type of chart is that it can be easily read and understood. It also shows the downward flow of delegation of authority, the chain of command, the functional relationships, and so forth.

One of the disadvantages is that the pyramid type of chart, can convey a wrong impression about the relative status of certain positions. This is due to the fact that some positions have to be drawn higher or lower on the chart, when in reality they are on the same organizational plane. For example, such an incorrect impression can result if one division of an organization has more levels than another. An organizational unit of say three levels may show a supervisor on the lowest level, whereas in a five-level unit he would be on the third level.

In addition to the pyramid type of chart, some hospitals may occasionally prefer a horizontal chart which reads from left to right such as that shown in Figure 8-6. Or a circular chart can also be used; it depicts the various levels on concentric circles rotating around the top administrator who is at the hub of the wheel (see Figure 8-7). Other hospitals prefer an inverted pyramid chart showing the chief administrator at the bottom and his associate administrators further up. This type tries to express the idea of the "support" given to each manager by his "superior."

No matter what type of charts are used, however, they can be a great help to all managers not only because they portray the existing organizational structure, but also because they can be useful in making for better communications and relations. And as pointed out above, charts can also be very valuable for future planning purposes. Indeed, a supervisor may want to have two charts for his department, one showing the existing arrangements and another depicting the ideal organization. He may use the latter in such a way that all the gradual changes he plans fall within the design of the ideal which represents the ultimate organizational goal of his department in the future.

There are a number of additional advantages in establishing charts of both the over-all organization as well as of each department's organization. As a graphic portrait is drawn up, the organization must be carefully analyzed. Such analysis might uncover structural

FIGURE 8-6

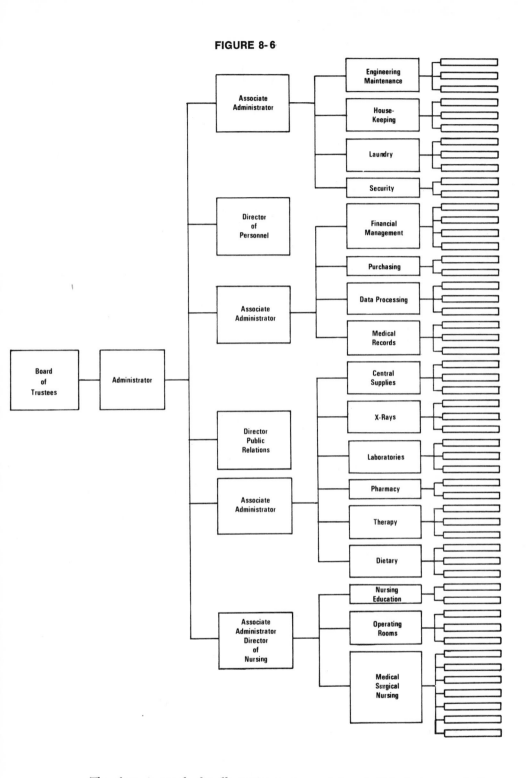

The above is merely for illustrative purposes; it is not all inclusive, nor is it a recommended organizational arrangement.

FIGURE 8-7

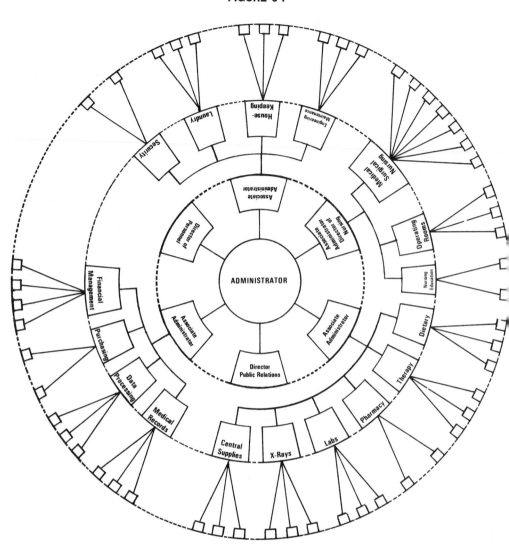

faults and possibly also duplications of effort or other inconsistencies. Or one might uncover cases where dual reporting relationships exist, where one person is reporting to two superiors, where there are overlapping positions, and so on. Moreover, charts might indicate whether the span of supervision is too wide or too narrow. An unbalanced organization can also be readily revealed. And charts can indicate possible routes of promotions for managers as well as for other employees. In addition, charts afford a simple way to acquaint new members of the organization with its makeup. It is only natural that most employees within the organization have a keen interest in knowing where they stand, in what relation their supervisor stands to the higher echelons, and so forth.

Of course, there are some limitations to charts, especially if they are not continually kept up to date. It is imperative that organizational changes be recorded at once because failure to do so makes charts as useless as yesterday's newspaper. Another shortcoming of charts is that the information they give is limited. A chart does not show the amount of authority and responsibility, it only shows what is on the surface. Moreover, it does not show any informal relationships or the informal organizations which we will discuss in another chapter. Nevertheless, charts are still a very useful tool for every manager.

ORGANIZATION MANUALS

The organization manual is another helpful tool for achieving effective organization because it provides in comprehensive written form the decisions which have been made with regard to the institution's structure as well as its major policies and objectives. The organization's manual, moreover, is a readily available reference defining the scope of authority and the responsibilities of managerial positions and the channels to be used in obtaining decisions or approvals of proposals. A manual will also be of great help in the indoctrination and development of managerial personnel. The manual should clearly specify for each manager what the responsibilities of his job are and how they are related to other positions within the organization. In addition, it reiterates for the individual manager the objectives of the enterprise and of his department, and it provides a means of explaining the complex relationships within the organization. Every supervisor will do well to familiarize himself with the contents of the institution's manual, especially with those parts which affect his own department.

Objectives and Policies

In the manual, as we have said, top management states the major objectives and goals which the institution seeks to reach. In the case of a hospital, the manual would state the institution's creed, its philosophies, and its broad policies in regard to patient care, the type of medicine practiced, social responsibility, and many other areas of responsibility. It would mention, for example, the hospital's objectives of the education of professional and paramedical people, of investigative studies and possibly research in the fields of medical services. It may state that one of the objectives is to be alert and responsive to the changing needs of the community, and so forth.

Job Descriptions

All manuals also contain job descriptions. There is some confusion, however, in the use of the term "job description" as compared to "job specification." Generally speaking, job descriptions objectively describe the elements of a position, that is, they indicate the principal duties and functions of the position as well as its scope and kind of authority. Job specifications, on the other hand, specify the human qualities required, the personal (man) specifications which are necessary to perform the job adequately; in other words, the education, training, experience, disposition, etc. In some enterprises, job descriptions are extended to include such man specifications. However, the latter do not necessarily have to appear in the organization manual. The job descriptions which are supposed to appear in the manual will vary depending upon the size of the departments and the type of work involved. For instance, in the manual section intended for nursing services, all jobs starting with the director of nursing services down to the jobs of aides and orderlies should be described. If a job is particularly complicated or if it involves numerous, activities, its description will probably be rather lengthy; otherwise, most descriptions are fairly short.

Initially, job descriptions should be written by the chief administrator and his staff as they go about the organizing process. However, at times a hospital will not have job descriptions and, if this is the case, the departmental supervisors should see to it that they are drawn up. To help them in this endeavor, the supervisors should be able to call upon the personnel department which has the necessary expertise to facilitate the job. Even when job descriptions are available, it is the supervisor's duty to familiarize himself with them in order to make sure they are realistic and up-to-date. Job descriptions have a tendency to become obsolete, and this can have serious consequences. Thus, it is necessary for the supervisor to check with the employees who hold the various positions in his department and to compare the descriptions they give of their own jobs to what it says in the manual. If the manual is outdated or incorrect, the supervisor must have it revised. Times are changing and in all likelihood the content of some jobs has changed without the administrator's being aware of it; furthermore, requirements for background, education, and training have undergone significant changes in many cases. All of this should be recorded on the job description.

If they are kept current, job descriptions will prove invaluable to many people throughout the organization. For instance, the personnel director will refer to the job description when he is asked by the supervisor to recruit applicants for an open position. He will use them in the preliminary interview. The supervisor will also keep the job description in mind when he interviews the applicants for positions in his department. And the new employee should, of course, have a chance to see the description of the job for which he has been hired. In many hospitals, it is a practice to hand the new employee a copy of it for him to keep and study. The job description is also used when the supervisor evaluates and appraises the employee's performance at regular intervals. And there are many additional occasions when references to job descriptions will be necessary. For all of these reasons, both the supervisor and the administrator should be vitally concerned that the content of the job description is proper and current.*

*Also see the various departmental charts and job descriptions in the Appendix at the end of the book.

CHAPTER 9

Delegating Organizational Authority

THE MEANING OF AUTHORITY

Authority is a difficult concept; it has many interpretations and meanings including the one we shall use in this chapter, namely, that authority is an attribute of the managerial position, that it is the key to the managerial job. In this sense, authority refers to the formal or official power of a manager to obtain the compliance of his subordinates with directives, communications, policies, and objectives. Such authority is associated with the manager's function in the organization. It is vested in organizational roles or positions. As long as an individual holds the position, he has the privilege of exercising the authority which is inherent in it. And since positions are meaningless unless they are occupied by someone, we generally speak of the authority of the manager, the authority that is delegated to him, and so forth. Although it would be more precise to speak of the authority of the managerial position itself or the authority delegated to that position rather than to the person who occupies it, the difference is generally regarded as semantic. As long as we understand that authority resides in the position, we may speak rather loosely of the authority of the manager, of the supervisor, etc.

Of course, there are other forms of authority which are not associated with organizational positions and roles. They come from expertise in a given field and from the personal qualities or attractiveness of an individual. This kind of authority involves a personal capacity to affect the actions of others which cannot be delegated. We will discuss such authority more fully as a form of influence later on in the book.

Limits of Authority

There are, of course, limitations to the authority that a manager has by virtue of his position in an organization. These limitations, which also help to define authority, can be either explicit or implicit. Moreover, some of them stem from internal sources and others from external sources. External limitations on authority would include such

114

things as our codes, folkways, and life style, along with the many political, legal, ethical, moral, social, and economic considerations which make up our society. For example, laws referring to collective bargaining and resulting contractual obligations are a specific example of external limitations on authority.

Internal limitations on authority would be set mainly by the organization's articles of incorporation and its by-laws. In addition to these over-all internal restrictions, each manager in a particular position is subject to the specific limitations spelled out by the administrator when he assigns duties and delegates authority. Generally speaking, there are more internal limitations on the scope of authority the further down one goes in the managerial hierarchy. In other words, the lower the rung on the administrative ladder, the narrower the area in which authority can be exercised. This is known as the tapering concept of authority as shown in Figure 9-1.

FIGURE 9-1

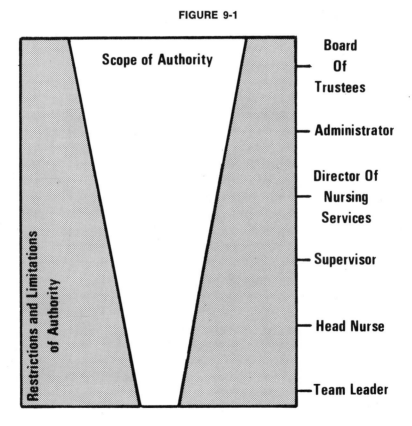

All of the above would be explicit, fairly obvious restrictions on authority. In addition to these, there are a number of more implicit limitations such as the biological restraints which exist simply because the human being does not have the capacity to do certain things.

No subordinate should be expected to do the impossible. Thus, physical and psychological restrictions on authority must be recognized and accepted. In today's society, considerations of this kind significantly limit the scope of authority of every manager.

Sources of Authority

It is important for understanding the meaning of authority to discuss its sources; that is, where authority originates, where it comes from. There are two different theories on this; namely, that authority originates at the top of the organizational hierarchy and that it is delegated downward from superiors to subordinates, or that authority originates at the bottom of the organizational pyramid and is conferred upwards from subordinates to superiors. Let us look at each of these theories more carefully in order to gain further insight into the difficult authority concept.

Formal Authority Theory

The formal authority theory is the top-down theory. It traces the delegation of authority downward from top management to subordinate managers. You can trace your own authority as coming directly from your boss who has delegated it to you. He, in turn, receives his authority, let us say, from an associate administrator who, in turn, receives his authority from the chief administrator, who, in turn, traces his authority directly back to the board of directors, who, in turn, receive their authority from the owners or the stockholders. In private corporations, therefore, we may say that the actual source of authority lies in the stockholders who are, loosely speaking, the owners of the corporation. These owners delegate their power to administer the affairs of the corporation to those whom they have put into managerial positions. From the top adminstrator, such power flows down through the channel of command until it reaches the supervisor.

This is the formal way of looking at the origin of authority as a power which results from our recognition of private property. According to this theory, then, the ultimate source of all managerial authority in America would be the constitutional guarantee of the institution of private property. Additional supporting authority would be bestowed by the laws interpreting and upholding the constitution. The formal theory thus considers the concept of authority as being transmitted from the basic social institutions to the individual managers.

Acceptance Theory

A large group of writers do not agree with the formal theory but maintain that management has no meaningful authority unless and until subordinates confer it. These writers claim that formal organizational authority is effective only to the extent that subordinates accept it. They state that unless your subordinates accept your authority you, as a manager, actually do not possess that authority. In reality, of course, subordinates often do not have a choice between accepting authority or not accepting it. The only choice they have is to leave the job. Nevertheless, this is a worrisome thought, one which indicates that there is considerable merit in looking at authority as something which must be accepted by your employees.

It should be pointed out, however, that the advocates of the acceptance theory state that in most instances a manager does not have a real problem since an employee, when he accepts a job, knows that the boss of his department has the authority to give orders, to take disciplinary action, and to do whatever else goes with the managerial position. It is likely that when some of the acceptance advocates discuss authority they are actually referring to another sort of authoritative influence, namely leadership. But leadership is a completely different concept from that of organizational authority as we are discussing it here. Leadership will be examined later in Chapter 17.

To repeat, then, the origin of authority can be considered from two viewpoints, namely, the formal way of looking at authority as something which originates with private property—formally handed down from the owners at the top to the lowest line supervisor; or, in contrast, looking at authority as something which is conferred upon the supervisor by his subordinates' acceptance of his authority. It is not our intention to go further into this academic argument here. We have touched on it, however, because in reality it significantly influences the practice of supervision, the manner and the attitudes with which supervision is approached.

This will become more obvious when we realize that adherence to the acceptance theory does not necessarily rule out the downward delegation of authority from upper to lower levels of management. The acceptance theory can be thought of as merely adding another dimension to the formal concept of organizational authority. That is, in addition to having formal authority delegated to him from above, the manager must also have such authority accepted from below. Every manager must be aware that he possesses formal authority and, if need be, he can resort to it as a final recourse. Obviously, in this day and age no one would want to rely exclusively on the weight of his authority to motivate workers to perform their jobs. However, there will be times and occasions when every manager will have to make full use of his authority and power. But, hopefully, these will be the exceptions and not the rule. And even when the manager does have to invoke his authority, the manner in which he does so will make a difference in whether it is resented or accepted without resentment. If it is accepted graciously most of the time, the manager will know that his subordinates have chosen to recognize and respect the authority which his superiors have delegated to him formally. We are now ready to discuss in greater detail just what this formal process of delegation means and what it involves.

THE MEANING OF DELEGATION

Just as authority is the key to the managerial job, so is delegation of authority the key to the creation of an organization. Although the formal structure of an organization may have been meticulously designed by the chief administrator and carefully explained in manuals and charts, the organization will still not have life or body until and unless authority is delegated throughout its entire structure. In other words, delegation of authority makes the organization operative. Through this process of delegation, *the subordinate manager receives his authority from his superior*. Without such authority, he would not be a manager. Without it, his job would not be real. In other words, if authority were not delegated, there would be no subordinate managers and hence no one to occupy the various levels, departments, and positions which comprise the organizational structure. Thus, we can truly say that only by delegating authority to subordinate managers is the organization actually created. Only by such delegation can the administration vest a subordinate with a portion of its own authority, thereby setting in motion the entire managerial process.

But delegation of authority does not mean that the boss surrenders all of his authority. The delegating manager always retains the over-all authority to perform his functions. He can, if need be, revoke all or part of whatever authority he has granted to a subordinate manager. A good comparison can be made between delegating authority and imparting knowledge in school. A teacher in school shares knowledge with his students who then possess this knowledge; but the teacher still retains the knowledge as well.

The Scalar Chain

Through the process of delegation, as we have said, formal authority is distributed throughout the organization. In flows downward from the source of all authority at the top, through the various levels of management, to the supervisor, and from him possibly to lower line supervisors. As with private industrial concerns the broad authority necessary to run a health care center is usually delegated by the board of directors or trustees to the administrator or executive director who in turn must delegate authority to subordinate managers who delegate further down the line, and so forth.

This line of direct authority relationships throughout the organization is commonly known as the scalar chain. It is a clear line from the ultimate source of authority to the lowest managerial ranks. This chain of command must be clearly understood by every subordinate, and it must be closely adhered to or else the risk exists of undermining authority. It is quite possible that by the time this "flow of authority" reaches the supervisory level it has pretty well narrowed down to a discreet "trickle" of delegation rather than a continuous stream. Nevertheless, it can be traced directly upward to the ultimate source.

Unity of Command

We are already aware that this delegation of authority flows from a single superior to a single subordinate and each subordinate reports to only one superior. He is accountable only to that superior from whom he receives his authority. This is what is known as unity of command, the important organizational principle to which we referred in Chapter 8. We also pointed out in Chapter 8 that the concept of functional authority is a violation of unity of command and that it is clearly an exception to the direct line of authority relationships encompassed in the scalar chain. Nevertheless, the scalar chain still provides the major route along which the process of delegation moves.

THE PROCESS OF DELEGATION

This process of delegation which is the lifeblood of an organization is something that every manager must be thoroughly familiar with. It consists of three components all of which must be present. These three components are inseparably related in such a manner that a change in one of them will require an adjustment of the other two. The three components of the delegating process are: 1) the assignment of duties by a manager to his immediate subordinates; 2) the granting of permission (authority) to the subordinates to make commitments, use resources, and take all the actions which are necessary to perform their assigned duties; and 3) the creation of an obligation (responsibility) on the part of each subordinate to the delegating superior to perform his assigned duties satisfactorily.

Unless all three of these component steps are taken, the success of the delegating process cannot be insured. This is true no matter which level of management is doing the delegating. It is important to realize that all managers from the chief administrator on down to the line supervisors must do their part in delegating authority throughout the entire organization. The chief administrator does the initial delegation when he groups activities, sets up line and staff departments, and assigns them their duties. Then the manager of each department or division must subdivide and reassign these duties within his own section, and at the same time delegate the appropriate amount of authority and responsibility to carry them out. But no matter whether it is the chief administrator who is delegating authority to his associate administrators and directors or the line supervisor who is delegating authority to his non-managerial subordinates, the steps in the process of delegation are the same. In the following discussion of these steps, we will approach the delegation process mainly on the departmental level rather than on the administrative level because it is for departmental supervisors that this book is primarily written.

Assignment of Duties

In the assignment of duties, the supervisor determines how the work in his department is to be divided among his subordinates and himself. He will consider all the tasks which must be accomplished in the department and will determine which of them he can assign to a subordinate and which he must do himself. There are some duties which are more routine, and there is no doubt that the manager would do best to assign these to his regular subordinates. There are other functions which he can only assign to those subordinates who are particularly qualified for them. And then there are the remaining functions which a supervisor cannot delegate but must do himself.

In all likelihood, however, a number of duties will be borderline cases which could fall into any of these groups. In such cases, much will depend upon the manager's general attitude and the availability of subordinates. But there are some logical guidelines which can aid the manager when he is assigning duties. It is better that his assignments be justified and explained on the basis of such logical guides rather than on the basis of personal likes and dislikes or hunch and intuition. This is important because the supervisor will be subject to pressures from different directions when he assigns duties. There will be those who wish to acquire more activities and those who feel that they should not be burdened with certain duties. Thus, in spite of the fact that there are guidelines available, it will often be difficult for the supervisor to decide where best to place a given activity.

One way of doing this is to assign the activity to those employees who will make most use of it most of the time. Or one may be inclined to assign an activity to employees who are already particularly skilled or primarily interested in it. If there is some special interest, then the likelihood is good that these employees will carry out the activity in the best manner.

By considering such factors, the supervisor should be able to assign work so that everybody gets a fair share and so that every employee can do his part satisfactorily. In order to achieve this, of course, the supervisor must clearly understand the nature and the content of the work to be accomplished. Furthermore, he must be thoroughly acquainted with the capabilities of his employees. All of this is not so simple as it might at first appear. The supervisor is often inclined to assign heavier tasks to those employees who are more capable because that is the easiest way out. However, in the long run it would be far more advantageous to train and bring up the less capable employees so that they also can perform the more difficult jobs. If too much reliance is placed on one or a few persons, the department will be in a bad spot if they are absent or if they should leave the employment of the enterprise. Thus, it is always a good idea to have a sufficient number of available employees who have been trained in the department's most difficult tasks. And the supervisor's problems of assigning various duties will become simpler as he builds up the strength and experience of all of his employees.

Of course, the manner and the extent to which the supervisor assigns duties to his employees will significantly affect the degree to which they respect and accept his authority. Much of the success of the manager will depend upon his skill in making assignments. This function will be discussed further throughout the text. Let it suffice at present to repeat that the first step in the process of delegating authority is that certain tasks or duties must be assigned to each subordinate; each must have a job to perform in order to warrant a delegation of authority.

Granting of Authority

The second component in the process of delegation is the granting of authority, the granting of permission to make commitments, to use resources, and to take all those actions which are necessary for the successful performance of the allocated duties. It is advisable to state again at this time that duties are assigned and authority is delegated to *positions* within the institution rather than to people. But unless these positions are staffed by people, all of this would of course be meaningless. That is why one commonly refers to the delegation of authority to subordinates instead of to subordinate positions.

To be more specific, this granting of authority means that a supervisor confers upon his subordinates the right and power to act and to make decisions within a pre-determined and limited area. It is always necessary for the manager to determine in advance the exact scope of authority which is to be delegated. How much authority can be delegated will, of course, depend upon the amount of authority that the manager himself possesses and upon the type of job to be done. Generally speaking, enough authority must be granted to the subordinate for him to adequately and successfully perform what is expected of him. There is no need for the degree of authority to be larger than necessary; but by all means it must be sufficient to get the job done. If you expect your employee to fulfill the tasks which you have assigned to him and to make reasonable decisions for himself within this area, he must have enough authority to do all of these things.

The degree of authority delegated is intrinsically related not only to the duties assigned but also to the results expected. Whenever management delegates authority, it must bear this in mind. Of course, it is also necessary to let the subordinate know the results that are expected of him, for example, how fast he is expected to accomplish his duties, how "perfect" his work is expected to be, etc. For this purpose, standards of performance are established to provide a basis for judging work done and to facilitate management's control. These standards will be discussed more fully in the control section of the book.

At this point, it is enough to say that you as a supervisor must be specific in telling each employee just what authority he has and what results are expected of him while he is exercising his authority. If you do not state this clearly, he will have to guess how far his authority extends, probably by trial and error and experimentation. As a supervisor, you may have found yourself in such a deplorable position when your own boss was not explicit as to how much authority you really had. You do not want this to happen to your subordinates. Therefore, it is necessary that the scope and the results of authority be clearly defined and explained to each subordinate. As time goes on, of course, they will know and less explanation will be necessary. But bear in mind that if you should change an employee's job assignment, you must at the same time check to see that the degree of authority you have given him is still appropriate. Perhaps it is more than he needs. Then you may have to revoke some of his delegated authority. Whenever conditions and circumstances of the job change, additional clarification of the scope of authority also becomes necessary.

Only One Boss

Throughout this process of delegation your employee must be reassured that all his orders and all his authority can come only from you, the only boss he has. In other words, in granting authority you must follow the principle of unity of command. It is very important that this principle be constantly stressed because situations do occur where two superiors try to delegate authority to one subordinate. Ever since biblical times it has been pointed out that it is difficult, if not impossible, to serve two masters. This sort of dual command is bound to lead to unsatisfactory performance by the employee, and it definitely results in confusion of lines of the formal authority. The subordinate does not know which of the two bosses has the authority that will contribute most toward his success and progress within the organization. Eventually such a situation will result in conflicts and organizational difficulties. It too may have to be resolved by revoking some of the delegated authority.

Revoking of Delegated Authority

As stated before, delegating authority does not mean that management has divested itself of its authority. The delegating manager still retains his own authority and he always has the right to revoke whatever part of that authority he has delegated to a subordinate. From time to time, as activities change, there is a definite need to take a fresh look at the organization and to realign authority relationships. Managers frequently speak of reorganizing, realigning, reshuffling, and so forth; what is meant by this is the revoking of authority and its reassignment elsewhere. Naturally such realignments of authority should not take place too often. But periodic reviews of authority delegations are not merely advisable, but necessary in any organization. This applies to the top administration as well as to the lowest level manager.

Accepting Responsibility

The third major aspect of the delegation of authority is the creation of an obligation on the part of the subordinate toward his boss to satisfactorily perform the assigned duties. The acceptance of this obligation creates responsibility. And without responsibility, the process of delegation would not be complete.

Of course, the terms responsibility and authority are closely related to each other. Both terms are often misunderstood and misused. Although it is common to hear such expressions as "keeping subordinates responsible," "delegating responsibility," etc., these expressions do not get at the heart of the matter because they imply that responsibility is handed down from above, whereas in actuality it is accepted from below.

Responsibility is the *obligation of a subordinate* to perform the duty as required by his superior. By accepting a job, by accepting the obligation to perform the assigned tasks, an employee implies acceptance of his own responsibility. But this responsibility cannot be arbitrarily imposed upon him, rather it results from a sort of mutual contractual agreement in which the employee agrees to accomplish his duties in return for rewards. Thus, it is clear that while the authority to perform duties flows from management to subordinate, the responsibility to accomplish these duties flows in the opposite direction, from the subordinate to management. This is still another manifestation of the way in which the formal theory of authority and the acceptance theory can be inextricably linked together.

It is essential to bear in mind, however, that responsibility unlike authority, cannot be delegated. It cannot be shifted. Responsibility is something which your subordinate accepts, but which you still have. The supervisor can assign a task and delegate to a subordinate the authority to perform a specific job. But he does not delegate responsibility in the sense that once the duties are assigned the supervisor is relieved of the responsibility for them. The delegation of tasks does not relieve the supervisor of his own responsibilities for these tasks. A manager can delegate some of his authority to a subordinate, but he cannot delegate any of his responsibility.

It is true that the administrator of a hospital must delegate to his associate administrators a great deal of authority in order for them to oversee the performance of the various tasks and services. These associate administrators, in turn and of necessity, have to delegate a large portion of their authority to the supervisors below them; but none of them delegates any responsibility. Each still accepts all the responsibility for the tasks originally assigned to him. Although subordinates may be granted the authority to actually perform these tasks, the superior is still responsible for seeing to it that the performance is satisfactory. This obligation cannot be shifted or reduced by assigning duties to another.

Similarly, when you as a supervisor are called upon by your boss to explain the performance within your department, you cannot plead as a defense that you have "delegated the responsibility" for such activity to some employee or some group. You may have delegated the authority, but you have remained responsible and you must answer to your boss. It is essential that every supervisor clearly understand this vital difference between authority and responsibility. You must understand that when a manager delegates the authority to do a specific job, he reduces the number of duties which he himself has to perform and he also conditionally divests himself of a certain amount of his own authority which, however, he can take back at any time if conditions are not fulfilled. But in this process he does not reduce the over-all amount of responsibility which he originally accepted from his superior. Although his own subordinates also accept a certain amount of responsibility for the duties he assigns them, this does not in any way diminish the manager's responsibility. What it does do is to add another layer or level to the over-all responsibility. thereby creating *overlapping obligations*. Such overlapping obligations serve to provide double or triple insurance that a job gets done and that it gets done correctly and responsibly.

Thus, the fact remains that although responsibility is something which you accept, you cannot rid yourself of it. This may be a worrisome thought for you. After all, delegations and re-delegations are necessary to get the job done. Although you as a supervisor will try to follow the best managerial practices, you cannot be certain that each and every one of your subordinates will use his best judgment all of the time. Therefore, allowances must be made for errors, and in evaluating your performance as a supervisor some attention will be paid to the degree to which you must depend on your subordinates to get the work of your department accomplished. Although the responsibility has remained with you, your boss will understand that you cannot do everything yourself. In appraising your skill as a manager, he will take into consideration how much care you have shown in the selection of your employees, in training them, in supervising them continuously, and in controlling their activities. All of these matters will become especially important in evaluating your ability in case something has gone wrong in your department.

Equality of the Three Components

Always bear in mind that the three components of the process of delegation must go together in order to make this process a success. Authority, responsibility, and duties must be commensurate. This means that there must be enough authority (but not more than necessary) granted to your subordinates to do the job, and that the responsibility which you expect them to accept cannot be greater than the area of authority which you have delimited. Your subordinates cannot be expected to accept responsibility for activities for which you have not handed them any authority. In other words, do not try to "keep your subordinates responsible" for something that you have not actually delegated to them.

Inconsistencies between delegated authority, responsibility, and assigned tasks will generally produce undesirable results. You may have been in organizations where some of the managers had a large amount of authority delegated to them but had no particular jobs to perform. This created misuse of authority and disturbance. Then again, you may have been in positions where responsibility was exacted from you when you did not have the authority to fulfill an obligation. This, too, is a most embarrassing and frustrating situation. Therefore, you must make certain that the three components necessary for successful delegation are of equal magnitude and that whenever you change one you must change the other two simultaneously.

THE DEGREE OF DELEGATION OF AUTHORITY

As discussed earlier, delegation of authority is the key to the creation of an organization. If no authority has been delegated, one can hardly speak of an organization. Hence, from an organizational point of view the problem is not whether or not to delegate authority, but rather *how much* authority will be delegated to the various subordinates on the different organizational levels. It is not a question of yes or no, instead it is a question of the *degree* of authority to be delegated.

This question of the degree of delegation is extremely important because it will determine the answer to another highly significant organizational question—that is, the extent to which the organization is decentralized. Variations in the extent of decentralization are innumerable, ranging all the way from a highly centralized structure where one can hardly speak of an organization to a completely decentralized organization where authority has been delegated to the lowest possible levels of management. In the first instance, the chief executive is in close touch with all operations, makes almost all decisions, and gives almost all instructions. He has delegated hardly any authority and, strictly speaking, it cannot be said that he has created an organization. There are many small enterprises which regularly operate along these lines. Often such one-man shows will collapse if their chief executive dies, becomes incapacitated, or for some other reason leaves the scene.

A much less extreme situation is found in organizations where authority has been delegated to a limited degree. In such organizations, the major policies and programs are decided by the top manager of the enterprise, and the task of applying these policies and programs to daily operations and daily planning is delegated down to the first level of supervision. In between the top manager and the supervisors, there are very few other or no other levels. This kind of arrangement is often found in medium-sized enterprises. It is obviously advantageous in that it limits the number of managers which the general manager must hire, and thus allows him to keep expenses down. Furthermore, it is advantageous in that the unusual knowledge and good judgment which the general manager possesses can be applied directly. There are probably quite a large number of enterprises in the United States which have this type of organization with a limited degree of delegation of authority.

At the other end of the spectrum, we find those organizations where authority has been delegated to the broadest possible extent and to the lowest levels of management. In order to find out if an organization is this decentralized, it is necessary to determine the kind of authority which has been delegated, how far down in the organization it has been delegated, and how consistent the delegations are. In other words, one must ask how significant a decision can be made by a manager and how far down within the managerial hierarchy. The more important the decisions that are made further down in the hierarchy, the more decentralization is prevalent. The greater the number of such decisions and the more functions affected by them also serve as indicators of decentralization. Furthermore, the less checking that is done by upper level management, the greater the degree of decentralization. The answers to all of these questions will indicate whether or not you are dealing with an organization which has delegated authority to the greatest extent possible.

It should be pointed out that timing is a very important factor in solving this degree of delegation problem. Although centralization of authority or limited decentralization may be the most logical organizational forms to use in the early stages of an enterprise, later stages will usually require the top administrator to face the problem of delegating more authority and decentralizing his organization to a greater extent. Such decentralization of authority becomes necessary when centralized management finds itself so burdened with decision-making that the top executives do not have enough time to adequately perform their planning function or to maintain a long-range point of view. This type of situation usually occurs when an organization expands. It should indicate to top management that the time has arrived to delegate authority to lower echelons. In other words, there should be a gradual development toward decentralization of authority commensurate with the growth of the enterprise.

Advantages and Disadvantages of Delegation

You are probably aware by this time that there are numerous advantages to delegating and decentralizing authority. Moreover, these advantages become even more important as the enterprise grows in size. For example, by delegating authority the senior manager is relieved of much time-consuming detail work. Subordinates can make decisions without waiting for approval of their decisions from their superior. This increases flexibility and permits more prompt action. In addition, such delegation of decision-making authority may actually produce better decisions, since the man on the job usually knows more about the factors involved than the manager at headquarters and since speedy decisions are often essential. Delegation to the lower levels, moreover, increases morale and interest and enthusiasm for the work. It also provides a good training ground. All of these advantages serve to make the organization more democratic and more responsive to the needs and ideas of its employees.

Of course, there are some possible disadvantages to considerable delegation. For example, the supervisor of a department may feel that he no longer needs the help of upper level managers and that he can develop his own supporting services. This could easily lead to duplication of effort and waste. Another disadvantage could be a possible loss of control, although the delegating manager can take steps to see that this does not happen. All in all, we must conclude the advantages of a greater degree of delegation far outweigh the disadvantages.

SUMMARY

In the foregoing chapter, we discussed the meaning of authority as that power which makes the managerial job a reality. This definition becomes more understandable when we consider the source of authority. One way of looking at the source is to state that all formal managerial authority emanates from the top of the organization. From there, it is delegated downward through an uninterrupted chain of command beginning with the chief administrator and ending with the supervisor on the lowest level of the managerial pyramid. According to the formal theory, then, managerial authority is conferred from above. However, this approach to the source of authority has been deeply shaken by what is commonly known as the acceptance theory. The acceptance theory postulates that a manager only has authority if and when his subordinates confer it upon him by accepting it. The superior manager does not possess authority until and unless this acceptance by his employees takes place. In reality, a choice between the formal theory and the acceptance theory does not have to be made. The two theories can be realistically combined by saying that the best managers are those who use their formal delegated authority in such a way that their employees accept and respect it without resentment. A good manager should not have to depend exclusively on the formal weight of authority to motivate his workers. As a matter of fact, this would probably be the least desirable and the least effective way of motivating them.

Nevertheless, a good manager must know how to use formal authority and how to delegate some of it to his subordinates. Through the process of delegation of authority, management actually creates the organization. This process of delegation is made up of three components, namely, the assignment of a job or duty, the granting of authority, and the acceptance of responsibility. All three are coexistent and a change in one will necessitate a change in the other two. Since this process of delegation is the only way to create an organization, the question is not whether top management will delegate authority, but rather how much or how little authority will be delegated. If much authority is delegated all the way down to the lowest levels of supervision, then one speaks of a highly decentralized organization; if most authority is more or less hoarded at the top, one refers to such an organization as being highly centralized. Although centralization might be appropriate when an enterprise is just getting started, there are greater advantages arising from decentralization or the broad delegation of authority, one of the most important being the increased motivation of subordinates.

CHAPTER 10

Organizing on the Departmental Level

Thus far we have discussed the organizing process mainly from an over-all institutional point of view. We have outlined how the chief administrator establishes the formal organizational structure, utilizes organizational charts and manuals, and delegates organizational authority. Although the process of delegation was approached more on the supervisory level, we have still not yet focused our full attention on how a supervisor actually goes about organizing and delegating within his own department. Logically, we could not really discuss the organizing process on the departmental level until we understood the basic organizational principles and how they are applied in the creation of the over-all structure. Now that we have (hopefully) gained this broad understanding, we are ready to approach the organizing function more specifically from the supervisor's point of view—in terms of his departmental goals and objectives, his daily operations and activities, and his existing personnel and resources. In other words, we shall now look at organization on a narrow scale, zeroing in on the microcosm known as the department.

Naturally, it should not be surprising to find that the organizing process is basically the same whether it is the chief administrator or the lowest line supervisor who is doing it. It involves grouping activities for purposes of departmentalization or subdepartmentalization on the supervisory level, assigning specific tasks and duties and, most important of all perhaps, delegating authority. In essence, this means that the basic organizational principles must be understood and applied by the supervisor when he is setting up his own department just as they were by the chief administrator when he was structuring the over-all institution. Let us see how a supervisor might actually go about applying these principles, using them on a day-to-day basis so that they are not just abstractions which one reads about in textbooks, but rather lifegiving parts of a healthy departmental body.

THE IDEAL ORGANIZATION OF THE DEPARTMENT

When designing the organizational structure of his department, the supervisor should plan for the ideal organization. The word "ideal" in this instance is not intended to mean "perfect," rather it is used to mean the most desirable organization for the achievement of stated objectives. It is the supervisor's job to design an organizational setup which will be best for his particular department. In so doing, he must observe the "principles" and guides of organization which have been developed over the years. Following these is no guarantee that the department will not have any problems from then on. But a significant number of problems will be avoided because the organizational network has been designed in such fashion that it will function smoothly in the majority of cases.

The manager must bear in mind, however, that certain organizational concepts and arrangements which work well in a very large institution may not be applicable to his institution if it is smaller. In other words, he must not blindly follow the idea that what is good for one enterprise is also good for the other. Moreover, it is not essential that the manager's organizational plans for his department look pretty on paper or that his organization chart appear symmetrical and well-balanced. Rather, his ideal design should represent the most appropriate organizational arrangement for reaching his particular departmental objectives. It should be uniquely tailored to suit the conditions under which he works, instead of some abstract image of what an "ideal" department should look like.

In planning this ideal but realistic organization, the supervisor must consider it as something of a standard with which he can compare his present organizational setup. The ideal structure should be looked upon as a guide to the short- and long-range plans of the department. Although the supervisor should carefully plan for the ideal structure as soon as he becomes the department's manager, this does not mean that he should force the existing organization to conform to the ideal immediately. But each change in the prevailing organization should bring the existing structure closer to the ideal. In other words, the ideal organization of the department represents the direction in which the supervisor will move as he carries out his organizing function.

INTERNAL DEPARTMENTAL STRUCTURE

At this point, you might be a little bit unclear as to exactly how a supervisor would go about the process of designing his ideal departmental structure. What does this involve, how is it done, and is the supervisor really equipped to do it? In most cases, he is because in essence what he is being asked to do is to subdepartmentalize, to establish subdivisions or subunits within his department just as the chief administrator established the over-all divisions or units for the whole organization. Two examples of how a Director of Nursing Service might subdepartmentalize or set up the internal departmental structure are shown in the organization chart on pages 133 and 134 (Figures 10-1 and 10-2.)*

More specifically, what the supervisor is being asked to do is to consider the groupings of activities in his department, to consider the various positions which exist, and the assignment of tasks and duties to these positions. Is what he finds the best possible arrangement for achieving departmental and institutional objectives? Are all the present positions necessary or could some be eliminated or combined with others? Does each position have a fair assignment of tasks and duties, commensurate with its status and salary? Are the positions related in such a way that there is no duplication of effort and that coordination and cooperation are facilitated? In other words, is the department well organized? Does it function in the most efficient manner? Are there any changes at all which the supervisor would like to see in the internal organizational structure of his department?

If there are any such changes, then these will become the basis for what we have been calling "the ideal organization of the department." They will become the organizational goals toward which the supervisor will strive as he goes about structuring his department.

Of course, if a supervisor is setting up a new department or working in a new institution he will probably be able to implement much of his ideal structure at the beginning. This would naturally be the most desirable situation. But generally such is not the case and the supervisor is forced to gradually implement his organizational goals while working within the existing departmental structure and with the existing personnel.

Organization and Personnel

It is important to realize that the supervisor should design his ideal organization based on sound organizational principles regardless of the people with whom he has to work. This does not mean that departments could exist without people to staff their various positions. Without people, of course, there can be no organization. However, the problems of organization should be handled in the right order — first comes the sound structure, then the people are asked to fulfill this structure.

If the ideal organizational setup is planned first around existing personnel, then existing shortcomings will be perpetuated. Due to incumbent personalities, too much emphasis may be given to certain activities and not enough to others. Moreover, if a department is structured around personalities, it is easy to imagine what would happen if a particular employee should be promoted or should resign. If, on the other hand, the departmental organization is structured

---

*Also see the various departmental charts and job descriptions in the Appendix at the end of the book.

FIGURE 10-1

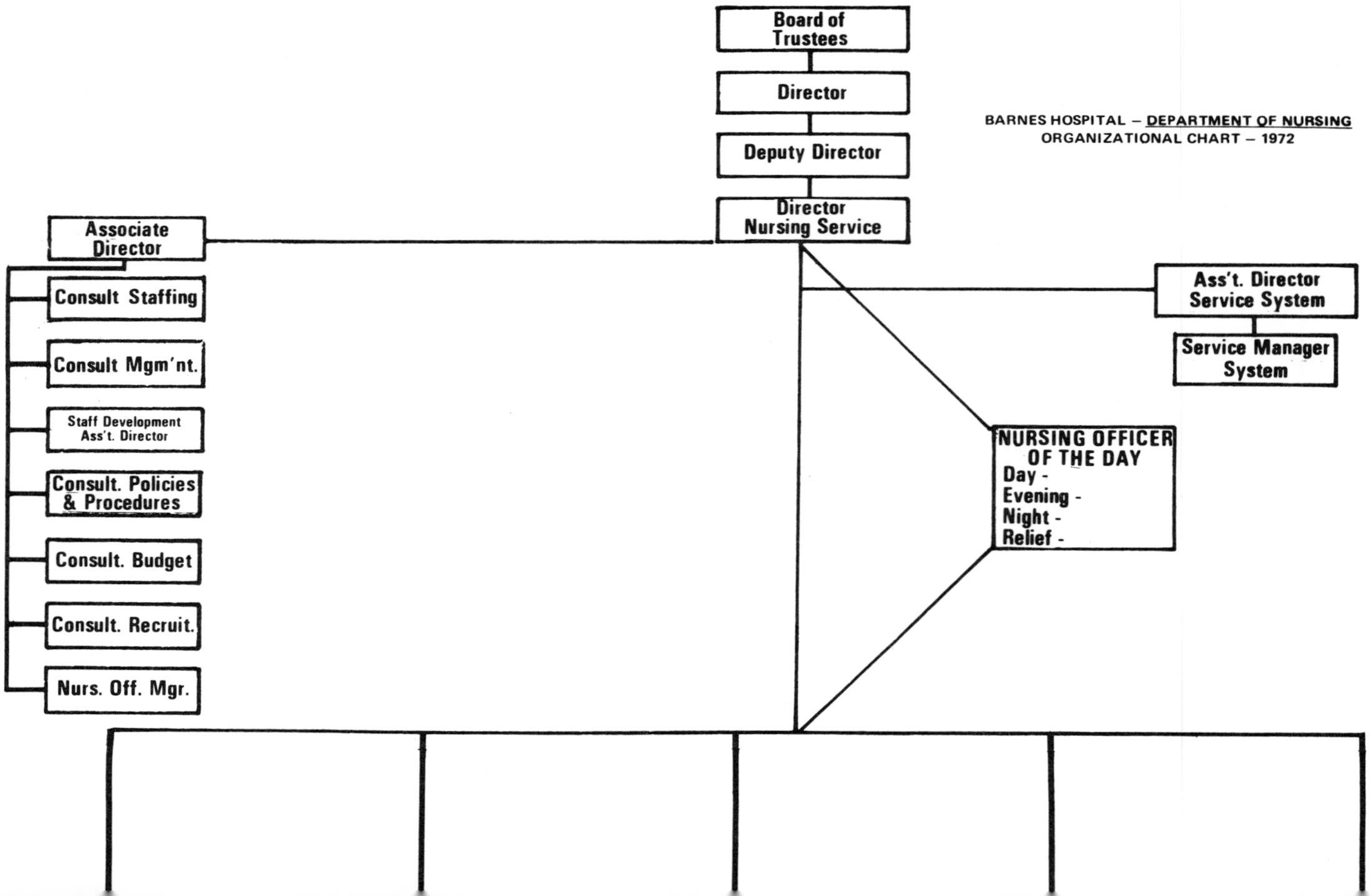

BARNES HOSPITAL – DEPARTMENT OF NURSING
ORGANIZATIONAL CHART – 1972

Board of Trustees

Director

Deputy Director

Director Nursing Service

Ass't. Director Service System

Service Manager System

NURSING OFFICER OF THE DAY
Day -
Evening -
Night -
Relief -

Associate Director

Consult Staffing

Consult Mgm'nt.

Staff Development Ass't. Director

Consult. Policies & Procedures

Consult. Budget

Consult. Recruit.

Nurs. Off. Mgr.

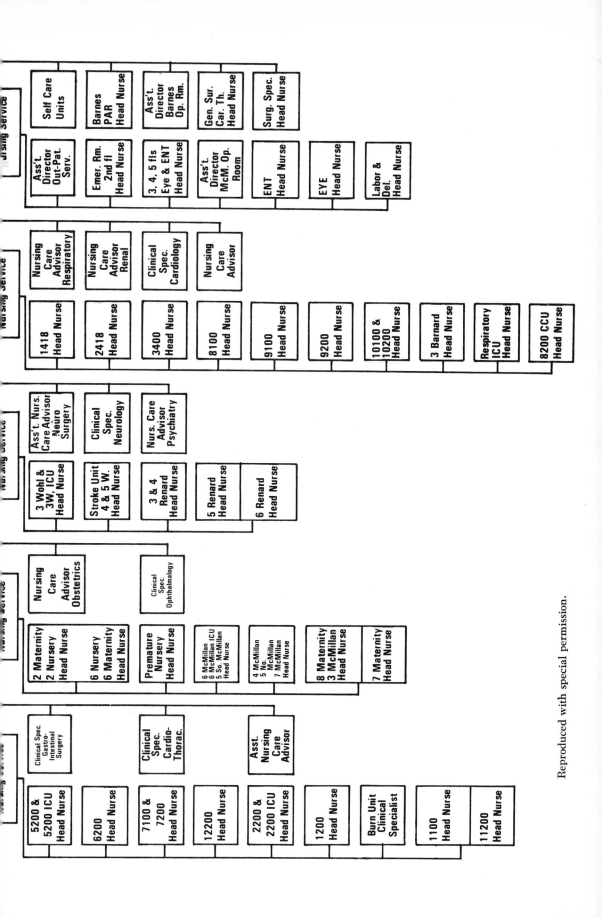

Reproduced with special permission.

FIGURE 10-2

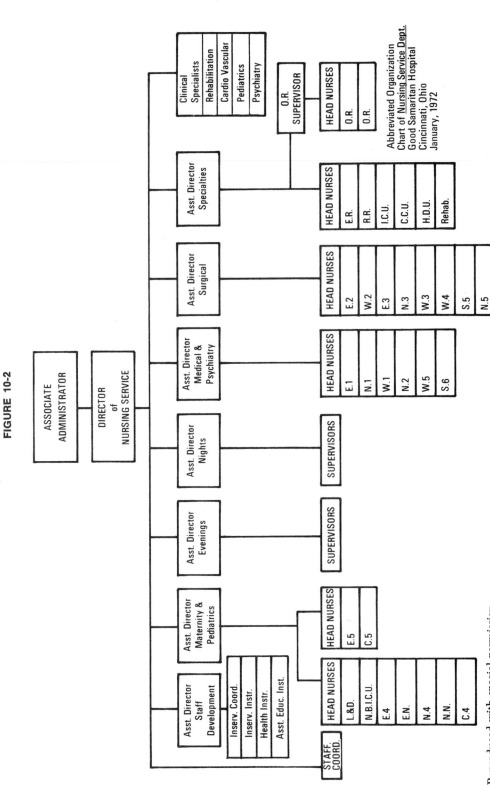

Abbreviated Organization
Chart of Nursing Service Dept.
Good Samaritan Hospital
Cincinnati, Ohio
January, 1972

Reproduced with special permission.

impersonally on the general need for personnel rather than on the incumbent personalities, it should not be difficult to find an appropriate successor for a particular position. Therefore, an organization should be designed first to serve the objectives of the department; then the various employees should be selected and fitted into departmental positions.

This, however, is easier said than done. It frequently happens, particularly in smaller departments, that the available employees do not fit too well into the ideal structure. Yet, they cannot all be overlooked or dismissed. In most instances, it is also true that the supervisor has been put into a managerial position in an existing and fully staffed department without having had the chance to decide on the present structure or personnel of the department. In such cases, the best the supervisor can do for the time being is to adjust the organization to utilize the capacities of the employees he has. He should realize that this is an accommodation of the ideal plan to fit present personalities, but he should regard it as merely a temporary arrangement. Such personal adjustments are sometimes necessary, but fewer of them will be required if the supervisor has already made a plan of the organization he would like to have if the ideal human material were available. Then, as time goes on, the supervisor will strive to come closer and closer to his ideal departmental setup. In other words, his ideal structure will become the basis for future changes in or reorganization of the department.

Reorganization

It must be kept in mind that organizational structure is not static. The organization is a living institution and therefore needs a certain amount of continuous adjustment. For this reason, the manager's organizing function is also continuous; he should be constantly checking, questioning, and appraising the soundness and feasibility of his departmental structure. Organization is not an end in itself, but rather a means to an end, namely, the accomplishment of the objectives of the department. A manager must continuously watch for new developments, practices, and thinking in the field of organization. He must be willing to *reorganize* his department if these developments warrant it or if he feels that the existing structure is too far from the ideal to permit effective functioning.

Of course, the term "reorganization" is used with all kinds of different connotations. However, in our discussion this term will refer to changes in the over-all organizational structure, in departmentalization, in the assignment of activities, and/or in authority relationships. There are various reasons which from time to time demand that a manager make such changes. These reasons may be due to technological advances, to the dynamic and changing nature of the department's activities, to a shift of supervisors or, as we noted above, reorganization may be necessitated by the need to overcome existing deficiencies.

Let us look, for example, at a sample case of reorganization to overcome existing deficiencies. Such a case will help us to better understand both the purpose of planning an ideal departmental structure as well as the means of implementing this ideal structure through the process of reorganization. For example, as time went on nurses found themselves burdened with a great amount of secretarial and clerical work which kept them away from actual patient care and bedside nursing. This was a poor situation since the thrust of their education and their purpose was the care of patients. Finally it became apparent that many of these functions could be performed by someone else just as effectively and this lead to the creation of positions which are now commonly known as unit managers, unit clerks, ward clerks and so forth. The care of "things" was assigned to them, whereas the actual care of "people" reversed back to where it should be, namely the nurses. The job of the ward clerk is to perform general clerical duties such as preparing, maintaining, and compiling patients' records in the nursing unit. He copies information from nurses' records, writes requisitions for laboratory tests, dispatches messages to other departments and so forth. He makes appointments for patients' services in other departments as requested by nursing staff, and he maintains an established inventory of stock supplies on the unit and makes requisitions. There are a multitude of additional duties he performs which heretofore the nursing personnel had to cope with. This was a case of reorganization where duties were reassigned, where new authority relationships had to be established between the clerks and the head nurses and so forth.

Once this or any other type of reorganization has been decided upon, it can be carried out either as a long-run, gradual, continued change, or as a one-time change covering only a short period. The latter approach has commonly been called the "earthquake" technique, indicating that the full shock of the reorganization is felt all at once. The long-run plan, on the other hand, provides for a period of more gradual adjustment to the organizational changes. No doubt this approach is less disturbing and creates fewer upsets than the earthquake approach. It must be kept in mind that changes are always disturbing to those who are affected by them, regardless of how well intended they are. A manager who frequently changes his department's organizational structure runs the risk of damaging the morale of his subordinates. To the supervisor suggesting the reorganization, it might seem trivial but to his subordinates it will probably appear frightening because it implies changes in their status and security. The wise supervisor will have to learn how to strike a happy medium in the desirable amount of organizational change. In most instances, he will probably find that his subordinates will quickly adjust to changes if they are properly explained and if the need for them is demonstrated. There will be a further discussion of the introduction of change in Chapter 19. In the meantime, it will suffice to repeat that regardless of the difficulties involved it is necessary for a supervisor to make organizational adjustments from time to time in order to keep his department as viable as possible.

DELEGATING AUTHORITY WITHIN THE DEPARTMENT

Delegation in a Medium or Large Department

Once a supervisor has organized or reorganized his department's internal structure, or at least planned the changes that are needed and recorded them in his ideal organizational design, he is ready to delegate or redelegate authority in accordance with the organizational structure that he has set up. We assume that the supervisor has himself been given sufficient authority and that he is in charge of all the activities within his section. Just as any other manager, the supervisor is faced with the necessity of delegating some of the authority that has been handed down to him. As mentioned previously, unless he does so he does not create any organization. He must certainly do this if he should be in charge of very many employees. In other words, the supervisor must assign tasks, grant authority, and create responsibility within each of the subunits and for each of the positions in his department.

Of course, if a supervisor is taking over an existing department he will probably find most of the delegation of authority already done. But he will have to check it carefully to see that it is consistent with his ideal organizational plans. Even if he is not reorganizing or making major changes at the moment, the supervisor should check the amount and type of authority delegated to each position in his department. He should ask himself whether the three component steps in the process of delegation were followed and whether there is quality and consistency of these three components. In other words, he should refer back to the specific procedure outlined in Chapter 9 in order to see that authority is delegated properly in his department.

Delegation in a Small Department

Let us now turn our observations to the situation in which the supervisor of a small department finds himself as a delegator of authority. We will be concerned with the supervisor's delegation of authority as a means of building a minimal organization structure within his own department, even if that department is too small to require subdivisions or subunits. Such a department would consist merely of a supervisor and a few employees (like three to six) working directly under him. The supervisor may wonder if under these circumstances it is necessary for him to delegate authority. The answer is yes. Even in a small department the supervisor will need someone whom he can ask to take over if he should have to leave either temporarily or for any length of time. Even in the smallest department there should be someone who can work as his backstop. It is a sign of poor supervision when there is no one in a department who can take over when sickness hits or the supervisor has to be away from the job. It can also happen that the supervisor himself misses a promotion because he has nobody to take over the unit he would leave. So sooner or later every supervisor needs a backstop, understudy, assistant, or whatever he may be called.

Availability of Suitable Subordinates

As a supervisor, you may have wanted to delegate more authority to some of your subordinates and to make one of them your assistant, but you had no one within your department who was willing to accept this authority and to take complete charge of an area of activities. Of course, the process of delegation assumes that there is someone available who is willing to accept the increased authority delegated to him. In reality, however, you may not have anyone working for you who is capable of handling more authority. In such a case, authority must be withheld and for the moment at least you cannot delegate it.

On the other hand, you may find yourself in a vicious circle, complaining that without better trained subordinates you cannot delegate but without delegating additional authority your subordinates will have no opportunity to obtain the necessary training. With additional experience and training, however, their judgment could be improved and they could become more capable subordinates. Although this lack of trained subordinates is often used by supervisors as an excuse for not delegating greater authority, the supervisor must always bear in mind that unless he makes a beginning in the delegation process he will never have a subordinate capable of being his backstop and of taking over the department if necessary. It is the supervisor's duty to develop and train such a person, and in the process it is very likely that the supervisor will find that he can delegate more authority not only to the individual selected as his backstop but also to his other employees as well. Moreover, this process of training for increased delegation will give the supervisor a much clearer view of his own duties, of the workings of the department, and of the various jobs to be performed. Bringing subordinates to the point where they can finally be given considerable authority is a slow and tedious process, but it is worth the effort. Naturally, in the early stages the degree of authority granted will be small, but as the subordinates grow in their capacities increasingly more authority can be delegated to them.

Selection of a Backstop

As we have said, this process of greater delegation of authority should include making one particular subordinate into an assistant or backstop for the supervisor. The first step here, of course, is to select the right person for the job. No doubt the supervisor knows which of his employees are more outstanding. These would be the ones to whom the other employees turn in case of questions and who are looked upon as leaders. The outstanding employee, moreover, is one who knows how to do his job very well, who seems to be able to handle problems as they arise, and who does not get into arguments. He should also have shown good judgment in the way he organizes and goes about his own job, he should have an open mind, and he should be interested in developing himself and moving into better positions. Without such ambitions on his part, even the best training would not achieve any results. The outstanding employee must have shown a willingness to accept responsibility and he must have proven his dependability. Sometimes a worker may not have had the opportunity to show all of this. But whatever qualities have remained latent will show up rather quickly during the actual training process.

If the supervisor has two or three equally good employees in his department, he should start training all of them for greater delegations of authority on an equal basis. Sooner or later it will be obvious which one has the superior ability and this individual will then become the major trainee for the backstop position. Once the selection of a single person is made (or in a large department there could be several assistant backstops), it is not necessary to come out with general formal announcements in this respect. Of course, the supervisor should discuss and explain his intentions fully to the employee chosen. And it is even more important for the supervisor to follow through by laying a thorough groundwork for good training so that the one who has been chosen will work out as an understudy.

Training of the Backstop

Although the phrase "training a subordinate" is frequently used, the term "training" is really not appropriate. It would be more appropriate to speak of the development or even self-development on the subordinate's part which is necessary in order for him to advance. By this we mean the subordinate's eagerness to improve himself and his initiative to be a self-starter.

If a subordinate has such initiative, he will gradually develop himself into a backstop with just a minimal amount of help from the supervisor. For instance, the supervisor should gradually let the understudy in on the workings of the department. He should explain some of the reports to him and show him how he gets the information he needs. He should tell him what he does with these reports and why it is done. The supervisor should also introduce his understudy to the people with whom he deals and he should have the understudy contact them himself as time goes on. It is advisable to take the understudy along to some of the hospital meetings after he has had a chance to learn the major aspects of the supervisor's job. On such occasions the supervisor should show him how the work of his department is related to that of the other departments in the hospital.

As daily problems arise, moreover, the supervisor should let the understudy participate in them and even try to solve some of them for himself. By letting the understudy come up with some solutions to problems, the supervisor will have a chance to see how well he analyzes and how much he knows about making decisions. In time, the supervisor should give his understudy some areas of activities for which he will be entirely responsible. In other words, he should gradually assign more duties and authority.

Of course, this whole process requires an atmosphere of confidence and trust. The boss must be looked upon by the understudy as a coach and friend, not as a domineering superior. The supervisor should caution himself that in his eagerness to develop the understudy as rapidly as possible, he does not overload him or pass problems on to him which are beyond his capability. The supervisor must never lose sight of the fact that it takes time to be able to handle problems of any magnitude.

Obviously, all of this will require much effort and patience on the supervisor's part. And it is conceivable that just about the time the understudy comes to the point where he can be of real help, he may be transferred to another job outside of the supervisor's department. This may be discouraging for the moment, but the supervisor may rest assured that the administrator will give him credit for a training job well done.

The Supervisor's Hesitancy to Delegate

We should not be surprised to find that often supervisors do not like the idea of creating a backstop. It is understandable that the supervisor may be reluctant to delegate so much authority because he knows that he cannot delegate his responsibility. He knows that in the final analysis responsibility remains with him, and may therefore think it is best to make all decisions himself. Thus, out of fear of their subordinates' mistakes many supervisors are not willing to delegate authority, and as a result of this they continue to overburden themselves. Their indecision and delay may often be costlier than the mistakes they hoped to avoid by retaining their authority. Always bear in mind that there is also a certain likelihood that the supervisor himself may make mistakes. Moreover, if employees are permitted to learn from some of their own mistakes, they will not resent the supervisor's authority and they will be more willing to accept greater authority themselves.

As stated above, the supervisor's reluctance in delegating such authority is understandable in view of the fact that he still remains accountable for the results. The old picture of a good supervisor was one who rolled up his sleeves and worked right alongside his employees, thus setting an example by his efforts. Such a description is particularly true of a supervisor who has come up through the ranks and for whom the supervisory position is a reward for hard work and technical competence. He has been placed in a managerial position without having been equipped to be a manager, and he is faced with new problems with which he cannot always cope. He therefore retreats to a pattern in which he feels secure and works right alongside his employees. There are occasions when such participation is needed, for instance, when the job to be performed is of a particularly difficult nature or when an emergency situation has arisen. Under these conditions, the good supervisor will always be right on the job to help. But aside from such emergencies and unusual situations, he should spend most of his time carrying out his supervisory job while his employees should be doing their assigned tasks. It is the supervisor's job not to do, but to see that others get things done.

Frequently, however, a supervisor will still feel that if he wants something done right he has to do it himself. Often he believes that it is easier for him to do the job than to correct his subordinate's mistake. And, even if he lets the subordinate do it, the supervisor may feel a strong temptation to correct any mistakes himself rather than explain to the subordinate what should have been done. It is frequently more difficult to teach than to do it oneself. Moreover, the supervisor often feels that he can do the job better than any of his subordinates, and chances are that he is right. But sooner or later he will have to get used to the idea that someone else can do the job almost as well as he can, and at that point he should delegate the necessary authority. In this manner, he will be able to save his own time for more important managerial jobs, for thinking, planning, and for more delegating. If the supervisor is willing to see to it that his employees become increasingly competent with every additional job, then his own belief and confidence in their work will also grow. This mutually advantageous relationship will permit the supervisor to carry out the basic underlying policy of delegating more and more authority as his employees demonstrate their capability in handling it.

In spite of the fact that a certain amount of authority must be delegated in order to create an organization, there are some supervisory duties which cannot be delegated. It should always remain to the supervisor to apply and interpret policies, to give the general directions for his department or division, to take necessary disciplinary action, to promote employees and to appraise them. Aside from these duties, however, subordinates should do most things for themselves.

The Reluctant Subordinate

The delegation of authority and especially the training of an understudy are, of course, two-sided relationships. Although the supervisor may be ready and willing to turn over authority, the subordinates may sometimes be reluctant to accept it. Frequently, a subordinate may feel unsure of himself, unsure that he will be able to handle the job assigned to him. Merely ordering him to have more self-confidence, of course, will have little effect. The supervisor himself, as we have said, must create this self-confidence by carefully coaching and training the subordinate to undertake more and more difficult assignments. Then, and only then, will the subordinate be able to accept the increased responsibility which goes along with harder tasks and greater authority.

Naturally, with increased responsibilities there should also be commensurate positive incentives. These may be in the form of pay increases, bonuses, a fancier title, recognized status within the organization, or other rewards of a tangible and intangible nature. Such rewards will, of course, include the self-satisfaction which the subordinate feels knowing that he is able to handle increased responsibility and that he has moved up in the organizational ranks.

DELEGATION AND GENERAL SUPERVISION

Now that we have discussed the delegation of authority to employees of a small department who work directly below their supervisor, we have reached the lowest rung of the organizational ladder and further delegation of authority is no longer possible. There is an end to delegation in the strict sense of the word when we reach the point of execution of daily duties, in other words when we reach the level of employees who are actually doing the work. Since we have reached this level, the question now arises as to how a supervisor can effectively reap the benefits of delegation, how he can take advantage of the motivating factors of delegation in the daily working situation. The answer to this question can be found at the point where the philosophy of delegation takes on the form of what is commonly referred to as loose or general supervision.

The Employee's Reaction to General Supervision

Most employees accept work as a part of normal, healthy life. Accordingly, most managers display the underlying managerial attitude of McGregor's Theory Y toward their employees. Such managers understand that in their daily jobs employees seek a satisfaction which wages alone cannot provide. Most employees also enjoy being their own bosses. They like a degree of freedom which allows them to make their own decisions in matters pertaining to their work. The question arises as to whether this is possible if one works for someone else, whether such a degree of freedom can be granted to an employee if he is to contribute his share toward the achievement of the enterprise's objectives. This is where the ideas of delegation of authority and general supervision can help. The desire for freedom, for being one's own boss can be enhanced by a delegation of authority which in a working situation means merely giving orders in broad, general terms. It means that the supervisor, instead of watching every detail of the employee's activities, is primarily interested in the results achieved. He permits his subordinates to decide how to achieve these results within accepted professional standards.

In other words, the delegation of authority in the daily working situation does not amount to more than a general form of supervision whereby the supervisor sets the goals and tells his subordinates what he wants accomplished, fixing the limits within which the work has to be done. But he lets his employees decide how to accomplish these goals. He gives each employee maximum freedom — naturally, within the constraints of the organization. This broad, general kind of supervision on the employee level has the same results as the delegation of formal authority on the higher levels of management.

Advantages of General Supervision

There are significant advantages which result from this approach to supervision, similiar to the advantages which have been cited in our discussion of the process of delegation. The supervisor who learns the art of general supervision will benefit in many ways. First of all, he will have more time to handle his own job as a supervisor. If he tried to practice close detailed supervision and tried to make every decision by himself, he would probably exhaust himself physically and mentally. With delegation, however, he will be freed from many of the details of his work and will thus have time to plan and control. In so doing, he will also have more time to receive and handle greater authority which his boss will then be able to delegate to him.

Moreover, the decisions which general supervision allows employees to make will probably be superior to those made by a harried supervisor trying to practice detailed supervision. We have already pointed out that the employee on the job is closest to the problem and therefore in the best position to solve it. Furthermore, this will give the employee a chance to develop his own talents and abilities. It is always very difficult for a supervisor to instruct his employees on how to make decisions without letting them actually make them. They can really only learn by practice.

This leads us to the third advantage of general supervision: that it enables employees to take great pride in the results of their decisions. As stated before, employees enjoy being independent. Repeated surveys have revealed that the one quality that employees most admire in a supervisor is his ability to allow them to be independent by delegating authority. Employees want a boss who shows them how to do a job and then trusts them enough to let them do it on their own. In this way, the supervisor provides on-the-job training for them and a chance for better positions. Thus, we can see that general supervision allows for the progress not only of the supervisor himself, but also of his employees, his department, and the enterprise as a whole.

Much more will be said about general supervision when we discuss the managerial function of influencing. Let us repeat at this time that practicing the broad, general approach to supervision, instead of an autocratic, dictatorial, detailed approach provides many of the satisfactions which employees seek on the job and which money alone does not cover. Because their needs are fulfilled, employees are motivated to put forth their best efforts in achieving the enterprise's objectives.

Attitudes Toward General Supervision

It seems appropriate at this stage to point out that the broad, general approach to supervision and the idea that it is necessary to provide positive motivation for employees was not always as widely accepted as it is today. There was a time when management believed that emphasis on negative authority was the best method of motivating employees. Those who depended upon the force of authority as their major means of motivation — and a few may still erroneously believe in this today — thought that managing consisted of forcing people to work by threatening to fire them if they did not. One of their assumptions was that the only reason people work is to earn money and that they will work only if they fear losing their jobs. This approach, of course, ignores the fact that employees want many other intrinsic satisfactions from their work besides the salary. It also assumes that people do not like work, that they try to get away with doing as little as possible. On this basis, the need for very close supervision is justified. The supervisor must tell the workers precisely what is to be done every minute of the day and not permit the worker any chance to use his own judgment. In brief, the older school of managerial thought was based on Theory X as its underlying assumption.

Such reliance on the sheer weight of authority has, of course, lost most of its followers. This kind of approach was possible in the early days of the industrial revolution when workers were close to starvation, when they would do anything in order to obtain food, clothing, and shelter. In recent years, however, employees have begun to expect much more from their jobs. This is particularly so when times are good and employment is high. We also find that the educational process of our children has had a significant influence on recent attitudes. Many years ago children were used to strict obedience toward their elders. But now schools and homes emphasize freedom and self-expression, and it is therefore becoming more and more difficult for the young employee to accept any kind of autocratic management on the job. In addition to this, the growth of unions has made it more difficult for a supervisor to fire an employee.

But perhaps the most important change in current attitudes is the increased awareness that the "be strong" form of "motivation" provides no incentive to work harder than the minimum which is required in order to avoid punishment and discharge. Under these conditions, employees will probably dislike work which, if they are not unionized, can lead to slowdowns, sabotage, and spoilage. To this, management will likely react by watching workers even more closely. This, in turn, will encourage the employees to try to outsmart management. Thus, a vicious circle is started with new restraints and new methods of evading them. Sooner or later such a circle will produce aggression, arguments, fights, and a general devastating effect on the entire organization.

ACHIEVING DELEGATION OF AUTHORITY

Of course, the new attitudes and the emphasis on broader delegations of authority are not always easy to put into practice. In order for such delegations of authority to be effective, a sincere desire and willingness to delegate must permeate the entire organization. Top management must set the mood by not only preaching but also by practicing broad delegation of authority. Although top management's intentions may be the best, it is still conceivable that at times the desired degree of decentralization of authority is not achieved. For instance, top management may find that authority has not been delegated as far down as it intended because somewhere along the line there is what is known as an authority hoarder, a person who simply will not delegate authority any further. He grasps all the authority which has been delegated to him without redelegating any of it.

There are a number of reasons why managers might resist decentralization of authority in this manner. To some, the delegation of authority may mean a loss of status, a loss of power and control. Others may think that by having centralized power they are in closer contact with the administrator. And yet other managers are truly concerned with the expenses involved in delegating authority. Moreover, it is difficult for any manager to part with some of his own authority, still to be left with full responsibility for the decisions made by his subordinates.

There are several ways to cope with this problem and to achieve the degree of decentralization which is desired by top administration. As stated before, the entire managerial group must be indoctrinated with the philosophy of decentralization of authority. They must understand that by carefully delegating authority they do not lose status, nor do they absolve themselves of their responsibilities. One way of putting this understanding into practice is to request that each manager have a fairly large number of subordinate managers reporting to him. By stretching his span of management, the subordinate has no choice but to delegate authority. Another way to achieve broader delegations of authority is for the enterprise to adopt the policy of not promoting a manager until he has developed a subordinate manager who can take over his position. By doing this, as we noted in our discussion of backstops, the manager is encouraged to delegate as much authority as he possibly can at an early stage. Moreover, in the process he creates an ideal organizational climate in which his subordinates can find maximum satisfaction of many of their most important needs.

SUMMARY

In this chapter, we considered the organizing process from the supervisor's point of view. Basically, organizing on the departmental level involves the same general steps as organizing the over-all institution, that is, grouping activities or subdepartmentalizing, assigning specific tasks and duties, and delegating authority. However, the supervisor should supplement these steps by designing an ideal organizational structure specifically for his department. Such a structure represents the way the supervisor would organize his unit if he could start from scratch with ideal resources and personnel. But in most cases the supervisor comes into an already existing department and he cannot immediately implement his ideal organizational design because for one thing the available personnel may not fit into his model. What he must do instead is to plan changes in or a complete reorganization of his department in order to make it come closer to the ideal. Such reorganization is a normal and important part of managerial life; however, it should not be so frequent that it undermines the security and morale of employees. Of course, organizational changes can be implemented either all at once or gradually depending upon the imminence of the need for them.

After reorganization has been accomplished or at least planned, the supervisor can proceed to delegate or to redelegate authority in accordance with the departmental structure he has set up. In a large or medium department, the process of delegation will be that outlined in Chapter 9: assigning duties, granting the authority to carry out these duties, and encouraging employees to accept responsibility for their duties. In a small department, the delegation of authority will take the form of developing a backstop, an understudy who can take over when the supervisor is not there. This is a long and tedious process because it involves careful training and progressively increasing delegations of authority. But it is well worth the effort since it will contribute to high motivation and morale among employees. Moreover, unless the supervisor does train someone to be his backstop and does grant authority to him, he will not have created any organization and his department is bound to collapse if he has to leave the scene.

However, this decentralization of authority is not as easily achieved as it might seem. Indeed, management frequently runs into obstacles which must be overcome in order to achieve broad delegation. These obstacles may be caused by an authority hoarder somewhere down the line, by a manager's reluctancy to shoulder authority and responsibility, or by the unavailability of suitable subordinates to whom authority can be delegated. Somehow or other, this vicious circle should be broken into and broader delegation should be instituted.

Of course, there comes a place in the organization where further delegation of authority is not possible. This is at the interface between the supervisor and the non-managerial employees as they go about performing their daily tasks. At this level, delegation of authority expresses itself in the practice of a general or loose kind of supervision which involves giving the employee a great amount of freedom in making his own decisions and in determining how to do his own job. In other words, general supervision is an application of Theory Y and not Theory X. It enables the employee to use his own judgment, and in so doing he will receive greater satisfaction from his job. Such general supervision is probably also the best way to motivate employees, whereas dependence on the sheer weight of authority would normally bring about the least desirable results. There might be occasions when the manager must fall back upon his authority, but with the new attitudes and expectations of our society the general trend is toward more freedom and self-determination in management as well as in other aspects of life.

CHAPTER 11

Committees as an Organizational Tool

As institutions grow in size and in the degree of specialization, it becomes more difficult for a single administrator to run their affairs. One way to cope with this difficulty is by establishing committees and turning over to them specific issues that can no longer be efficiently settled by one person. A committee is *a group of people who function collectively*. Committee members normally have regular duties in the organization and devote only part of their time to committee activities.

Yet, the amount of time spent in committee activities is increasing. There is definitely a growing emphasis on committee meetings within today's organizations. This is true for several reasons. First of all, as most enterprise activities have become more complex and specialized, there is an increased and more urgent need for coordination and cooperation. Conferences and meetings have proven to be a good means of answering this need. Another reason for the emphasis on meetings is the growing realization that people are more enthusiastic about carrying out the directives and plans that they themselves have helped to devise than they are about carrying out those that are handed down from above. Thus, committees are an additional means for effectively combining the formal and the acceptance theories of authority, for giving employees more freedom and greater delegations of authority, and for motivating them. In other words, committees are another proven tool for carrying out the general approach to supervision .

As we know, the job of a supervisor is to get things done through and with the help of the employees in his department. If he is skilled in establishing, running, and participating in committee meetings, it will significantly help him in achieving this objective. Although it is a common complaint that there are too many meetings and that they take up too much time, committees are still a widely used device in all organizations, especially in health care centers. There seems to be no substitute for them. Without committee meetings it would be almost impossible for an organization of any size to operate efficiently and effectively. There are many other ways of obtaining the ideas and opinions of employees on how to handle certain problems, but there is really no better way than by holding a meeting. The real criticism of meetings is probably not that there are too many of them, but that the results produced often do not warrant the time and effort invested.

No doubt you have sometimes been annoyed when you found yourself tied up in a meeting which the chairman allowed to amble along in all directions, "covering the waterfront" without any purpose whatsoever. In the meantime, more important work was accumulating on your desk. It is very likely that the chairman had not properly prepared the meeting, and that his performance did not increase your respect for his managerial ability. If you have had an experience of this type, you can quickly see how important it is for a supervisor to acquaint himself with committee meetings and with the committee or conference leadership technique. In other words, he should learn how to run committees well and how to obtain effective participation. Meetings will then become increasingly interesting and stimulating because the participants will have the satisfaction of knowing that the meeting is accomplishing something.

It must be pointed out that with the growing importance and number of committee meetings, it will not be just the occasional supervisor who comes in contact with them. Every supervisor must familiarize himself with the workings of a committee. There may be occasions when the supervisor will find it necessary to establish an interdepartmental committee or when he will have to be the chairman of such a committee. At other times, he may only be an ordinary member of the committee. And there will definitely be many instances when the supervisor will have to act as a conference leader or chairman of a committee made up only of employees of his own department.

THE NATURE OF COMMITTEES

Definitions

A committee is a group of people to whom certain matters have been committed. They meet for the purpose of discussing those matters that have been assigned to them. As stated above, committees function collectively and their members normally have other duties, making their committee work merely a part-time assignment. Because committees function only as a group, they differ considerably from other managerial devices.

Committees can be classified as *standing* or *temporary*. A standing committee has a formal permanent place in the organization. Typically, it deals with problems which are recurring in nature; in a hospital, for instance, the tissue committee, the infection committee, the joint committee and many others would be considered standing committees. A temporary committee, on the other hand, is one which has been appointed for a particular purpose and will be disbanded as soon as it has accomplished its task.

Functions of Committees

The Committee as a Place to Inform or to Discuss

Most management committee meetings may be described as either informational or discussion. The *informational* type of meeting is the kind where the leader or chairman does most of the talking in order to present certain information and facts. Assume, for example, that a supervisor wants to make an announcement and a meeting is called as a substitute for posting a notice or speaking to each employee separately. It may be expensive to take the whole work force away from the job; but, on the other hand, it guarantees that everyone in the department is notified of the new directive at the same time. Such a meeting also gives subordinates a chance to ask questions and to discuss the implications of the announcement. Care should be taken, however, that questions from participants are largely confined to further clarification of the supervisor's remarks so that the meeting will not stray from its purpose.

In the *discussion* type of meeting, the chairman encourages more participation of the members in order to secure their ideas and opinions. The supervisor could ask the individuals singly for suggestions on how to solve a problem, but it is probably better to call a meeting to allow them to make recommendations. Although it is up to the supervisor to make the final decision and to determine whether or not to incorporate some of the employees' suggestions, the employees will nevertheless derive great satisfaction from knowing that their ideas have been considered and that some of them may even be used. It is likely that good suggestions will be offered, and in all probability the implementation of suggestions will be more enthusiastic if the employees of the department have participated in finalizing them. In this case the committee acted in a staff capacity.

The supervisor can also go further than merely asking for suggestions. He may call a meeting for the sole purpose of having the employees of his department fully discuss and handle a problem themselves, that is, come up with their own decision. As we shall see below, this involves using the committee as a sort of collective managerial decision-maker.

The Committee as a Decision-Maker

In addition to committees whose purpose is to spread information and/or merely discuss a matter and make recommendations, there are those committees to which formal authority has been delegated to make decisions. Just as a supervisor can delegate decision-making authority to an individual subordinate, so he can form a committee and delegate authority to the group to decide on a solution to a problem that involves them all. In these instances the committee has decision-making power, in other words, line authority.

There are many questions in a health care center which are of such magnitude and which affect so many departments that it is far better to have the decision made by a committee consisting of representatives of many functions than by the administrator or one of his associate administrators alone. The same situation can exist within a department. For example, it frequently happens that employees are dissatisfied with the allocation of overtime, week-end work, and so forth, regardless of the supervisor's efforts to be fair. Naturally, the supervisor can make a decision for his employees on this matter; but it would be better if they could find a solution themselves. In such a case, management is not really concerned with precisely what decision is made so long as it falls within the limits set; for example, that the time allotted for overtime is not exceeded. By letting the group make this type of decision, they will come up with a solution which they accept. Even if such a solution is only adequate and not necessarily the best, it is still better if it is implemented by the group with great enthusiasm than a perfect decision which meets with their resistance. There are many of these problems and areas where management is not concerned with the details of the decision as long as it remains within certain boundaries.

Benefits of Group Discussion

There is little doubt that a group of individuals exchanging opinions and experiences often comes up with a better answer than any one person thinking through the same problem alone. It is an old saying that two heads are better than one. Various people will bring to a meeting a wide range of experience, background, and ability, which would not be available if the subject had been committed to an individual decision-maker. Indeed, many problems are so complicated that a single person could not possibly have all the necessary knowledge to come up with a wise solution. The free oral interchange of ideas among several persons will stimulate and clarify thinking and chances are that the recommendation made by the group as a whole will be better than that made by any single member. This is perhaps the major benefit of group discussion.

Group deliberation can also be a real help in promoting coordination. Members of the committee become more considerate of the problems of other employees and of the manager. They become more aware of the advantages of working together and of seeking cooperative solutions. Moreover, as we already stated, an individual who has participated in the formulation of a plan is more likely to be motivated to see that it is properly executed than if he had not been consulted. In reality, it matters little how much he actually contributed to the plan, as long as he was a member of the committee and sat in on the meeting. In this respect, group meetings are advantageous in establishing the proper climate for coordination, cooperation, and motivation.

Limitations of Committees

In spite of all of these beneficial features, the committee device has often been abused. Sometimes committees are created to delay action, and many people have come to think of the committee as a debating society. Jokes about committees are numerous. They have been defined as a group that "keeps minutes but wastes hours;" as a group "where the unwilling appoint the unfit to do the unnecessary." Remarks are often made that there are meetings all day long without leaving any time to get the work done. Indeed, one of the most often-voiced complaints about committees is that they are exceedingly *time-consuming*. This is true since each member is entitled to have his say and often certain individuals use up a great amount of time trying to convince other members of the validity of their points of view.

In addition to their costliness in time, committees also cost *money*. It is clear that time spent in committee meetings is not spent otherwise. Hence, every hour taken up by a meeting costs the institution a certain amount of dollars. Furthermore, there might be travel expenses involved and additional expenses for the preparation of meetings. Obviously, a single executive could reach an answer in a much shorter time and at less expense; but the problem is whether his decision would be as good as the one reached by group deliberation.

Another shortcoming of committees is that there are limitations to the *sense of responsibility* that they evoke. When a problem is submitted to a committee, it is submitted to a group and not to individuals. Responsibility does not weigh as heavily on the group's shoulders as it would on one individual's. In other words, the committee's problems become everybody's responsibility which in reality means they are nobody's responsibility. It is difficult to criticize the committee as a whole or any single member if the solution proves to be wrong since each person is quick to answer that it was the "committee" which made the decision. This thinning-out of responsibility is natural and there is no way of avoiding it.

Another shortcoming of committees is the danger of a *weak compromise decision* or *tyranny of the minority*. It has often become a tradition to reach decisions of unanimity based on politeness, cooperative spirit, mutual respect, and other considerations. However, this often leads to committee action which is a weak, watered-down compromise solution, frequently utilizing the lowest common denominator. It also can happen that in their desire for unanimous or nearly unanimous conclusions, committees are tyrannized by a minority holding out as long as possible. Finally, the majority might allow itself to be dominated by such a minority because of lack of time, interest, or sense of responsibility.

THE EFFECTIVE OPERATION OF A COMMITTEE

After management has considered the advantages and shortcomings and has decided to establish a committee, it must familiarize itself with the means for insuring effective committee operation. It is not easy to make committee meetings and conferences a success because the goals are numerous and difficult to achieve. As we have already suggested, the goals of a committee meeting are: first, to come up with the best suggestions or solution for the problem under consideration; second, to do this hopefully with unanimity; and third, to accomplish it in the shortest period of time. It is a challenge for any committee to fulfill these goals, but the task will be made easier if the following discussion is used as a guide for effective committee operation.

Delineating the Committee's Scope, Functions, and Authority

The first thing a committee must know in order to operate effectively is its scope and functions. The executive establishing the committee must define the subjects to be covered and the functions that the committee is expected to fulfill. This will prevent the committee from floundering around and will enable the manager to check on whether it is doing what is expected of it.

In addition to functions and scope, the degree of authority conferred upon the committee must be specified. It must be clearly stated whether the committee is to serve in an advisory (staff) capacity or whether it is to serve in a decision-making capacity (line authority). In the case of a formal standing committee, all such information should be set down in writing in the organization manual. For a temporary committee, scope, functions and authority must also be explicitly stated but perhaps not so formally. It is extremely important that temporary committees only be established for a subject worthy of group consideration. If a topic can be handled by one person or over the phone there is no need to call a meeting.

Composition of the Committee

Since the quality of committee work is only as good as its members, care should be exercised in choosing people to serve on committees. Members should be capable of expressing and defending their views, but they should also be willing to see the other party's point of view and be able to integrate their thinking with that of the other members. Hopefully, they should be independent of each other so that their deliberations will not suffer from any connotations of a direct superior-subordinate relationship. If committee members are chosen from different departments, the problems of rank are more easily overcome.

Indeed, the committee device is a good opportunity for bringing together the representatives of several different interest groups. Specialists of different departments and activities can be brought together in such a way that all concerned parties have proper representation. This will result in balanced group integration and deliberation. The various representatives will feel that their interests have been heard and considered. Of course, the top administrator should see to it that this concern with proper representation is not carried too far. It is more essential to appoint capable members to a committee than merely representative members. The ideal solution, of course, is to have a capable member from each pertinent activity on the committee.

Number of Members

No definite figure can be given as to the ideal size of a committee for effective operation. The best that can be said is that the committee should be large enough to provide for thorough group deliberation and broad resources of information. However, it should not be so large that it will be unwieldy and unusually time-consuming. If the nature of the subject under consideration is such that a very large committee is needed, it might be wise to form subcommittees which will consider various aspects of the problem. Then, the entire committee can meet to hear subcommittee reports and decide on a final solution.

Effective Conference Leadership

Even after the above-mentioned requirements are fulfilled, the success of any meeting will depend largely upon the chairman's ability to handle it. It is necessary for him to be familiar with effective conference or committee leadership* techniques in order to guide the meeting to a satisfactory conclusion. There is no doubt that the individual members of a committee bring to the meeting their individual patterns of behavior and points of view. The chairman must know how to handle the membership in such a way as to fuse the individual viewpoints and attitudes so that teamwork will develop for the benefit of the group. It will take considerable time and patience on the chairman's part to create a closely knit group out of a diverse membership, but that is generally the best way to achieve integrated group solutions. Let us look a little more carefully at just what the chairman's role is.

---

*The term "conference leadership" is generally used in the literature. We have used it here to be synonomous with "committee leadership."

The Role of the Chairman

It is only human nature for committee members to think first of how a new proposition would affect themselves and their own working environment. This kind of egotistical thinking can easily lead to unnecessary frictions. People tend to see the same "facts" differently. Words mean different things to different people. The first necessity in a group situation, therefore, is to find agreement on the basic nature of the problem under discussion so that everybody understands what the issues are. The task of the chairman is to try to find out from the participants what they *think* the issues are in order to learn whether or not they understand them as they actually are.

This, however, is easier said than done. A frequent comment about committees is that the issues on the conference table are really not as difficult to deal with as the people around the table. Individuals at a meeting will often react toward each other rather than toward their ideas. For instance, just because A talks too much, everything he suggests may be rejected. Or B might be a person who automatically rejects whatever someone else is for. And then there is C, that member of the committee who keeps his mouth shut all the time.

It is the chairman's job to minimize these personality differences by using the legitimate tools of parliamentary procedure. As we shall see when we discuss a typical committee meeting, he can arrange for the speaking time of each participant to be limited so that one person will not monopolize the entire meeting. And he can be especially careful to call on people who seldom speak. Sooner or later, with the help of such leadership techniques the committee will start reacting toward the content of the meeting, the issues involved, and not the individuals around the table. For a meeting to be successful, it is necessary that the various members forget about their personalities and their outside allegiances and work together as a team in a manner that will move the meeting toward a meaningful solution of the problem at hand. In all of this, the chairman plays a critical role.

Of course, the quality of the solution will also depend to some extent upon the amount of time spent in reaching it. Too much haste will probably not produce the most desirable solution. On the other hand, most meetings are under a time limit. If they were not, the members would become bored and frustrated with a meeting that lasts too long. It is the chairman's job to give every member a chance to participate and to voice his suggestions and opinions. This is especially important when the committee members are also expected to execute the decisions that they make. Then, it may be necessary for the chairman to use persuasion in order to induce a minority to go along with the decision of the majority. Or, on other occasions, he might have to persuade the majority to make concessions to the minority. All of this takes time, and may result in a compromise which does not necessarily represent the best possible solution. However, if the solution has been arrived at democratically, the chairman's leadership abilities will have been demonstrated and the major purpose of the meeting will have been accomplished.

Should the Chairman Express His Own Opinions?

It has often been stated that the function of a good chairman is to help the members of the group reach their own decisions, to work as a catalyst to bring out the ideas present among the committee members. There is no doubt that if the chairman expresses his views, the members of the committee may hesitate to argue with him or to make known their opinions especially if they disagree; this is particularly so if the chairman also happens to be their boss. On the other hand, there are many occasions when it would be unwise and completely unrealistic for the chairman not to express his views. He may have some factual knowledge or sound opinion, and the value of the deliberations would be lessened if these were left unknown to the members of the committee.

On the whole, it is best for the chairman to express his opinions, and at the same time clearly let it be known that he is willing to subject them to constructive criticism and suggestions. After all, silence on the leader's part may be interpreted to mean that he cannot make a decision himself or that he does not want to do so for fear of assuming responsibility. On certain occasions, however, the chairman must use his sensitive judgment as to whether or not or to what extent he will express his own opinions.

The Style of Leadership

There also is the question of how much of a formal leadership role the chairman should display. The variations of the chairman's role can run anywhere from the one extreme of an autocratic dictator to the other extreme of a democratic moderator. At times, however, it may be necessary for even a very permissive, democratic chairman to use tight control over the meeting, while on most occasions he will employ the loosest sort of control. Indeed, it has often been found that if the group of participants consists of mature managers from the upper administrative echelons, no formal control and no formal chairman are really necessary.

Although this may be true for the highest level committee meetings, normally on the lower levels there is a need for a stable structure and strong leadership from a chairman. If the group has a formally elected or appointed chairman, they will naturally look to him to keep the meeting moving along so that it will come to an efficient conclusion. Under most conditions, the formal leadership of the chairman is necessary to ensure that group decision-making is effective.

The Agenda

The best means of keeping a meeting from wandering off into a discussion of irrelevant matters is a well-prepared agenda. The chairman must carefully outline his over-all strategy, his agenda, before the meeting. Topics to be discussed should be listed in the proper sequence, and often it is advisable to set up a timetable. Establishing an approximate time limit for each item assures better control of the situation. If possible, the agenda should be distributed to the members before the meeting so that they can better prepare themselves for the coming discussion.

Although the agenda designs the over-all strategy, it must not be so rigid that there is no means for adjusting it. The chairman should apply the agenda with a degree of flexibility, so that if a particular subject requires more attention than originally anticipated, the time allotted to some other topic can be reduced. In other words, staying close to the agenda should not force the chairman to be too quick to rule people out of order. What seems irrelevant to him may be important to some of the other committee members. As a matter of fact, some irrelevancies at times actually help to create a relaxed atmosphere and to relieve tension which has built up.

Since it is the chairman's job to keep the meeting moving along toward its goal, it is a good idea for him to pause at various points during the meeting to consult the agenda and remind the group of what has been accomplished and what still remains to be discussed. A good chairman will learn when the opportune time has arrived to summarize one point and to move on to the next item in the agenda. If past experience tells the chairman that his meetings have a tendency to run overtime or not to complete all the agenda items, it might be advisable to schedule them shortly before the lunch break or just before quitting time. This seems to speed up meetings; somehow the participants seem to run out of arguments around those hours of the day.

A TYPICAL COMMITTEE MEETING

Now that we are familiar with the guidelines for effective committee operation, we are ready to examine how these guidelines would be applied in a typical committee meeting. In other words, we want to see how a diverse group of people can, with the help of an effective leader, hold a meaningful discussion and arrive at satisfactory answers to the questions under consideration.

General Participation in the Discussion

After a few introductory remarks and social pleasantries, the chairman should make an initial statement of the problem to be discussed. This will open up an opportunity for all members of the meeting to participate freely. Any member should be able to bring out those aspects of the problem which seem important to him, regardless of whether or not they seem important to everyone else. Sooner or later the discussion will simmer down to those points which are relevant.

There are always some members at the meeting who talk too much and others who do not talk enough. One of the chairman's most difficult jobs is to encourage the latter to speak up and to keep the former from holding the floor for too long. There are various ways and means for the chairman to do this. For example, after a long-winded speaker has had enough opportunity to express his opinions, it may be wise to conveniently overlook him and not recognize him, giving someone else the chance to speak. It might also help to ask him to please keep his remarks brief. Or arrange his seat on the conference table in a blind spot where it is easy not to recognize his request to have the floor. Most of the time, moreover, the other members of the committee will quickly find subtle ways of censoring those members who have too much to say.

Of course, this does not mean that all members of the meeting must participate equally. There are some people who know more about a given subject than others, and some who have stronger feelings about an issue than others. The chairman must take such factors into consideration, but he should still do his best to stimulate as much over-all participation as possible. In this endeavor, his general attitude with regard to participation will be extremely important. He must accept everyone's contribution without judgment and must create the impression that he wants everyone to participate. He may have to ask controversial questions merely to get the discussion going. Once participation has started, the chairman should continue to throw out provocative, "open end" questions, questions which ask why, who, what, where, and when. However, questions that can be answered with a simple yes or no, should be avoided.

Another technique which can be used by the chairman is to start at one side of the conference table and ask each member in turn to express his thoughts on the problem. The major disadvantage of this technique is that instead of participating in the discussion spontaneously whenever they have something to say, the rest of the group will tend to sit back and wait until called on. But the skilled chairman will watch the facial expressions of the different people in the group. This may very well give him a clue as to whether someone has an idea but is afraid to speak up. He can then make a special effort to call on such a person.

If a meeting is made up of a large number of participants, it may be advisable for the chairman to break it up into small groups, commonly known as "buzz sessions." Each of the small subgroups will hold their own discussions and report back to the meeting after a specified period of time. In this way, those people who hesitate to say anything in a larger group will be more or less forced to participate and to express their opinions. Buzz sessions are usually advisable whenever the number of participants is greater than twenty or thereabout.

Of course, in using all of these techniques to evoke general participation in the discussion, the chairman should try to stick to his agenda and to see that the discussion is basically relevant. It sometimes happens that a chairman who is inexperienced at holding meetings is so anxious to have someone say something that there will be a lot of discussion for discussion's sake. Most of the time, this is not desirable because it confuses the issues and delays the even more important decision-making phase of the meeting.

Group Decision-Making

Once a problem has been pretty well narrowed down and understood in the same sense by all members of the group, it is advisable to get to the facts in as objective a manner as possible. Only by ascertaining all the relevant facts will the group be able to suggest alternative solutions. The chairman knows that the best solution can only be as good as the best alternative which was considered. He will make certain that no solution is overlooked by urging the members of the meeting to contribute as many alternatives as they can possibly think of.

The next step is to evaluate the alternative solutions and to discuss the advantages and disadvantages of each. In so doing, the field can eventually be narrowed down to two or three alternatives on which general agreement can be reached. The other alternatives can probably be eliminated by unanimous consent. Those which remain must be discussed thoroughly in order to bring about a solution. The chairman should try to play the role of a middleman or conciliator by working out a solution which is acceptable to all members of the group, possibly even persuading some members that their opinions are wrong.

The best procedure would probably be to arrive at a solution which is a synthesis of the desirable outcomes of the few remaining alternatives. By the process of integration, all important points can be incorporated into the most desirable solution. Throughout this process, the chairman has the difficult job of helping the minority to save face. It is easier to conciliate the minority if the final decision which the group comes up with incorporates something of each person's ideas so that everyone has a partial victory. Of course, this can be a long and tedious process and, as we have said, such a compromise may not always be the strongest solution.

Sometimes, however, the group may not be able to reach a compromise or to come to any decisions on which the majority agrees. This will frequently happen if the chairman of the meeting senses that he is confronted by a group which is hostile. In such a situation, it is necessary for him to find out what is bothering the group, to bring their objections out into the open and discuss them. It is not uncommon for participants in a committee meeting to think first of what is objectionable about a new idea rather than to think of its desirable features. A discussion of such objections may dispel unwarranted fears and may allow participants to perceive the positive aspects of a certain alternative. Or, by the same token, the objections may be strong enough to void the proposition. In any case, it is necessary for the group to have a chance to voice their negative feelings before a positive consensus can be reached.

Taking a Vote

The chairman is often confronted with the problem of whether a vote should be taken, or whether he should keep on working until the group reaches a final unanimous agreement regardless of how long this would take. Off hand, many people would say that voting is a democratic way to make decisions. But voting does accentuate the differences among the members of the group, and once a man has publicly committed himself to a position by voting it is often difficult for him to change his mind and yet save face. Also, if he is a member of the losing minority he cannot be expected to carry out the majority decision with great enthusiasm. Therefore, wherever possible it is better not to take a formal vote and to work toward a roughly unanimous agreement.

However, as pointed out above, one of the disadvantages of reaching a unanimous conclusion is that it can cause serious delay in the meeting. It also is true that the price of unanimity is often a solution which is reduced to a common denominator and which may not be as ingenious and bold as it would have otherwise been. Of course, it will depend on the situation and the magnitude of the problem involved whether or not unanimity is desirable. It should be pointed out that in most instances it is not as difficult as one might think to come up with a unanimous decision. The skilled chairman can usually sense the feeling of the meeting, and all he should do then is say that it seems to him that the consensus of the group is that such and such be the solution. At this point, especially in a small meeting, parliamentary procedure and a formal vote can probably be dispensed with. In a large meeting, of course, unanimity may be an impossible goal and decisions should be based on majority rule.

Follow-up of Committee Action

Regardless of whether a committee was acting merely to come up with a recommendation or whether it has final decision-making authority, its findings need a follow-up. After the chairman has reported the committee's findings to the superior who originally channeled the subject to the committee, it is the latter's duty to keep the committee posted as to what action he has taken. Indeed, the practice of good human relations and ordinary courtesy will tell the superior that he owes the committee some explanation. Inadequate statements or no statements at all from him will cause the committee to lose interest in its work. Of course, when the committee has had authority to make a final decision, then the problem of carrying out the decision usually belongs to the committee itself. The chairman will generally be asked to oversee this or the particular executive who normally deals with the subject matter may execute the decision himself. In any event, the committee members must be kept informed as to what has happened.

SUMMARY

There is probably no supervisor who has not been involved in committees either as a member or as an organizer. Indeed, committees are becoming an extremely important device for augmenting the organizational structure of an enterprise. They allow the enterprise to adapt to increasing complexity without a complete reorganization. They permit a group of people to function collectively in areas which a single individual could not handle. Obviously, the advantages of committees are offset to a certain extent by their limitations and shortcomings, one of the most important being that responsibility cannot be pinned to any individual member of the committee. In spite of this and other criticisms leveled against committee meetings, they can be of great value if properly organized and lead.

Because the increasing complexities of today's society are making more and more committees necessary, it is essential for the supervisor to familiarize himself with the workings of a committee. Committee meetings are called either to disseminate information or to discuss a topic. If discussion is involved, a distinction should be made between whether the committee is to arrive at a final decision on the question under discussion and whether it is to take action based on this decision, or whether it is to merely make recommendations to the line manager who appointed the committee.

Regardless of the purpose of the committee, it is likely that group deliberation will produce a more satisfactory and acceptable conclusion than one which was formally handed down from above. Decisions will be carried out with more enthusiasm if employees have had a role in making them or in making recommendations through committees. However, in order for group decisions and recommendations to be of high quality, it is necessary that the committee members be carefully selected. In the composition of a committee, it is essential that as many interested parties as possible be represented. The people chosen as representatives should be capable of presenting their views and of integrating their opinions with those of others. As to the size of a committee, it is advisable that there be enough members to permit thorough deliberations, but not so many as to make the meetings bulky and cumbersome.

In addition to the above factors, the success of committee deliberations depends largely on effective committee or conference leadership. This means that the chairman's familiarity with effective group work will make the difference between productive and wasteful committee meetings. The chairman's job is to produce the best possible solution in the shortest amount of time and hopefully with unanimity. In trying to achieve these goals, the chairman is constantly confronted with the problem of running the meeting either too tightly or too loosely. If his control is too tight, he may frustrate the natural development of ideas, force conclusions before all alternatives have been considered, and in general create resentment. If his control is too loose, he may give the members of the meeting the feeling of aimlessness and confusion. In practice, he will have to depend upon a keen perception of the "mood of the meeting" in order to know exactly how to lead it and bring it to a successful conclusion. Thus, the chairman will have to sense when there has been enough general participation in the discussion, when alternative solutions have been properly evaluated, and when and if a vote is necessary in order to arrive at a group decision. In all of these matters, the leadership abilities of the chairman will be of utmost importance.

CHAPTER 12

Informal Organization

Closely related to the workings of committees and to the phenomenon of group participation, yet quite different in origin, is the informal organization found in most enterprises. The informal organization is a powerful source of influence which interacts with and modifies the formal organization. Although many managers would like to conveniently overlook its existence, they will readily admit that in order to fully understand the nature of organizational life it is necessary to "learn the ropes" of the informal organization. In almost every institution such an informal structure will develop. It reflects the spontaneous efforts of individuals and groups to influence the conditions of their existence. Whenever people are associated, social relationships and groupings are bound to come about. The informal organization has a positive contribution to make to the smooth functioning of the enterprise and to this extent the manager must understand its workings, respect it, and even nurture it.

To be a bit more specific, informal organization arises from the social interaction of people as they associate with each other. Such interaction may be accidental or incidental to organized activities, or it may arise from personal desire or gregariousness. At the heart of informal organization are people and their relationships, whereas at the heart of formal organization is the organizational structure and the delegation of authority. A manager can create or rescind a formal organizational structure which he has designed; but he cannot rescind the informal organization since he did not establish it. As long as there are people working together in a department, there will be an informal organization consisting of the informal groupings of employees.

THE INFORMAL GROUP

At the base of all informal organization is the small group. And the first question which comes to our minds is why people join such groups. We may wonder what advantages they gain from them since they are already members of a department where their duties are specifically assigned, where channels of communication exist, where a line of authority has been established, and where they are a significant part of a formal organizational structure. The answer to this question is that employees have certain needs which they would like to satisfy, but which apparently the formal organization leaves unsatisfied. People have a basic need to associate with their fellow men in groups small enough to permit intimate, direct, and personal contact among individuals. The satisfactions which are derived from these kinds of relationships generally cannot be obtained from working within a large organization. Thus, the small group provides the individual with satisfactions which are uniquely different from those that he can get from any other source.

Benefits Derived From Groups

First of all, group participation provides a sense of *security* and *self-assurance*. An individual in a group is usually surrounded by others who share similar values with him. This reinforces his own value system and gives him confidence since it is always more comfortable to be among people who think the same way we do. There is also the need for *friendship* and *companionship* which the group fulfills. The employee needs and enjoys the social contact with his fellow workers, sharing experiences, joking, finding a sympathetic listener and an opportunity to get some of his troubles off his chest. The group will, furthermore, fulfill the need for *belonging*, the need to associate with others who have the same purposes and goals. Informal groups, like more formal committees, help employees to accomplish tasks which may be impossible to accomplish alone. They also serve to bring the goals of these tasks more into the realm of the employee. There are, of course, objectives and goals in the formal organization. But these may appear remote and meaningless to the average employee. It is much simpler to identify with the objectives and goals of one's immediate work group. And often an employee will readily forego some of his own goals and replace them with the goals of the group.

Another need which is satisfied by belonging to a small group in many instances is the need for *protection*, namely, protection from what the members may think of as an imposition or an encroachment by management. We are all familiar with the old saying that there is strength in unity. In this respect, the small group is a source of support. Often when people enter an organization for the first time they have feelings of significant anxiety. The surroundings are unfamiliar and a great deal of uncertainty exists. When several people are in the same circumstance, a small group may arise on this basis alone. An additional need which a small group fulfills is the need for *status* because the group enables an employee to belong to a distinct little organization which is more or less exclusive. It also gives the individual an opportunity for self-expression, a kind of audience before generally sympathetic listeners. A further reason why people join groups is in order to secure *information*. Groups tend to form around an individual who seems to be the focal point in a communications network. An individual who has information is able to satisfy the communication needs of others, even though the information trans-mitted by him may be false or distorted by the grapevine.

It is important for the supervisor of a department to be aware of all of these needs which his employees want satisfied. Then, he will understand why employees tend to join informal groups and in his daily supervision he can attempt to use these groups constructively rather than being suspicious and trying to destroy them.

INFORMAL GROUPS AND THE INFORMAL ORGANIZATION

Small informal groups, as we said, are at the basis of informal organization and all small informal groups have the potential to be-come informal organizations. The informal organization develops when a small group acquires a more or less distinct structure and a set of norms and standards as well as a procedure to invoke sanctions in order to assure conformity to the norms. The informal organiza-tional structure is determined largely by the different status posi-tions which people within the small group hold.

Status Positions

Generally speaking, there are *four* status positions; the group's informal leader, the primary members of the group, the members who have only *fringe status,* and those who have *out status*. The informal leader of the small group is the person around whom the primary members of the group cluster; their association is close and their in-teraction and communication is intense. This is normally considered the small nucleus group of which newcomers would like to become members. These newcomers are usually new employees of the de-partment. They remain on the fringe of the group while they are be-ing evaluated by the small nucleus for acceptance or rejection. Eventually these individuals will either move into the nucleus and be-come a bonafide member of the small group or they will move into the outer shell because they have been rejected. The people in the outer shell are still a part of the informal organization even though they have not been accepted as members of the core group. Such re-jection, however, can have serious behavioral effects especially if a person wants badly to belong to the nucleus group. This is true be-cause in essence the group represents a system of interaction which causes members to modify their own individual behavior and to have a marked impact on the behavior of persons on the fringe shell or the outer shell.

Of course, the person who plays the role of the informal leader is usually the dynamic force of the group. Like the committee chairman, he is the one who crystalizes opinions, sets objectives, and so forth. This group leader is generally democratically chosen. He acquires his leadership role by a consensus of the group he leads. He is normally a dominant personality who functions in such a way as to facilitate the satisfaction of most of the needs of group members. From time to time, one might find small groups where the aspects of leadership are shared, in other words, where there are different leaders who perform different functions. For example, one leader may deal with administration, whereas another may deal with the union, and a third one may try to maintain internal cohesiveness. Most of the time, however, there is only one informal leader with whom the supervisor will have to deal.

Norms and Standards

In addition to status positions, there are norms and standards within the informal organization. The norms set the standards of behavior between group members, the standards for quality and quantity of work, and the standards that cover such things as squealing to management about a co-worker, etc. The standards governing work output are particularly important in almost every informal organization. They tell exactly how many salads a salad girl in the nutrition department will fix per hour, how many records will be processed in the medical records department during a day, and so forth, regardless of what the supervisor would like to have accomplished. And these norms often are far from what the supervisor would like to have.

In order to be admitted to the group, the employee must be willing and eager to accept such standards in lieu of his own. Since groups are capable of granting or withholding the advantages of membership, the individual must modify his behavior so that it corresponds to that of the group. This is the reason that informal organization has such a significant influence over the behavior of employees who are group members.

Sanctions

Along with norms and standards, there must be an effective procedure for invoking sanctions in case the group member does not conform with the norms set. These sanctions can range all the way from being elusive and evasive on the one hand to being quite visible on the other hand. The most powerful sanction is, of course, that of rejection and ostracism. The employee who consistently does not comply with the group's norms will soon find himself on the outside. His life can then be made miserable, his work can be sabotaged, and eventually he may want to leave the institution completely. But sanctions can also be very mild, perhaps in the form of a friendly talk or excluding someone from social activities such as lunching together. All of these sanctions of the informal organization, whether subtle or strong, serve to see that group members adhere to the group's idea of correct on-the-job behavior.

Additional Characteristics

In addition to the above characteristics, the informal organization also creates its own channel of communication, namely, the unofficial channel known as the *grapevine*. This manifestation of the informal organization has already been fully discussed in the chapter on Communication. Let it suffice to repeat here that the grapevine is the major connecting link of the informal organization just as communication through regular channels serves to link the formal organizational structure. As stated above, the informal organization influences the behavior of employees regardless of the status they occupy within the informal group. This is important for a supervisor to remember because he cannot hope to understand individual behavior without understanding the behavior of the organizational forces which shape it.

One such force is the tendency of the informal organization to *resist change*. It resists especially those changes that could be interpreted as a threat to the informal group. Over time, the small group has developed a very satisfying social relationship and any change that may challenge its equilibrium and stability will be greeted with resistance. This resistance can take the form of complaints, slowdown of work, excessive absenteeism, reduction in the quality of the job performed, and so on. It is essential for a supervisor to understand the dynamics of these types of group behavior in order to introduce change successfully. This will be discussed further in Chapter 19.

RELATIONS BETWEEN THE INFORMAL AND FORMAL ORGANIZATIONS

Often it might appear that the functioning of the informal organization makes the job of the supervisor a more difficult one. Because of the interdependence between informal and formal organizations, the attitudes, goals, norms, and customs of one affect the other and vice versa. Informal organizations do frequently give life and vitality to the formal organization. But this is not always the case. Indeed, informal organizations can have *either* a constructive or a hindering influence on the formal organization and on the realization of departmental objectives. In the final analysis, the supervisor's basic attitude will have much to do with whether that influence is positive or negative.

It is important for the supervisor to be aware of the fact that these informal groups are very strong, and that they may often govern the behavior of employees to an extent that interferes with formal supervision. Sometimes it can even go so far that the pressure of the informal group frustrates the supervisor in carrying out the policies which his superior expects him to enforce. The wise supervisor, therefore, should make all possible efforts to gain the cooperation and goodwill of the informal organization and the informal leader, and to use them wherever possible to further the departmental objectives. In practice, if properly handled by the supervisor, the informal organization can be useful as an effective channel of communication and as an efficient means of getting the departmental job done.

How the Supervisor Can Use the Informal Organization

One way the supervisor can put the informal organization to the best possible use is to let his employees know that he accepts and understands its existence. Such an understanding will enable him to group employees so that those most likely to comprise a good team will be working with each other on the same assignments. The supervisor's understanding of how the informal organization works will also help him avoid activities which would unnecessarily threaten or disrupt the informal group. He should do his utmost to integrate the interests of the informal organization with those of the formal organization.

The supervisor should exhibit such a positive approach because he knows that there are positive attributes in a cohesive informal group. Morale is likely to be high, turnover and excessive absences tend to be low, and the members tend to work smoothly as a team. This can make supervision much easier because the supervisor escapes a lot of bickering; it can also ease the burden of communication since the group provides its own effective, though informal, channels. Therefore, the supervisor should emphasize the positive by "communicating" informal responsibility to the informal leader and by allowing the group — naturally within limits — to go about the job as much on their own as possible.

A supervisor can do even more to bring out the positive aspects of informal groups by sharing his decision-making authority with them. In effect, he is turning the informal group into a sort of self-contained committee. As we know, decisions arrived at by a group or committee usually turn out to the advantage of all involved. They enable the group to exercise control over their own activities, and to make certain that all their interests are taken into account with the result that no one comes out a loser.

However, the supervisor must make sure that he establishes certain ground rules for this group decision-making process. Otherwise, it could bring about opposite results. First of all, the supervisor must sincerely believe in group decision-making and want it. Second, he must set clear limitations to the area of deliberation. For instance, if he lets the group arrange its own holiday schedule, he should state how many employees with a special skill must be present on holidays, what the time limits are, and so forth. Third, he must make it clear whether he is asking the group merely for suggestions or whether he is actually delegating to it the authority to find a solution and make a decision. And last but not least, the supervisor should choose a problem where the enthusiastic acceptance and execution is at least as important — if not more important — than the specifics of the decision itself. Under these conditions, group decision-making can be an additional means of accentuating the positive aspects of informal organization.

The Supervisor and the Informal Group Leader

It is also very important for the supervisor to maintain a positive attitude toward the informal group leader. Instead of looking at him as a "ringleader," the supervisor will do better to consider him as someone "in the know," to respect him, and to work with him. In his efforts to build good relations with the informal leader, the supervisor can pass information on to him before giving it to anyone else. He can ask his advice on certain problems, and particularly if he is considering a rearrangement of duties, he may want to discuss it with the informal leader first to get his reaction. Or he may ask him to "break-in" a new employee of the department, knowing full well that he would do it anyway.

In taking this approach, however, the supervisor must be careful not to cause the informal leader to lose his status within the group because working with the supervisor means working with management. In other words, the supervisor should not extend too many favors to the informal leader as this would ruin the latter's leadership position within the group at once. Of course, all of the foregoing assumes that an informal group leader is easily visible in every department. But often it is difficult for a supervisor, and especially for a new supervisor, to identify the informal leader of a group. Observation is probably the best means to find out. The supervisor should look for that person to whom the other employees turn when they need help, the person who sets the pace and who seems to have influence over them. The supervisor must continually and closely observe this because the informal group will occasionally shift from one leader to another, depending upon the purposes to be pursued. But regardless of who the leader is, the supervisor should do all in his power to work *with* him instead of against him.

It would, however, be unrealistic to think that such a positive approach is the sinecure to all conflicts between the informal and the formal organizations. No doubt, there will be occasions when agreement and harmonious interaction may be impossible. There are situations where every supervisor must go contrary to the desires of the group he supervises. In those instances, the dictates of formal authority will probably be the decisive factor.

SUMMARY

In addition to the formal organization, there exists in every enterprise an informal organization based on informal groups. These groups satisfy certain needs and desires of their members which apparently are left unsatisfied by the formal organization. For example, an informal group can satisfy the members' social needs. It gives them recognition and status and a sense of belonging. Informal information transmitted through the grapevine provides a channel of communication and fulfills the members' need and desire to know what is going on. The informal organization also influences the behavior of individuals within the group and requests them to conform with certain standards and norms which the group has set up. Informal organization can be found on all levels of the enterprise from the top to the bottom. It exists in every department regardless of the quality of supervision.

Informal organization can have either a constructive or a destructive influence on the formal organization. In order to make the best possible use of informal organization, the supervisor must understand its workings and must be able to identify its informal leaders. Then he can work with them in a way that will help accomplish the objectives of his department. For example, he can use the informal group and its leader to train new employees or to transmit messages. Instead of dwelling on the informal organization as a source of conflict, the supervisor should remember that both the formal and the informal organizations are part of a complex system interacting with each other. Instead of viewing it as something antagonistic, he should approach it positively and emphasize its potential for the good of the enterprise. After all, informal groups are similar in many respects to more formal committees and they have many of the same advantages.

PART FIVE

Staffing

CHAPTER 13

The Staffing Process

Staffing is the function which supplies the human resources to fulfill the institution's plans and objectives. Once goals have been determined, departments set up, and duties and task relationships established, people must be found to give life to what would otherwise be only a paper structure. It is the manager's responsibility to vitalize his own department by staffing it properly. He must staff it in a manner that the capability of the employees in his department matches their authority and responsibility. This is very important because if an employee's capabilities exceed the challenges and authority of the position, he is not employed to his full capacity and he will not derive the necessary satisfaction from his job. If, on the other hand, the employee's capability is beneath the demands and authority of the position, he will probably not be able to perform his job satisfactorily. The purpose of the staffing function, then, is to achieve the optimum use of human resources which is only possible when job authority and demands match the employee's capability. And, of course, this matching process is the essence of the managerial staffing function.

More specifically, the staffing function of the manager includes the selection, placement, development, training, and compensation of the subordinates in his department. It is every manager's and every supervisor's job to evaluate and appraise the performance of their employees, to promote them according to their effort and ability, to reward them, and, if necessary, to discipline or even discharge them. Only if a manager performs all of these duties can it be said that he is truly fulfilling his managerial staffing function.

In checking the above list of activities, however, many supervisors may be inclined to think that some of them are more properly the responsibility of the personnel director and the personnel department. It is true that in certain hospitals and related health care facilities some of the above-mentioned activities are performed by the personnel department. In such institutions, the personnel department has very broad jurisdiction. Nevertheless, good management still considers the above-mentioned duties as part of the supervisor's legitimate functions. Although the supervisor may be assisted in the performance of these functions by the personnel staff, they are still primarily his responsibility.

THE STAFFING FUNCTION AND THE PERSONNEL DEPARTMENT

Throughout the following discussion, it will be assumed that within the organizational structure of the institution the personnel department is considered a staff department as defined in our discussion of line and staff. The usefulness and effectiveness of the personnel department will depend largely upon its ability to develop a good working relationship with line supervisors, that is, on the quality of the line-staff relationship that exists. This, of course, will be governed in part by how clearly and how specifically the administrator has outlined the activities and authority of the personnel department. In determining its scope and its relationship to the staffing function of line supervisors, it is necessary for the administrator to understand the historical place of the personnel department in the institution. Only then will he be able to establish a structure which is meaningful in terms of current needs and patterns.

Historical Patterns

The personnel department started primarily as a record-keeping department. It kept all employment records for the employees and managers, all correspondence pertaining to their hiring, application blanks, background information, date hired, various positions held within the enterprise, dates of promotions, salary changes, leaves of absences granted, disciplinary penalties imposed, and other kinds of information which describe the employee's relationship to the enterprise. Of course, the proper maintenance of these clerical records is still of great importance today, especially with the growing emphasis on pension and insurance programs, unemployment claims, seniority provisions of all kinds, and promotional and development programs. By assigning such clerical service activities to the personnel staff, the administrator knows that they will be handled with high technical competence and efficiency due to the specialization of the department. If such a service were not provided by the personnel department, each and every supervisor would have to keep these records himself for his own department. Obviously, this would be a cumbersome and time-consuming task with which to be burdened in addition to the daily chores of getting the job done. Therefore, line supervisors are happy to have the personnel staff perform these complicated clerical services for them. The line supervisors are just not interested in doing this work themselves, and very often they may not even have the ability to do so.

As we said, most early personnel departments concerned themselves only with these record-keeping activities. Then as time went on, mainly during the 1920's, many managers in industry felt that the threat of unionization might be thwarted if efforts were made to give employees cafeterias, better rest rooms, bowling teams, company stores, etc. Although most of these benefits have a strong flavor of "paternalism," management thought that they would make the employees happier and less resentful in the existing organizational setup. Since none of these activities fitted into the regular line departments of the enterprise, however, the personnel department took responsibility for an increasing number of them.

During the 1930's, another shift in the emphasis of the personnel department took place. With the increase of union activities, the personnel department was expected to take direct charge of all employee and union relations. It often assumed full responsibility for hiring, firing, handling union grievances, and dealing with general labor problems. In other words, management thought that by having a personnel department all personnel questions could be handled by them, leaving the line supervisors with practically no staffing function.

However, this lead to serious difficulties for while the duties and power of the personnel department increased significantly, the standing of the supervisor as a manager decreased. The more power the personnel director acquired, the weaker the supervisor's relationship became with his own employees. The demoralized supervisor justifiably complained that it was impossible for him to effectively manage his department without having the power to select, hire, discipline, and reward his employees. The employees no longer regarded the supervisor as their boss. Because someone in the personnel department hired the employees, established their wages, and promoted, disciplined and fired them, employees looked to someone in the personnel department as their supervisor. Since this obviously led to a bad state of affairs in many organizations, good management now clearly delineates between the functions of the personnel department in a staff capacity and the supervisor's role as a manager of his department.

Present Pattern

Sound management principles advocate that the job of the personnel department is to provide the line supervisors with advice and counsel concerning personnel problems, and to help the line supervisors in every possible respect. Going beyond this would lead to a fragmentation of the supervisor's job, and would make it impossible for the supervisor to be an effective manager within his department. Naturally, the line supervisor should take full advantage of the expert advice and assistance which is available within the personnel department; but the line supervisor must retain the basic responsibility for managing his department.

The supervisor and the personnel department must work together and their activities must intertwine. But their roles and areas of authority should not be permitted to shift. Since it is the supervisor's job to get out the work within his department, he must make the managerial decisions which concern the people who work under him. Generally speaking, this means that it is up to the supervisor to define the specific qualifications he expects from an employee who is to fill a specific position. It is the personnel department's function to develop sources of qualified applicants within the local labor market. This means that the personnel department must let the community know what jobs are available and, in general, create an image of the organization as an employer. The personnel department can accomplish this by fostering good community relations, and recruiting in high schools, training schools, colleges, and other sources of employees.

The personnel department should conduct preliminary interviews with those who apply, to determine whether or not their qualifications match the requirements as defined by the supervisor. Necessary reference checks as to previous employment dates and past records should be made by the personnel department and those applicants who do not meet job requirements should be eliminated from consideration. Those candidates who meet the stated requirements should be referred to the supervisor.

It is up to the supervisor to interview, select, and hire from among the available candidates. It is the supervisor who does the actual hiring — no one else. The supervisor assigns the new employee to a specific job, and it is his responsibility to judge how he can best utilize and develop this new employee's skills. It is the personnel department's job to give the new employee a general indoctrination about the hospital, about the benefits, general hospital rules, shifts, hours, etc. But it is the supervisor's job to introduce the employee to the specific details of his job — wages, departmental rules, hours, rest periods, etc. It is the supervisor's job to arrange compensation within the pattern of remuneration, to instruct and train the new employee on the job, and to assess the employee's performance to determine, as time goes on, whether or not he should be promoted into a better job. If the need to take disciplinary measures should arise, it is clearly the supervisor's duty to do so, and, if necessary, even to fire the employee. During all the time an employee is with the organization, his complete employment record is maintained by the personnel department.

In carrying out the staffing function the supervisor will be greatly aided by the personnel department. They maintain all the clerical services for him, keep the records, and are there to provide advice, counsel, and guidance whenever personnel problems arise. The supervisor, however, in making his decisions, can follow, reject or alter the personnel department's advice and counsel. In reality, of course, it is often difficult to draw such a fine line of distinction between the advice, counsel and guidance of the personnel department and the supervisor's decision-making.

The following example will illustrate how blurred the distinction can be between providing information and giving advice, and, on the other hand trying to make decisions for the supervisor. When the staff man merely provides information, he furnishes the facts which help the supervisor make a sound decision. For instance, he might inform the nursing director that those applying for an open position are expecting a starting salary which is higher than the institution's starting rate. Or, he might advise that if the director of nursing were to hire a nurse at a certain salary, the director may have some dissatisfied older employees in the department. In the latter remark the staff man is providing not only information but also advice. By selecting the facts carefully and by phrasing his advice, he may actually sway the line supervisor's decision one way or the other. He may even advise paying the new nurse X amount per month. And before anyone realizes it, the information becomes advice and the advice becomes a decision. This may have come about not because of a desire on the personnel man's part to broaden his authority or to reduce the supervisor's authority: the line supervisor himself may have encouraged this growth of staff activity.

It sometimes happens that the supervisor will welcome the personnel department's willingness to help him out of a difficult situation. Frequently many a supervisor will ask the personnel department to make a decision for him so that he won't become burdened with so-called "personnel problems." He gladly accepts the staff man's decision because he feels that if the decision is wrong, he can always excuse it by saying that it was not his decision but that of the personnel man. In other words, the line supervisor is only too ready to capitulate to the personnel man in many instances. In so doing he can "pass the buck" to the personnel department.

Although it is understandable that the supervisor is reluctant to question and disregard the advice of the staff expert, the supervisor must bear in mind that the staff man sees only a small part of the entire picture. The staff man is not responsible for the performance of the department. There are usually many other factors involved in the over-all picture which will affect the department, factors with which the staff man is not as familiar as the line supervisor. The supervisor cannot separate his functions between clear areas of personnel problems and performance problems. Every situation has certain personnel implications, and it is impossible to separate the various components of each problem within the department. Only the supervisor is likely to know what the broad picture is.

If the supervisor capitulates and has the personnel department make his decisions, his relationship with his employees will sooner or later be damaged. His subordinates will decide that it is the personnel department and not the supervisor who has the real power which will influence their jobs within the hospital. The supervisor's leadership position will slowly deteriorate if his employees detect that the personnel staff determines salaries, and hiring and firing practices. They will discover that the supervisor does not control rewards and penalties and that, in reality, he does not make the decisions in the department.

The supervisor must make it clear that it is he who makes the decisions and takes the responsibility for their consequences. Although there are occasions when it may seem convenient to "pass the buck" to the personnel department, such practices sooner or later will backfire. It is not uncommon for supervisors to say that they would gladly give their employees a certain raise but that "they" (the personnel department) will not let them do so. Although this may be expedient for the moment, practices of this type lead eventually to erosion of the supervisor's authority. In the above situation the supervisor has to state that *he* has explored all possible alternatives and that much to his regret there is nothing *he* can do at this time for the employee, that he will keep trying, etc.

At times a supervisor may see the necessity of discharging an employee, but the personnel department "advises" him not to do so. If in the future this particular employee's performance leads to additional difficulties within the department, the supervisor is apt to shrug off his responsibility by merely saying that he wanted to fire the person a long time back, but that the personnel man "advised" him not to do so. The supervisor is thus disclaiming all responsibility for this particular employee, and all of this leads to untenable conditions within a department. It is up to the supervisor to make managerial decisions and to take the responsibility for them, regardless of the difficulty or risks involved. He is the only boss in his department.

As was stated in the beginning of Chapter 13, all of the above remarks refer to an organizational arrangement where the personnel director is attached to the organization in what is strictly a staff position. However, there are a number of health care institutions where the chief administrator has decided that all discharges have to be approved by the director of personnel. The top administrator has the authority to make such a provision and in this instance he has conferred upon the personnel director what is known as functional staff authority as discussed in Chapter 8. In other words, he wants the director of personnel to make the final decision as to whether or not an employee who has been working in the hospital longer than the probationary period of three months or so should be fired. The administrator is removing this part of the supervisor's authority and conferring it upon the director of personnel.

There must be strong reasons behind such a decision, since it clearly runs counter to the principle of unity of command and weakens the authority of the supervisor's position. The chief administrator may have done this in order to protect the hospital from excessive unemployment compensation claims which result from too many firings. Or the decision may have been based on the administrator's desire to comply with all possible fair employment practices and regulations so as not to expose the hospital to embarrassing situations.

There may be other reasons as to why an administrator may want to delegate this final authority to the director of personnel. In such situations it is desirable for the personnel director to disseminate as much information as possible to all first line supervisors. For example he should inform supervisors as to how unemployment compensation claims affect the over-all wage bill of the hospital. Also, he should familiarize them with the latest government provisions regarding fair employment practices. The various possibilities of engaging in conscious or unconscious discriminatory practices should be brought to the attention of the supervisors. The chief administrator should explain how important documentation is and he should urge the line supervisors to keep meaningful records which they and the hospital can refer to in case of need. If the supervisor is familiar with this type of thinking, it is doubtful that he will discharge an employee unless he has considered all the possible ramifications. Under these circumstances it is likely that the director of personnel will go along with a proposed discharge, since the supervisor has a well documented and substantiated case which can become a valid defense. It is desirable, therefore, that the director of personnel who has been given the final authority on discharges will use this authority with much discretion and in a manner of "consultation" with the various supervisors and not use it as if he were the "supreme power."

THE SUPERVISOR'S STAFFING FUNCTION

The staffing function is a continuous activity for the supervisor. It is not something which is required only when the department is first established. As a matter of fact, it is much more realistic and more typical to think of staffing as a situation where a supervisor is put in charge of an existing department with a certain number of employees already in it. Although there is a nucleus of employees to start with, it is likely that before too long changes in personnel will take place. Since every supervisor is dependent upon his employees for the operating results of the department, it is his responsibility to make certain that there is a supply of well-trained employees to fill the various positions.

Determining the Need

In order to make certain that the department can perform the jobs required of it, the supervisor must determine both the number and kind of employees who will be needed for his department. If the supervisor has set up the structure of the department, he has tentatively designed an organizational structure where the functions and jobs are shown in their proper relationships. If the supervisor takes over an existing department, he should orient himself by drawing a picture of the existing jobs and functions within his department. For example, the supervisor of the maintenance department may find that he has a group of painters, a group of electricians, carpenters, and other skilled *persons* within his department. After taking this inventory of personnel, he should determine how many skilled *positions* there are or should be within his department. The working relationships between these positions should be examined and defined by the supervisor. After determining the needs of his department, the supervisor may have to adjust the ideal setup to existing necessities. Or he may have to combine several positions into one if there is not enough work for one employee. It is only by studying the organizational setup of the department that the supervisor can determine what employees are needed to perform what jobs.

Job Description

In order to fill the various positions with appropriate employees, it is necessary to match the available jobs in the department with the credentials of prospective employees. This can only be done with help of job descriptions (Figures 13-1 and 13-2; see also the examples cited in the Appendix at the end of the book). The job description tells exactly what duties and responsibilities are contained within a particular job. It describes the content of the job by listing as completely as possible every duty and responsibility involved. In many instances the supervisor will find a set of job descriptions available to him. If none are available, he will find the personnel director to be of great help in establishing a set of job descriptions. But no one is better equipped to describe the content of a job than the supervisor himself. It is the supervisor who is responsible for the accomplishment of the tasks of the department, and he more than anyone else knows or should know the content of each position. Although the final form of the job description may be prepared in the personnel office, it is the supervisor who determines its specific content.

Only by describing the job requirements in great detail is it possible to ascertain the skills which are necessary in order to perform the job satisfactorily. Even if the position is one that is already in operation, it is still advisable to follow this procedure of determining the major duties and responsibilities. After this has been done it is advisable to compare this list with the current job description and

FIGURE 13-1 *
Job Description

November 11, 1972
(New)

JOB TITLE: Supervisor, Pharmacy Manufacturing
DEPARTMENT: Pharmacy
JOB CODE NO: 022   JOB GRADE: 18

JOB SUMMARY

Under the direct supervision of the Chief Pharmacist, supervises Pharmacist Technicians and Aides in manufacturing area of Pharmacy. Assists in directing Pharmacy policies and procedures in accordance with established policies of department and Hospital. Implements decisions of Administration pertaining to the Pharmacy. Manufactures and dispenses medicines and preparations according to formulas developed by department and utilized in the institution. Prepares and sterilizes injectible medication manufactured in Hospital, and also manufactures pharmaceuticals. Performs related duties as required.

OPERATIONAL GUIDELINES

1. Responsible for the preparation and sterilization of injectible medication, including irrigation solutions, manufactured in Hospital.
2. Supervises the manufacture of pharmaceuticals, dispensing of drugs, chemicals, and pharmaceutical preparations.
3. Supervises the filling and labeling of all drug containers issued to services.
4. Maintains a perpetual inventory of injectible medications, irrigation solutions, and manufactured pharmaceuticals as well as which drugs, chemicals, and pharmaceutical preparations have been dispensed.
5. Maintains file of specifications for purchase of chemicals.
6. Establishes and maintains, in cooperation with Accounting Department, a system of records and bookkeeping in accordance with policies of Hospital for charges to patients, and control over requisitioning and dispensing of drugs and pharmaceutical supplies.
7. Plans, organizes, and directs Pharmacy policies and procedures in accordance with established policies of Hospital.
8. Must be accurate in use of chemical and pharmaceutical equipment for compounding and dispensing drugs and medicines.
9. Must be accurate in accounting for, diluting, and handling of alcohol.

QUALIFICATIONS

1. Must have completed four year course in an accredited college leading to a degree of Bachelor of Science.
2. One year previous experience in a Pharmacy desirable. On-the-job orientation can be accomplished.
3. Good physical and mental health.
4. Must be willing to work with realization that errors may have serious consequences to patients.
5. Must be able to give undivided attention to details over extended periods of time.
6. Must have a memory for details and be alert to detect errors in compounding.
7. Must be able to cooperate with other employees and have the ability to supervise subordinate workers.
8. Must be able to plan operation and work schedule of department.
9. Follows standard formulas, but makes frequent decisions in a variety of technical matters.
10. Must be familiar with professional and commercial phases of pharmacy and have the ability to utilize all necessary reference books and textbooks related to medicine and pharmacy.
11. Must know pharmacy and chemical technique.

This description is for illustrative purposes only.

FIGURE 13-2 *

Job Description

July 19, 1972
(New)

JOB TITLE: Clinical Specialist
DEPARTMENT: Nursing Service
JOB CODE NO: 012   JOB GRADE: 21

JOB SUMMARY

Is directly responsible to the Associate Director of Nursing Service. Submits monthly activity reports. With the general support of an Associate Director of Nursing Service, the Clinical Specialist plans for, implements, and evaluates the care of a specific group of patients and their families. Responsible for developing and improving techniques and standards of patient care in relation to both physical and psychological needs. Functions as an independent nurse practitioner and makes competent nursing decisions as related to patient care management based on clinical judgment. Acts as consultant to other Clinical Specialists and to nursing staff needing assistance.

OPERATIONAL GUIDELINES

The Clinical Specialist's primary function is the management of nursing care for a specific group of patients and their families within a specialized field of nursing. To accomplish this will:

1. Carry a patient case load and direct nursing care. Not bound by geography and/or hours, sees patients in clinic and hospital.
2. Utilizes all resources to provide continuity in the patient's nursing care.
3. Makes nursing diagnosis, writes nursing orders, plans and implements intervention and evaluates nursing care. Makes final decision regarding nursing care in conjunction with the Head Nurse.
4. Available as a consultant to Staff Development, School of Nursing, and to Nursing Service Administration.
5. Consults with, and refers patients to other Clinical Specialists as the need arises.
6. Functions as a liaison person between the various disciplines involved in patient care.
7. Develops the competence of nursing personnel who co-work in providing patient care.
8. Functions as a team leader and/or team member to serve as a role model for teaching and guiding staff in planning, implementing, and evaluating patient care.
9. Alert to limitations or restraints on nursing practice and works toward their modification or removal.
10. Keeps informed about scientific progress in particular field and adopts sound and appropriate means for incorporating new findings into nursing practice whenever this is feasible.

QUALIFICATIONS

1. Graduate of an accedited school of professional nursing.
2. Master of Science in Nursing, preferably with a major in the defined clinical specialty.
3. Minimum of two years nursing experience, preferably with one year in the area of specialization.
4. Current licensure with the Missouri State Board of Nursing.

This description is for illustrative purposes only.

with what the employee is actually doing. The older job description may no longer fit the current content of the job, and should be corrected. The supervisor may find that some of the duties assigned to the job really do not belong to it. Even if the job in question is a new position, the supervisor should proceed along similar lines. He should decide what the duties and responsibilities of the job are, and with the help of the personnel department draw up a job description. Once the content of the job has been specified, the supervisor should then specify the knowledge, education, degrees, experience and the skills which are required of the prospective employee who applies for this particular job assignment.

In every job there are certain things which an employee must know before he can perform his job effectively. For example, it may be necessary for him to be able to read simple blueprints or, perhaps, the employee should be familiar with mathematics. To elaborate on this last instance, if a knowledge of mathematics is needed for a certain job, the specific type of mathematics required should be clearly defined. The word "mathematics" could imply knowledge far beyond a working knowledge of simple arithmetic, and a knowledge of simple arithmetic might be all that is required in the job. The more precisely defined the required job knowledge is, the easier it will be to select from among available applicants.

When stipulating the skills needed for a particular job, the supervisor should not ask for a higher degree of skill than is absolutely necessary. One way to avoid this is to check the requirements drawn up with the qualifications of employees who are doing the same or similar kinds of work. Such investigation may quickly reveal that for a certain job, a high school education is not necessary. The supervisor may discover that an older person without a high school diploma can perform this kind of work.

The supervisor should realize that by setting employment standards unrealistically high the task of finding the person to meet these specifications will become unnecessarily difficult. There is no need to specify a certain number of years of formal education and experience if all that is required is simple job know-how. This does not mean that the job specifications should ask for less than what is actually needed. However, it should specify the requirements realistically. If the requirements are set too high, people will be placed on the job who are over-qualified for the particular job. The likely result of this is that the particular employee may prove to be troublesome because he will find that his capacities are not completely utilized. By the same token, it is just as disasterous to ask for less than necessary. Once placed on the job, the employee may turn out to be unsatisfactory. Many of these difficulties can be avoided if the supervisor analyzes the job content diligently and specifies the job knowledge and the job skills required in a realistic manner.

The personnel department will prove to be of great help in drawing up these job descriptions. But the supervisor should be cautioned not to turn over the job of doing this to the personnel man. The content must definitely be specified by the supervisor and by no one else. Once these job descriptions have been drafted, the supervisor should consult with some of the people who are holding these jobs, so as to compare the job descriptions with the actual positions in question. Once all difficulties have been ironed out, these job descriptions are maintained in the personnel department and, also, in the supervisor's file. Whenever the supervisor needs to fill a certain job, he informs the personnel department that such and such a job is open and the personnel man will try to recruit suitable applicants to fill this job. The personnel man can quickly screen out those applicants who are obviously unfit because they do not have the knowledge or necessary skills or cannot fulfill any of the other requirements. But all of those who seem to fulfill the requirements will be referred to the supervisor for his acceptance or rejection.

Since job descriptions should be kept up to date, the supervisor must review the contents of the job from time to time. Without regular reviews there is a danger that they may become incorrect because of changing requirements, education and advances in technology. The supervisor must continually audit the job descriptions in his department. Many activities in the health care field change considerably through new technology, scientific advances and sometimes due to the creative efforts of the person occupying a position. The extent and character of change must be determined so that accurate information is contained in the job description. This is necessary because the job description is constantly referred to when the personnel department recruits candidates, when the supervisor hires new employees, when he appraises their performance and when he attempts to establish an equitable wage pattern within his department.

How Many to Hire

Normally, the supervisor is not confronted with the situation where a great number of employees have to be hired at the same time. Such a situation could exist when a new department is created and the supervisor has to staff it completely from scratch. It is more typical that the question of hiring an employee will occur only occasionally. Of course, there are some supervisors who continuously ask for additional employees in order to get a job done. In most of these cases their problems are not solved even if they get more help. As a matter of fact, the situation may become worse; and instead of reducing the supervisor's problems they are actually increased.

Normally, a supervisor will need to hire a new worker when one of his employees leaves the department either due to voluntarily quitting or to dismissal or to some other reason. In such instances there is little doubt that the job must be filled. Occasionally, changes in the technical nature of the work take place and manual labor may be replaced by machinery or sophisticated instruments. In such a case a replacement may not be needed. But normally, a new employee has to be hired to replace the one who left.

There are other situations when additional employees have to be added. For example, when departmental activities have been enlarged, or when new duties are to be undertaken and no one within the department possesses the required job knowledge and skill, the supervisor has to go out into the open market and recruit employees. Sometimes a supervisor is inclined to ask for additional help if his work load is increased, or if he finds himself under added pressure. But before he requires additional employees under those conditions, he should make certain that the persons currently within the department are fully utilized and that additional people are absolutely necessary.

If there are vacancies within the department the supervisor should inform the personnel department, and the personnel manager in turn should see to it that a number of suitable candidates for the jobs are made available. The personnel department accomplishes this task by consulting the various job descriptions. Those applicants who are obviously undesirable and unfit for the position in question can quickly be screened out. Those who seem to be generally acceptable and fulfill the required knowledge and skills should be passed on to the supervisor. The actual hiring decision is not to be made in the personnel office; it is to be made by the supervisor in whose department the employee is to work. Although the supervisor may feel that this is not necessary in filling an unskilled job, he should not relinquish his prerogative and duty to hire the people who are to work in his department. It does not matter if it is a nonskilled, skilled or semiskilled job which is to be filled. It is up to the supervisor to hire the employee. Since all applicants are prescreened by the personnel office, the supervisor knows that all of those who are sent to him possess the minimum qualifications which are prescribed for the job. It is the supervisor's job to pick out the one who will probably fill the job best. This is not an easy task, but as time goes on the supervisor will gain more and more experience and it will become easier for him to make the right decision. All of this will be discussed in the following chapter.

SUMMARY

Staffing is one of the managerial functions every supervisor has to perform. It means to hire, train, evaluate, promote, discipline and appropriately compensate the employees of his department. All of this is the supervisor's line function. In fulfilling this duty he is significantly aided by the services of the personnel department. In most enterprises the personnel department is attached to the organization in a staff capacity and its purpose is to counsel, advise, and service all other departments of the enterprise. In its eagerness to be of service to the line manager, the personnel department may be inclined to take over line functions such as hiring, disciplining, setting wages, and so on. The supervisor must caution himself not to capitulate any of his line functions to the personnel department although at times it might seem expedient to let them handle the "dirty" problems.

Before the manager can undertake the staffing function he must clarify the number and kinds of employees needed in the department. The organizational chart combined with job descriptions will specify the kinds of workers necessary to fill the various jobs. In addition to this, the supervisor must take into consideration the amount of work to be performed and the positions allocated in the budget. In all of this he may call on the help of the personnel department. But it is his function to select and hire *all* the employees within his department.

CHAPTER 14

Conducting the Employment Interview

After all of the preliminary work has been performed by the personnel department, it is the supervisor's job to see the applicants, talk to them, and to select the one who will best fill the job which is vacant. This is a decisive step for the employee and for the supervisor. This is the moment when the supervisor must match the applicant's capability with the demands the job makes, with the authority and responsibility inherent in the position, with the strain of the working conditions, and the rewards and satisfactions it offers. The personal interview between supervisor and applicant is an essential part of the selection process. It is not an easy task to make an appropriate appraisal of someone's potential during a brief interview. Interviewing is much more than a technique, it is an art which can and must be developed by every supervisor. It can be acquired better by practice than merely by reading articles on it.

INTERVIEWS

Over a period of years the supervisor will learn that there are several kinds of interviews. There are pre-employment interviews between the supervisor and prospective employees, there are discussions when employees are fired, and there are counseling sessions during which the abilities and deficiencies of an employee are discussed. In addition, there are interviews when an employee voluntarily leaves his job, as well as when employees want to discuss complaints, grievances, and any other problem situations. Generally speaking, all of these can be grouped into two different kinds of interviews, directive and nondirective. Throughout our discussion we will separate these two approaches, but it should be noted that there are some interviews which have some aspects of both categories. For example, the appraisal interview is to a large extent a directive interview. But it may happen that the discussion may take on some aspects of a nondirective, counseling interview.

Directive Interviews

Normally, a directive interview is a discussion where the interviewer knows beforehand what particular facts will be discussed, and what the goals, objectives and limits of the discussion are. The interviewer will try to get the necessary information by encouraging the interviewee to volunteer as much as possible, and, if need be, by asking the interviewee direct questions. The employment interview where the supervisor selects one applicant over the other is an example of a directive interview.

Nondirective Interviews

Although we will be primarily concerned with the directive interview, it is advisable to call the supervisor's attention to what it means to conduct a nondirective or counseling interview. This kind of interview is usually applied to problem situations where the supervisor is eager to learn what the interviewee thinks and feels. The nondirective or counseling interview is employed in problem situations such as complaints and grievances, or it may take the form of an exit interview when the employee voluntarily leaves the job. Affording your subordinates the opportunity of counseling interviews is a vital aspect of good supervision.

The principal function of the nondirective interview is to give the supervisor a clue as to what the interviewee really thinks and feels and what lies at the root of a particular problem. In addition, it serves to give the interviewee a feeling of relief, and it helps the subordinate develop greates insight into his own problems, often finding his own solutions while "thinking out loud." There are many sources of frustration within and without the working environment and unless frustration is relieved it may lead to all kinds of undesirable responses.

The ground rule is to let the interviewee say whatever he wants to say and to encourage him to freely express feelings and attitudes. To carry on a nondirective interview is more difficult than to carry on a directive interview. It demands the concentrated and continuous attention of the supervisor. The supervisor must exert self-control and hide his own ideas and emotions during the interview. The supervisor should not express approval or disapproval even though the employee may request it of him. This may prove exasperating, but it is essential. In such a nondirective counseling interview the employee must feel free, perhaps for the first time in his life, to express how he feels about everything. The fact that the troubled employee can pour out his troubles has therapeutic value. In all likelihood as soon as he has expressed all his negative feelings, he may start to find some favorable aspects of the very same things which he has been criticizing. When the employee is encouraged to verbalize his problems, he may gain a greater insight into them. In fact, he may come up with some kind of answer or some course of action which he plans to take to solve his difficulties. It is essential that the employee is permitted to work through his difficulties himself without being interrupted and without being advised by the counselor regarding the best course of action. It should come from the employee.

The supervisor should exercise great care not to give advice or to let himself become burdened with the task of running the subordinate's personal life. Most of the time the interviewee wants a sympathetic and emphatic *listener* and not an advisor. The average supervisor is not equipped to do counseling and it is not a part of his job. If need be, he can help the subordinate by referring him to trained specialists. This may be necessary when sensitive areas and deep-seated personality problems are involved.

At first the nondirective counseling interview is difficult to conduct, but as time goes on a good supervisor will learn to exercise self-control, and by concentrated listening to grasp the feelings of the employee. The counseling interviews can often be very time-consuming. Although the supervisor is under many pressures and may not have much time for listening, he should make the time for such interviews. He will find out that by listening his relationships with his subordinates will be better and he probaby will have fewer personnel problems to cope with. He must encourage his subordinates to come to him and show that he is always willing to hear them out.

A common purpose of both directive and nondirective interviews is to promote mutual understanding and confidence. It is an experience in human relations which will permit the interviewer and the interviewee to obtain greater understanding. The following discussion will be primarily concerned with the directive employment interview, where the supervisor is interested in getting the necessary information from the interviewee by letting him volunteer as much as possible and by asking the interviewee direct questions.

Preparing For the Directive Employment Interview

Since the purpose of the directive employment interview is to collect facts and to come to a decision, the supervisor should prepare for it as thoroughly as possible. First, it is essential that the supervisor acquaint himself with the available background information. By studying all the information that has been assembled by the personnel director the supervisor can sketch a general impression of the interviewee in advance. The application blank itself supplies a number of facts such as the applicant's age, schooling, previous experience and other relevant data. While studying the application blank the supervisor should keep in mind the job for which the applicant is going to be interviewed. If some questions arise while studying the application blank, the supervisor should write them down so that he will not forget to ask about them. There may be some questions concerning results of previous tests given by the personnel department, and any questions in this area should be clarified by the supervisor before the interview takes place.

Since the purpose of the employment interview is to gather information in order to make a hiring decision, the supervisor should prepare a schedule or a plan for the interview. The interviewer should jot down all the important items about which he has no information. He also should write down all those points about which he would like to have further clarification. Once he has written all of these key points down, he is not likely to forget to ask the interviewee about them. It is conceivable that during the interview the supervisor may be interrupted, and he might dismiss the applicant before he has had a chance to ask about those points about which he still lacks some information. Writing them down beforehand will prevent such an occurrence. Having thought out the various questions in advance, the supervisor can devote much of his attention to listening and observing the applicant. A well prepared plan for the employment interview is well worth the time spent on it.

In addition to getting background information and making out a plan for the interview, the supervisor should be concerned with the proper setting for conducting the interview. Privacy and some degree of comfort are normal requirements for a good conversation. If a private room is not available, the supervisor should create an aura of semiprivacy by speaking to his applicants in a corner or in a place where other employees are not within hearing distance. That much privacy is a necessity. If it can be arranged he should take precautions so that he will not be interrupted during the interview by phone calls or other matters. This gives the interviewee additional assurance of how much importance the interviewer places on this interview.

Conducting the Interview

After having made preparations, the supervisor is ready to conduct the employment interview. The supervisor should make certain that he creates a leisurely atmosphere and that he puts the applicant at ease. The wise supervisor will think back about his own experience when he applied for a job and recall the stress and tension under which he found himself. After all, the applicant is meeting strange people who ask searching questions, and he is likely to be under considerable strain. It is the supervisor's duty to relieve this tension which is certain to be present in the applicant, and possibly, in the supervisor himself. He should create a feeling of leisure and put the applicant at ease by opening the interview with a brief, general conversation, possibly about the weather, the heavy city traffic, the World Series, or some other general topic of broad interest. Any general topic which does not refer to his eligibility for the job will be relaxing. The applicant may want to smoke a cigarette, and the supervisor may employ any other social gesture which may come to his mind. The feeling of leisure brought about by an informal opening of the interview will put the applicant at ease, and his tensions, stresses, and fears will diminish.

In addition to getting information from the applicant, the interviewer should see to it that the job seeker learns enough about the job to help him decide whether he is the right person for the position. The supervisor, therefore, should discuss with him the details of the job, such as, working conditions, wages, hours, vacations, who his immediate supervisor would be and how the job in question relates to other jobs in the department. The supervisor must describe the situation completely and honestly. The supervisor must caution himself against overselling the job by telling the applicant what is available for exceptional employees. If the applicant turns out to be an average worker this will lead to disappointments. In his eagerness to make the job look as attractive as possible, it is conceivable that the supervisor may state everything in terms better than they actually are.

After having outlined the job's details, the supervisor should ask the applicant what else he would like to know about the job. If the interviewee has no questions, the supervisor should proceed to question him in order to find out how well qualified he is. The supervisor will have some knowledge about his background from the application blank; but he will need to know exactly how qualified he is in relation to the specific job in question. By this time the applicant has probably gotten over much of his tension and nervousness, and he will be ready to answer questions freely. Most of this information will be obtained by the supervisor's direct questions. The interviewer should caution himself to put these questions in words which will be clear to the applicant. In other words, he should use terms which conform with the applicant's language, background, and experience. The interviewer should take care not to put questions in the form of leading questions which would suggest a specific answer. He should ask his questions in a slow and deliberate form, one at a time, in order not to confuse the applicant. The supervisor should never use trick questions as such procedure can only lead to antagonism.

All questions the supervisor asks should be pertinent and ones which are relevant to the work situation. This brings up the area of those questions which, although they are not directly related to the job itself, can become relevant to the work situation. It is helpful to know whether a married woman has young children and what arrangements she can make for them to be cared for. Problems of this nature, although only indirectly connected with the job, are relevant to the work situation, and therefore they are within the area of discussion. A supervisor will have to use good judgment and tact in this respect as the applicant may be very sensitive about some of the points to be discussed. By no means should the supervisor pry into personal affairs which are irrelevant and removed from the work situation, merely to satisfy his own curosity.

Recent developments of federal and especially state laws against discrimination have made the pre-employment interview more difficult. Some regulations clearly state that it is an improper pre-employment inquiry for a supervisor to inquire about marital or family status. If the supervisor has to comply with strict regulations frequently issued by Human Rights Commissions or similar state and federal agencies the interviewer will have to devise other means for obtaining the necessary information, and he may have to resort to questions such as: "Can you be away from home overnight if the job requires it?" or "Will your home responsibilities permit you to work unusual hours?"

Sizing-Up the Applicant

The chief problem in employment interviews which the supervisor faces is how to interpret the candidate's employment and personal history. It is impossible for a supervisor to completely eliminate all his preferences and prejudices. But he should take great care to avoid some of the more common pitfalls in interpreting the facts while sizing-up a job applicant.

One of the pitfalls is commonly known as the "halo" effect. This means basing the over-all impression of the applicant on only part of the total information and using this impression as a guide in rating all the other factors. This may work either favorably or unfavorably for the job seeker. In any event it is bad. It would be wrong for the supervisor to form an over-all opinion of the applicant on a single factor, for instance his ability to express himself fluently. If an applicant is articulate, there is no reason to automatically project a high rating for all his other qualifications. A glance at the employees in the department will remind the supervisor that he has some very successful employees whose verbal communications are rather poor. Another common pitfall is that of over-generalization. The interviewer must not assume that because an applicant behaves in a certain manner in one situation that he will automatically behave the same way in all other situations. There may be a special reason as to why he may answer a question in a rather evasive manner. It would be wrong to conclude from this evasiveness in answering one question that the applicant is underhanded and probably not trustworthy. People are apt to generalize quickly.

Another pitfall is that the supervisor will tend to judge the applicant by comparing him with current employees in the department. The supervisor may wonder how this applicant will get along with the other employees and with the supervisor himself. He may feel that any applicant who is considerably different from current employees is undesirable. As a matter of fact, this kind of thinking may do great harm to the organization as it will only lead to uniformity and there-after to mediocrity. This should not be interpreted to mean that the interviewer should make it his business to look for oddballs who obviously would not fit within the department. But just because a job applicant does not resemble exactly the other employees, there is no reason to conclude that he will not make a suitable employee.

Another hazard for the interviewer to avoid is that in his eager-ness to get the very best person for the job the supervisor may look for qualifications which exceed the requirements of the job. Although the applicant should be qualified to fulfill the requirements, there is no need to look for qualifications in excess of those required. As a matter of fact, an overqualified applicant would probably make a poor employee for a job.

The above are some of the more commonly known pitfalls in in-terpreting the facts brought out during an interview. The super-visor should make an all-out effort not to fall into these traps when assessing the qualifications of the applicant.

Concluding the Interview

At the conclusion of the employment interview the supervisor is likely to have the choice of one of three possible actions: to hire the applicant, to defer the decision until later, or to reject him. The appli-cant is eager to know which of these actions the supervisor is going to take and he is entitled to an answer. There is no particular prob-lem if the supervisor decides to hire this applicant. Under those con-ditions he will tell him when to report for work and may give him some additional instructions.

It is conceivable that the supervisor may consider it best to defer a decision until he has interviewed several other applicants for the same job. Under those circumstances it is necessary and appropriate for the supervisor to tell the interviewee this and to inform him that he will be notified later. Preferably the supervisor will give him a time limit within which the decision will be made. Such a situation occurs frequently; but it is not fair to use this tactic to dismiss the applicant in order to avoid telling him the truth. There are some su-pervisors who do this in order to avoid the unpleasant task of telling the applicant that he is not acceptable. Under such circumstances tell-ing the applicant that the supervisor is deferring action gives him false hopes, and while waiting for an answer he may not apply for another job and, consequently, let some other opportunities slip by. Of course it is unpleasant to tell an applicant that he is not suitable for the job. But if the supervisor has decided that he will not hire a cer-tain applicant, the applicant should be told by the supervisor in a clear but tactful way. Although it is much simpler to let the rejected appli-cant wait for a letter which never arrives the applicant is entitled to an honest answer. If he does not fulfill the requirements of the job, it is preferable to tell him the reason why. Some applicants may even use this criticism in a constructive way. If the supervisor does not want to go this far, the least he should do is to tell the applicant that he is not the right man for the job.

The supervisor should always bear in mind that the employment interview is an excellent opportunity to build a good reputation for the institution. The applicant knows that he is one of several candidates and that only one person can be selected. The only contact the applicant has with the organization is through the supervisor during the employment interview. Therefore, the supervisor should remember that the interview will leave either a good or a bad impression of the institution with the applicant. It is necessary, therefore, that an applicant leave the interview, regardless of its outcome, at least with the feeling that he has been courteously treated and that he has had a fair deal. Every supervisor should bear in mind that it is his managerial duty to build as much good will and good reputation for the health care center as possible, and that the employment interview presents one of the rare opportunities for him to do so.

It is advisable that the interviewer put down in writing the reasons he did not hire a certain applicant, and/or why he hired the one in preference to the others. It is essential to have documentation of this sort as the supervisor could not possibly remember the various reasons, and he may be questioned about his decision at some later time. A few notes on the back of the application, or even better, on a separate piece of paper to be attached to the application will serve the purpose.

Temporary Placement

It may sometimes happen that although the applicant is not the right man for a particular job, he would be suitable for another position for which there is no current opening. The supervisor might be tempted to hold this desirable employee by offering him temporary placement in any job which is available. The applicant should be informed about this prospect by the supervisor. It sometimes happens, however, that such temporary placement in an unsuitable job causes misunderstanding and disturbance within the department. It is usually strenuous for an employee to mark time on a job which he does not care to perform, while hoping for the proper job to open up. Normally, such strain causes dissatisfaction after a certain length of time, and this dissatisfaction is usually communicated to other employees within the work group. Therefore, generally speaking, interim placements are ill-advised and unsound.

SUMMARY

There are two ways of filling available job openings: to hire someone from the outside, or to promote someone from within the organization. In hiring from without, the supervisor is aided by the personnel department since it performs the services of recruiting and pre-selecting the most likely applicants. However, it is the supervisor's function and duty to appropriately interview the various candidates and to hire those who promise to be the best ones for the jobs which are open. In order to accomplish this it is necessary for the supervisor to acquire the skills needed to conduct an effective interview. The employment interview is primarily a directive interview, in contrast to the nondirective interview often encountered in the supervisor's daily work.

During the employment interview the supervisor tries to find out whether the applicant's capability matches the demands of the job. The purpose is to hire the person most suitable for the position open. In order to carry out a successful employment interview, the supervisor should familiarize himself with background information, he should prepare a list of points to be covered, and provide the proper setting. In addition to securing information from the applicant, the interviewer should discuss with him as many aspects of the job as possible. There will be a number of additional questions and answers before the interviewer is ready to size-up the situation and conclude the employment interview.

In addition to conducting directive interviews, the supervisor is often called upon to carry on nondirective, counseling interviews. This kind of interview usually covers problem situations and gives the employee the opportunity to freely express his feelings. There are many sources of frustration within and without the working environment which can easily lead to many kinds of undesirable responses. To give the subordinate the opportunity of a counseling interview is another vital duty of the supervisory position.

CHAPTER 15

Promotions, Transfers, and Appraisals

PROMOTION FROM WITHIN

No organization can rely completely on recruiting employees from the outside. Organizations depend heavily on promoting their own employees into better and more promising positions. The policy of promoting from within the organization is one of the most widely practiced personnel policies today. It is a policy which will help to achieve the organizational objective of being a good employer and a good place to work. The latter is undoubtedly one of the many goals of all health care centers.

The policy of promotion from within vs. recruitment from without is of considerable significance to the enterprise and to the individual employee. For the enterprise it insures a constant source of trained people for the better positions; for the employees it provides a powerful incentive to perform better. After an employee has worked for an enterprise for a period of time, much more is known about him than even the best potential candidate from outside the organization. Additional job satisfaction will result when the employee knows that with proper efforts he can work himself up to more interesting and more challenging work, higher pay, and more desirable working conditions. Most employees like to know that they can get ahead in the enterprise in which they are working. All of this provides strong motivation. There is little motivation for an employee to do a better job if he knows that the better and higher paying jobs are always reserved for outsiders.

Whenever Possible

The internal promotion policy should be applied whenever possible and feasible. However, there will be some occasions when strict adherence to internal promotion would do harm to the organization. For instance, if there are no qualified candidates for the better jobs, the internal promotion policy cannot be followed. If no one with the necessary skill is available, then someone from the outside has to be recruited for the position.

At times the injection of "new blood" into an organization may be very important as it will keep the members of the enterprise from becoming conformist and repetitious. Such a threat is important primarily in managerial jobs and less important in hourly paid jobs. Another reason the enterprise may have to recruit employees from the outside is when the organization cannot afford the expense of training and schooling current employees. A particular position may require a long period of expensive training and the hospital simply cannot afford this kind of upgrading program. Only large organizations can afford such expenses.

On the other hand, the supervisor should remember that not every employee wants to be promoted. There are some employees who are quite content with what they are doing and where they are within the enterprise. They prefer to remain with the employees whom they know and the responsibilities with which they are familiar. These employees should not be coerced into better positions by the supervisor.

The supervisor should also bear in mind that what he may consider a promotion may not seem like a promotion to the employee. A nurse may feel that a "promotion" to administrative work is a hardship and not an advancement. She may find the administrative activities less interesting than the professional duties, and she may be concerned about her professional future. The supervisor will have to provide promotional opportunities which do not entail compromises of professional feelings.

At times, the supervisor may be inclined to bypass someone for promotion because the promotion would cause the supervisor some extra work in replacing the promoted employee and training a new employee. He may fear that the productivity of the department will suffer. This, of course, is shortsighted since promotion from within is one of the prime motivators. Supervisors who are tempted to think this way should ask themselves where they would be today if their former superiors had had this attitude.

Basis of Promotion

In spite of the objections stated above, there are usually more applicants for promotions than there are openings within the organization. Because of this it is important for a supervisor to formulate a sound basis on which employees are to be promoted. Since promotions are considered an incentive for employees to do a better job, it would follow that the employee should be promoted who has the best record of quality, productivity, and skill. But in most situations it is difficult to objectively measure some employees' productivity, although a continuous effort in this respect is made by supervisors in the form of merit ratings and performance appraisals. (There will be further discussion of this later in this chapter.)

Length of Service

Since there are many factors beyond the control of an employee which may affect his productivity and performance, it would be unfair to base a promotion solely on these factors. Since it is difficult to find objective criteria which would eliminate favoritism and possible discrimination, it has been stated that the only objective criterion is length of service. Unions have put the greatest stress on seniority; and this sort of thinking is now regularly accepted even by those enterprises which do not deal with unions or where jobs are not covered by union agreements. Regardless of unions, managers have come to depend heavily on this concept of seniority as a basis for promotion. If management is committed to promotion based on length of service, it is likely that the initial selection procedure of a new employee will be a more careful one, and he will get as much training as possible in his various positions. Some managers feel that an employee's loyalty is expressed by his length of service and, consequently, this loyalty deserves the reward of promotion. Basing promotion on the length of service also assumes that the employee's ability increases with his service. Although this may be questionable, it is likely that with continued service his ability to perform is increasing.

Merit and Ability

Most unions have begun to recognize that length of service cannot be the only criterion for promotion. In most instances it is agreed that promotion should be based on seniority coupled with merit and ability. In all likelihood this is a provision which most union contracts incorporate. But then management will run into the difficulty of deciding what the trade-off should be between ability and seniority. In other words, how much more ability is necessary to make up for less seniority. Therefore, it frequently happens that even in those union contracts which require competence as a co-determinant for promotion, the only objective criterion which sooner or later wins out is the criterion of length of service.

Striking a Happy Medium

Good supervisory practice will attempt to draw a happy medium between the concepts of merit and ability on the one hand and the length of service on the other. When the supervisor selects from among the most capable subordinates he will no doubt choose the one with the longest service. Then again, the supervisor may decide that the employee who is more capable but has less seniority than another employee stands "head and shoulders" above the one with longer service. If this is not the case, then the one with more seniority will be promoted. Obviously, these decisions become increasingly difficult and it is easy to see why many supervisors have finally resolved the matter by making length of service the sole determinant of selection for promotion. The ideal solution, of course, is to combine both factors. It is on very rare occasions that a supervisor will choose a person with the greatest merit and ability from all eligible candidates without giving any weight to length of service.

Selection for promotion will also depend on the type of work involved, the demands of the position to be filled, the degree requirements prescribed by the accrediting association and many other factors. It is likely that increasingly more emphasis will be placed on merit and ability when the position to be filled is a demanding and sophisticated position on a higher level, whereas more weight can be given to seniority when it comes to promotion into a lower level position. Every organization must decide on the relative weight of these factors when deciding who is to be promoted.

TRANSFERS

Transferring an employee from one position to another within the hospital often results in placing an employee in a position where he will get greater job satisfaction. It is conceivable that a nurse's aide may consider a job as an aide in the operating room to be more prestigious than being an aide on the nursing floor. In reality the pay may be the same and one cannot speak of a promotion in the proper sense of the word. But to the aide such a transfer means greater job satisfaction and constitutes an achievement. It is necessary, therefore, that a health care institution have sound transfer policies and procedures so that those who desire a lateral transfer will be given the possibility of doing so. The personnel director together with the various line managers should design these policies and procedures and see to it that employees are prepared to make successful transfers.

It is probably best for the employment office to act as a clearance center for interdepartmental transfers. If the responsibility for interdepartmental transfers is given to the supervisor, the subordinate may be reluctant to ask him. Some supervisors may be understanding in these matters, while others may be resentful and not give their consent. In whatever procedures are instituted there must be provisions that the employee inform his immediate supervisor of his desire to transfer. It is only fair that the present supervisor should be familiar with what the employee intends to do. In case the immediate supervisor does not recommend the transfer, the employee should be able to appeal this decision to a higher line officer or possibly to the personnel director.

There must be provisions as to whether transfers are to be made only within departments or between departments. There must be a statement as to whether the employee carries his previous seniority credit with him or not, provisions as to the basis upon which the transfer decision will be made in cases where two or more persons desire transfer to the same job. For example, should length of service be the sole determinant or should capacity to handle the job be taken into consideration also. There are many additional aspects which good transfer policies and procedures must cover. But in any event there must be the opportunity for an employee to be transferred as this will provide more job satisfaction for him and will motivate him in much the same way as a promotion.

THE PERFORMANCE APPRAISAL SYSTEM

The appraisal of an employee's performance holds a key position in the supervisor's staffing function. It helps management identify those employees who have the potential to be promoted into better positions, it points to the need for further development and shows how effectively various subordinates contribute to departmental goals. Obviously, it is important for a supervisor to be in a position to objectively assess the quality of the performance of his employees in his department. Therefore, most organizations request that their supervisors periodically appraise and rate their employees.

The performance appraisal system serves a dual purpose. It is a guide for possible promotion and further development, and it provides a basis for merit increases. Appraisal is done with the help of a formalized system of evaluation, often also called a merit rating. The purpose of such a formal rating system is to translate into objective terms the performance, experience, and qualities of an employee and to compare these items with the requirements of the job. The appraisal system is designed to take into consideration such criteria as job knowledge, ability to carry through on assignments, judgment, attitude, cooperation, dependability, output, housekeeping, safety, and so on. Such a system of evaluation helps the supervisor to take all factors into account when considering merit increases or a promotion. It also gives him a rational basis for decision, since it reduces the chances for personal bias. Such a formal appraisal system forces the supervisor to observe and scrutinize the work of his subordinates not only from the point of view of how well the employee is performing his job, but also from the standpoint of what can be done to improve his performance. Since an employee's poor performance and his failure to improve may be due to the supervisor's own inadequate supervision, a formal appraisal system is bound to improve the supervisor's own supervisory qualities.

In addition to these reasons, a formal evaluation system serves another purpose. Every employee has the right to know how well he is doing and what he can do to improve his work performance. It can be assumed that most employees are eager to know what their supervisors think of their work. In some instances the employee's desire to know how he stands with his boss can be interpreted as his asking for reassurance about his future in the organization. In other instances this expressed desire can be interpreted in several other ways. For example, a subordinate may realize that he is doing a relatively poor job but hopes that his boss is not aware of it and the subordinate is anxious to be assured in this direction. On the other hand, another subordinate who knows that he is doing an outstanding job may wish to make certain that his boss is aware of it and this subordinate will want to receive more recognition.

The mere existence of regular appraisals is an important incentive to the employees of an organization. It is only too easy in a large complex organization for an employee to have the feeling that he and his contribution are forgotten and lost. With regular appraisals he has the assurance that there is the potential for improving himself in his position, and that he is not lost within the enterprise. It gives him the assurance that his supervisor and the entire organization care about him.

Therefore, the supervisor should appraise all the employees within his department on a routine basis — at least once a year. One year is normally considered a sufficiently long period of time, although if an employee has just started in a new and/or more responsible position, it is advisable to make an appraisal within six months. These periodic appraisals will assure the employee that whatever improvement he has made will be noticed, and that he will be rewarded for his progress. As time goes on, these periodic ratings and reviews will become an important determinant of an employee's morale. It reaffirms the supervisor's interest in him and in his continuous development and improvement.

Normally it is best for the immediate line supervisor to make the evaluation, since he is in the best position to judge the subordinate's performance. In some instances it may be necessary for the first line boss to call on the help of the next higher supervisor or the director of personnel. In some institutions the appraisal is made by a committee made up of the first line supervisor, his boss and possibly one or two other supervisors who are in a position to rate the employee. This has the advantage of eliminating any of the immediate supervisor's personal prejudices. On the other hand, this method is very time consuming. For all practical purposes, appraisal done by the immediate supervisor should suffice.

In summary, performance appraisals are beneficial in the following ways. They help management in decisions about compensation. They help in the area of the training and developmental needs of the employees. They provide an inventory of human resources suitable for promotions. They aid the supervisor since they show whether an employee is in the right job or not. They identify for him those employees who are going ahead and those who are not progressing satisfactorily. They show him whether or not he is succeeding in his job as a coach and teacher. As far as the employee is concerned, an appraisal program has many advantages. It tells him what quality of work he is doing and gives him a sense of being treated fairly and of not being overlooked. He knows what he can do in order to be promoted to a better job. It gives him an opportunity to complain and criticize; it gives him a chance to express his personal goals and ambitions. In this respect appraisals are motivational because they create a learning experience for subordinates that inspires them to improve. Performance appraisal consists of two distinct steps: first, the performance rating itself, and second, the evaluation interview which follows.

Performance Rating

In order to minimize and overcome the difficulties in appraising an employee, most enterprises find it advisable to use some kind of appraisal form. These appraisal forms are prepared by the personnel department often in conjunction with the supervisor's suggestions. Although there are innumerable types of appraisal forms available, most of them include factors which serve as criteria for objectively measuring job performance, intelligence, and personality traits. The following are some of the factors which are most frequently measured in appraisal forms: job knowledge, ability to carry out assignments, attitude, judgment, supervision required, conduct, cooperation, safety, housekeeping, adaptability, absenteeism, tardiness, personal appearance, and so on. For each of these factors the supervisor is supposed to select the degree of achievement attained by the employee. In some instances a point system is provided in order to arrive at a gross score. The form is usually of a "check the box" type and reasonably simple to fill out (see Figures 15-1 and 15-2).

In spite of the outward simplicity of these rating blanks, the supervisor will probably run into a number of difficulties. First of all, not all supervisors agree on what is meant by the terms good, excellent, or fair. It is advisable, therefore, that the form contain a descriptive sentence in addition to each of these adjectives, or in place of the adjective, and the supervisor can pick the one which most adequately describes the employee. For example, in rating the degree of emotional stability of a nurse, the appraiser may have the following choices: first, "unreliable in crises, goes to pieces easily and cannot take criticism"; second, "unrealistic, her/his emotions and moodiness periodically handicap her/his dealings, she/he personalizes issues"; third, "usually on an even keel, has mature approach to most situations"; fourth, "is realistic, generally maintains good behavior balance in handling situations"; fifth, "self-possessed in high degree, has outstanding ability to adjust to circumstances, no matter how difficult"; and so on.

FIGURE 15-1 *

JOB PERFORMANCE EVALUATION (Management and Professional Employes)

BARNES HOSPITAL
14067-3 — Pers 22
Rev. 6/70

NAME	EMPLOYE NUMBER	ACCOUNT NUMBER

1. To be completed in duplicate and attached to a Pers-8 at time of Periodic Review, Promotion, Demotion, Interdepartmental Transfer, etc.

2. Evaluate employe's performance since hire, last merit pay increase, promotion, transfer, etc., as applicable.

3. Check one block after each factor, decide the exact level of effectiveness (e.g., Average Contributor 74-83, decide which is most appropriate, 74, 75, or 76, etc.) then record under "Scoring Column".

4. To evaluate employes other than department heads and supervisors, complete first 7 factors only and divide the gross score by 7 to arrive at net rating score.

5. To evaluate department heads and supervisors (exempt employes), complete all 10 factors (front & back of form). Divide the gross score by 10 to arrive at net rating. Rounding to the nearest decimal may be necessary.

6. On the other side, "Suggestions for Improvement" section to be completed as applicable in each individual employe case. Use "Remarks" section to justify extremely high or low rating or to cover any factor not listed.

NO.	FACTOR AND DESCRIPTION	Borderline Contributor 50-62	Below Avg. Contributor 63-73	Average Contributor 74-83	Above Avg. Contributor 84-92	Outstanding Contributor 93-100	Scoring Column
1	**QUALITY:** Work meets or exceeds established standards for thoroughness, care, and lack of mistakes. Decisions when made, are sound and based on all available facts. Performs work within framework of existing hospital policies and procedures, and supervisor's instructions.						
2	**QUANTITY:** Personally produces a large volume of work. Rate of progress on assignments meets or exceeds expected progress. Meets assigned deadlines.						
3	**KNOWLEDGE:** Knows job well. Has an excellent understanding of all aspects of the position, and its proper relationship to other operations. Understands hospital policies and procedures relating to his work. Actively keeps informed of current developments in his own and related fields (where applicable).						
4	**DEPENDABILITY:** Is always on the job; seldom absent or tardy. Makes efficient use of working time while on the job.						
5	**INITIATIVE:** A self-starter; requires little supervision in completing routine duties or special assignments. Assumes responsibility when orders are lacking. Consistently seeks to bring about improvements. Sees problems and recommends solutions rather than requesting directions on how to proceed (where applicable). Follows through on own, always doing a little more than required.						
6	**WORKING RELATIONSHIPS:** Maintains effective working relationships with people (including subordinates, where applicable) without compromising the responsibilities of the job.						
7	**ATTITUDE:** Maintains an excellent attitude toward the hospital and his job, his superiors, peers, subordinates, patients and visitors; is loyal and tactful; has a good disposition.						

FOR EMPLOYES OTHER THAN DEPARTMENT HEADS & SUPERVISORS, GROSS SCORE _____ ÷BY 7, EQUALS NET RATING _____	Gross Score:

*Reproduced with special permission from Barnes Hospital, St. Louis, Mo.

FIGURE 15-1 **(Continued)**

This Section is for Department Heads and Supervisors (Exempt Employes) Only

NO.	FACTOR AND DESCRIPTION	Borderline Contributor 50-62	Below Avg. Contributor 63-73	Average Contributor 74-83	Above Avg. Contriubtor 84-92	Outstanding Contributor 93-100	Scoring Column
8	**PRODUCTIVITY OF GROUP SUPERVISED:** Group Performance has met or exceeded established quantity, quality, and cost standards during the review period.						
9	**APPRAISAL:** Rates employe's performance realistically, thoughtfully, thoroughly in relation to their contributions and progress. Conducts job performance evaluations and appraisal interviews within established time limits and in a way which has a positive, constructive influence on employe's desire to improve performance.						
10	**DEVELOPMENT:** Effectively motivates subordinates to work to maximum of their abilities, and to prepare themselves for greater responsibility. Delegates to each in proportion to his ability to benefit from and handle duties successfully.						

(FOR DEPARTMENT HEADS AND SUPERVISORS)   **GROSS SCORE** _____ **÷ BY 10, EQUALS NET RATING** _____ .

Gross Score, this side _____

Plus Items 1 — 7 _____

TOTAL GROSS _____

SUGGESTIONS FOR IMPROVEMENT (refer to each factor by number):

REMARKS:

(CHECK ONE BLOCK ONLY)

☐ This employe is being recommended for a pay increase on the basis of this evaluation and such increase is reflected on the attached Pers-8 form.

☐ This employe is NOT being recommended for a pay increase due to _____

_____ . Please change

periodic review date to and resubmit for reevaluation on (date) _____ .

after comparing this employe's performance with that of others in similar or like positions of responsibility, I feel his to be an impartial evaluation of his/her performance.	I have read this evaluation of my job performance (both sides of this sheet). Should I not agree with this appraisal, I understand that I may make my own explanation on a separate sheet and have it become a part of this evaluation
_____ Date	Signature of Employe Date

gnature of Evaluator   Date

FIGURE 15-2 *

V- EMPLOYEE PERFORMANCE EVALUATION (NON-SUPERVISORY PERSONN

INSTRUCTIONS

1. Complete Section 1 - EMPLOYEE IDENTIFICATION, other side.

2. Evaluate employee's performance since hire, last merit pay increase, or promotion, etc. as applicable.

3. Disregard your own personal stereotyped feelings, judge this employee on the factors listed below.

4. Try to remember specific instances that are typical of employee's work and behavior.

5. Using supportable, careful judgment, check the ONE BLOCK after each factor that best describes this employee.

6. Check ONE BLOCK only AFTER each factor and total the points near the bottom of page.

7. Use "REMARKS" section below to justify extreme high or low rating, and also to cover any factor not listed below.

REASON FOR EVALUATION ☐ Periodic Review ☐ Promotion ☐ Merit Pay Increase ☐ Transfer

☐ Other (Specify)_____

FACTOR	POINT RANGE				
1 **QUANTITY OF WORK** (WORK OUTPUT)	**2 POINTS** Slow - output is seldom in required amount.	**6 POINTS** Occasionally turns out more than required amount.	**4 POINTS** Turns out required amount but never more.	**10 POINTS** Exceptionally fast; high output.	**8 POINTS** Usually turns out more than expected.
2 **QUALITY OF WORK**	**8 POINTS** Errors rare.	**4 POINTS** Just gets by.	**10 POINTS** Exceptionally high quality.	**2 POINTS** Careless.	**6 POINTS** Does a good job.
3 **DEPENDABILITY**	**5 POINTS** Always dependable; no checking required.	**4 POINTS** Very little checking needed.	**1 POINT** Continual checking and followup required.	**3 POINTS** Follows instructions satisfactorily with some checking required.	**2 POINTS** Frequent checking required.
4 **COOPERATIVE ATTITUDE**	**8 POINTS** Cooperative.	**2 POINTS** Highly uncooperative; argumentative.	**10 POINTS** Gets along exceptionally well; a good team member.	**6 POINTS** Gives satisfactory though limited cooperation.	**4 POINTS** Passive resistance.
5 **UNAUTHORIZED ABSENTEEISM AND TARDINESS**	**1 POINT** Excessively absent; hardly ever on time.	**3 POINTS** Occasionally absent and generally on time.	**2 POINTS** Absent more than necessary and/or frequently late.	**5 POINTS** Rarely absent- Excellent punctuality record.	**4 POINTS** Rarely absent and/or occasionally tardy.
6 **PERSONAL APPEARANCE**	**3 POINTS** Average	**1 POINT** Unsatisfactory	**4 POINTS** Above average	**2 POINTS** Below average	**5 POINTS** Excellent

Improvement suggested as follows:_____

_____

REMARKS _____

_____

_____

☐ EMPLOYEE STATES ADDRESS SHOWN UNDER SECTION II IS CORRECT; OTHERWISE, I HAVE CORRECTED IT UNDER SECTION III, OTHER SIDE.

TOTAL POINTS ➡	
CLASSIFICATION	POINTS
Unsatisfactory	Up to 9
Borderline Acceptable	10 - 18
Average	19 - 27
Above average	28 - 36
Outstanding	37 - 45

(Check ONE BLOCK only)

☐ This employee is being recommended for a pay increase on basis of this evaluation and such increase is reflected on other side of sheet.

☐ Employee is NOT being recommended for a pay increase at this time due to _____

Please change periodic review date to _____ and resubmit for re-evaluation on _____ (Da

After careful consideration and comparing this employee's performance with that of other employees in similar or like jobs, I feel the above to be a fair and impartial evaluation of his/her performance. This employee has been advised of areas where improvement may be needed and how to go about making such improvement.

I have reviewed my performance evaluation above and have been advised by my evaluator how to go about making any improvements as may be suggested above.

Signature of Evaluator	Date	Signature of Department Head	Signature of Employee

*Reproduced with special permission from Barnes Hospital, St. Louis, Mo.

It is also common for one supervisor to be more severe than another in grading an employee. Some supervisors are afraid that they might antagonize their subordinates if they rate them low, thus making them less cooperative. A low rating for a subordinate may also reflect on the supervisor's own ability to encourage subordinates to improve themselves. The supervisor should also caution himself not to let the rating of one factor influence him in rating the other factors. If the supervisor feels that an employee is not good in one area he might tend to rate him low on most factors. One way to avoid this "halo" effect is to rate all the employees on a single factor before starting on the next factor. In other words, the supervisor only rates one factor of each employee at a time and then goes on to the next employee for the same factor, and so on. While filling out the form, the supervisor must be careful to exclude any personal bias he may have. As time goes on, the supervisor will hopefully improve his ability to fill out appraisal forms.

The appraisal should be made within the context of the employee's particular job. The supervisor's judgment must be based on the total performance of the employee. It would be unfair to appraise a subordinate on the basis of only one assignment which he had done particularly well or particularly poorly. The supervisor must caution himself not to let random impressions of an employee influence judgment which should be based on the employee's total record of performance, reliability, initative, skills, resourcefulness, and capability. In this way, the rating will be based on objective evidence and not on subjective evaluation. Therefore, the supervisor will do well to record and document certain specific incidents which he otherwise is likely to forget. This should not lead to a "little black book," but merely serve as a reminder for some unusual incidents — good and bad — when appraisal time comes around.

Although the results are by no means perfect, many human errors can be avoided and counteracted by top administration's continuous emphasis on training for those who do the appraising. In spite of all shortcomings, the above means are far more objective than any other form of evaluation.

The Evaluation Interview

The second step in the appraisal procedure, the evaluation interview, takes place when the immediate superior who has performed the evaluation sits down with his subordinate to discuss his performance. Many supervisors shy away from the idea of having to tell their subordinates how they stand in the department and what they should do to improve. They are afraid that this type of interview will lead to hostility and even greater misunderstanding.

Since evaluation interviews are not easy to conduct and, if they are poorly handled, can lead to considerable hostility and misunderstanding, it is essential for a supervisor to acquaint himself with the best possible way of carrying out such an interview. It is also essential for top administration to spend a great deal of effort in teaching supervisors how to carry them on, to impart to supervisors the necessary skills of directive and nondirective interviews, and to show that in the final analysis this is a part of every supervisor's coaching function. Although it would be better not to follow a formalized system, administration often suggests that supervisors follow a standardized outline. According to this outline, the supervisor should first state the purpose of the evaluation procedure and the interview. Next, the supervisor should go on to a discussion of the evaluation itself, first stating the subordinate's strong points and then his weak points. Next, there should be a general discussion giving the employee an opportunity to state his case and say what is on his mind. Another possible procedure is to let the subordinate appraise himself first. This gives him the opportunity to state his side of the story first; it is easier for him to criticize himself than to take criticism from the supervisor. Hopefully the interview will end with a discussion of what the subordinate can and wants to do about his deficiencies and what the supervisor will do for him in this connection. Although such suggested schemes will help some supervisors, it is better not to formalize this process. As the supervisor gains experience he will devise his own plan and it is likely that he will treat each subordinate in an individual manner.

Everything regarding general techniques of interviewing is applicable to the evaluation interview. But additional skills are necessary since the direction of evaluation interviews cannot be predicted. At times it may be very difficult for the supervisor to carry on this interview, especially if the subordinate shows hostility when the supervisor discusses some negative evaluations. Positive judgment can be communicated effectively, but it is difficult to communicate criticisms without generating resentment and defensiveness. It will take much practice and insight to acquire skill in handling this evaluation interview. Therefore, many administrators provide practice sessions and role playing experiences for supervisors to aid them in effectively carrying out appraisal interviews.

Some supervisors feel that there is no need for an evaluation interview because they are in daily contact with their employees and these supervisors claim that their door is open at all times. This, however, is not enough. The employee knows that he has been formally appraised, and it is understandable that he might be eager to have a first-hand report on how he made out. Also, he may have some things on his mind which he does not want to discuss in his everyday contacts with his supervisor.

The appraisal interview should be held shortly after the appraisal has been performed, and the supervisor should refresh his memory regarding his reasons for the opinions which he has expressed in the appraisal. At the outset the supervisor should state that the main purpose of the interview is to help the employee improve, for his own benefit and that of the enterprise. It is often suggested that the supervisor ask the employee to appraise his own performance. This will give the supervisor a chance to refer to the progress which the worker has made since the preceding counseling interview, compliment him on his achievements, and then go into the areas which need improvement. The formula of starting with praise, following it up with criticism, and ending the interview with another compliment is not necessarily the best method. As a matter of fact, good and bad may cancel each other out and the worker may forget about the criticism. An adult, mature employee is able to take deserved criticism when it is called for. By the same token, when he merits praise he should get it. It is not always possible to mix the two together.

Since the idea of being rated imposes some extra tensions and strains, a feeling of friendliness and the privacy of the interview is more important than probably at any other time. The supervisor should stress the fact that everybody in the same job in the department is rated according to the same standards, and that the particular worker has not been singled out for the special scrutiny. The supervisor should be in a position to document his rating by citing specific illustrations and actual instances of good and poor performance. The supervisor should be careful to relate the measured factors to the actual demands of the job. He must gear the rating to the present qualities of the employee's performance. This is particularly important if an employee is already doing good work and the supervisor is tempted to leave well enough alone. These are probably the very employees who are likely to make further progress, and to simply tell them to keep up the good work is not sufficient. These employees may not have major problems, but nevertheless they deserve thoughtful counseling. Such an employee is likely to continue to develop and the supervisor should be specific as far as future development plans are concerned. He must be familiar, therefore, with the opportunities available to the employee, requirements of the job, and the employee's qualifications. However, whenever discussing a subordinate's future, the supervisor should not make promises for promotion which he may not be able to keep.

Although we have assumed that every member of the department is eager to advance, this is not always the case. The supervisor will run into some subordinates who have no particular desire to advance any further. This sometimes happens with women employees who do not want the prospect of added responsibility. They feel that the increase in pay and status would demand too much of their time and energy which they would prefer to devote to their families.

The interview should also give the employee an opportunity to ask questions so that the supervisor can answer them fully. Any misunderstanding cleared up at this time may avoid future difficulty. The supervisor should also make it clear that there will be further performance ratings and interviews, that this is a regular procedure with the enterprise. The supervisor should always bear in mind that the purpose of the appraisal interview is to help the employee to see his shortcomings and to aid him in finding solutions to them. The real success of the interview lies in the employee's ability to see the need for his own improvement and to stimulate in him a desire to do so.

Since the performance interview is the most important part of the appraisal procedure, the supervisor should do all in his power to make certain that at its termination, the employee has a good objective view of his performance, the ways in which he can improve, and a desire to improve. Hopefully the employee will establish goals which are mutually satisfying to both the supervisor and the subordinate. A commitment on the part of the employee will provide some quantitative measurable goals against which future performance can be judged. At the end of the next period, both supervisor and subordinate will meet to evaluate how well the goals have been achieved and what the next objectives will be. This will give the subordinate a custom-made standard of evaluation. It provides him with a specified goal within a specified period. He will be so much more motivated, since the goal was a commitment on his part.

As a matter of formality it is customary to have the subordinate sign the evaluation form. But it should be made very clear that the employee's signature confirms merely the fact that the interview has taken place and that he in no way approves or disapproves of the statements contained in the evaluation. With this understanding the subordinate will sign. If however, he would like to state his views, no harm is done in letting him do so. The real purpose of the signature is that the supervisor's own boss can be certain that the evaluation interview has taken place. As stated above, many supervisors have mixed reactions about the evaluation interview. However since it is essential as feedback in the entire evaluation procedure, the administration must make certain that it takes place and the signature is the simplest way to ascertain this.

It takes great skill and practice for a supervisor to conduct a mutually satisfying evaluation interview. It will be necessary for him to adapt his approach to the individual employee's reaction during the interview. In reality it is a form of coaching.

PROPER COMPENSATION

Part of the supervisor's staffing function is to make certain that the employees of his department are properly compensated. There is no doubt that in most health care centers wage rates and schedules have been set by top administration and the supervisor's authority is severly limited and handicapped. Nevertheless, he should do the best he can under the circumstances to see to it that the employees in his department are compensated appropriately. It is every manager's job to offer the kind of compensation which will retain competent employees in his department, and, if necessary, attract good workers from the outside. Monetary rewards are an exceedingly important factor for most employees. Many employees are much more concerned about how their salaries compare to the earnings of others than they are about their absolute earnings. No doubt many of the wage rates and schedules have followed historical patterns and others are often accidental. For instance, the problem of personalities has frequently distorted certain wage rates. In the long run such a situation cannot be tolerated. It is the supervisor's duty to see to it that the wages paid in his department are properly aligned *internally* and *externally*. *Internal alignment* means that the jobs within his department are paid according to what they are worth. *External alignment* means that the wages offered for the work to be performed in his department compare favorably with the going rate within the community. If they do not, the supervisor knows that he will lose the most experienced workers he has, and that he will be unable to attract new ones from the outside.

Job Evaluation

In order to pay the various jobs within his department according to what they are worth, the supervisor should call on the help of the personnel department to conduct a job evaluation. In such a procedure the jobs are evaluated according to various factors and an appropriate wage rate can be devised based on the worth of each job. Based on the results of what the jobs are worth, an appropriate wage schedule can be instituted. Of course, there will be some questions about what to do with some exceptional cases, namely, those employees who are receiving either excessively high or exceedingly low salaries in relation to others. But once a plan has been designed, it is necessary to maintain it properly, so that no new inequities arise.

The job evaluation program is usually administered by a committee under the general guidance of the personnel department. It is a procedure with which the personnel department is acquainted, and if it has not been performed at a recent date for the entire hospital, the supervisor should request a job evaluation at least for his own department. Sometimes the help of an outside consultant is used.

Wage Survey

In order to determine whether or not the rates which the department offers are attractive to outsiders, it is advisable to request the personnel department to undertake what is commonly known as a wage and salary survey. A wage and salary survey involves collecting data on wages paid in the community for similar jobs in similar or related enterprises. In other words, it might be a wage and salary survey of all the hospitals and related health facilities of one local area. Very frequently such information is already available from a local hospital association and can be obtained easily. Then by comparing this information with his wage patterns, the supervisor can determine whether or not his wages are properly aligned externally.

A sound wage and salary pattern should always be of great concern to the administrator; it is a subject in which the supervisor has very little direct authority. However, the supervisor's awareness of inadequacies and inconsistencies will often cause the administrator to investigate. In most instances the supervisor himself will not have enough authority to make wage and salary adjustments except within the framework of the departmental wage scale. But he should definitely plead his case with top administration. However, in order to make an intelligent presentation, it is necessary for the supervisor to know the value of the various jobs within his department and the going rates within the community. As every supervisor knows, proper compensation of employees is a significant aspect of the employee's continuing satisfaction and motivation. Without a sound wage and salary pattern, it is almost impossible for a supervisor to recruit competent employees or to keep his subordinates motivated.

Most enterprises also provide fringe benefits for employees, such as, vacations with pay, retirement plans, insurance and health services, low cost meals, etc. In general, they are incentives to do a better job. Most of these additional benefits are established by the administrator as institution-wide measures; the supervisor has little to do with them other than to make sure that his subordinates understand how they operate and to be sure that each subordinate receives his fair share of these benefits.

SUMMARY

A second important source of employees for certain positions is the reservoir of employees who are currently with the institution. Promotion from within whenever possible is one of the most rewarding personnel policies any enterprise can practice. It is of great benefit to the enterprise and to the morale of the employees. Although it is difficult to clearly specify the various bases for promotion, it is normally acknowledged that a happy balance between ability and merit on the one side, and length of service on the other, should be used. However, in order to be able to clearly assess the ability and the merit of the employee, it is necessary that the supervisor remain continuously aware of the employee's achievements. In order to do this the supervisor must regularly appraise the performance of the employees of his department. An evaluation system consists of the process of rating the employee and the evaluation interview which regularly takes place thereafter. Although the appraisal interview between the supervisor and the employee may prove to be a difficult situation, the entire performance appraisal system is of no use, if this aspect is ignored or not carried out appropriately.

In addition to all these duties, the staffing function includes making certain that the employees of the department are properly compensated. Although much of this is out of the domain of the supervisor, it is his function to make certain that within his department there is good internal wage alignment, meaning that each job is paid in accordance with its worth and difficulties. To achieve this end, a job evaluation is necessary. In addition to good internal alignment between the various jobs, it is also essential that the enterprise have a sound external alignment. This means that the wages paid must be high enough to attract people from without the organization, and to prevent present employees from leaving for higher wages. In order to do this, it is essential to be familiar with current rates being paid in the community in similar occupations. Such information can be obtained by wage and salary surveys conducted by the personnel department.

PART SIX

Influencing

CHAPTER 16

Motivation

The influencing function is that managerial function by which the supervisor evokes action from others in order to accomplish organizational objectives. It is the process that management uses to achieve goal-directed action from subordinates and colleagues in the organization. In other words, it is a human resources function particularly concerned with behavioral responses.

The influencing function is also known as motivating, directing, and actuating. Regardless of the terminology, however, it is that managerial function which the supervisor exercises in order to get the best and most out of his subordinates and at the same time create a climate in which the subordinates find as much satisfaction of their various needs as possible. In the past, managers depended largely upon negative persuasion, disciplinary action, and a few incentive programs to influence their employees. The notion of organizational hierarchy dominated managerial thinking until the behavioral sciences brought about new understanding of human motivation and taught us better methods of influencing. Today every manager must be aware of the human activities of which he is an essential part and of the potential he has for influencing them. That is, he must understand some of the psychology involved in interpersonal relations.

As we have said before, it is the role of every manager, of every supervisor, to influence in order to get the work done through and with the help of his employees. Influencing is the managerial function which *initiates* action. Without it, nothing, or at best very little, is likely to be accomplished. Planning, organizing, and staffing can be considered preparatory managerial functions; the purpose of controlling is to find out whether or not the goals are being achieved. But the connecting and actuating link between these functions is the managerial function of influencing. This function includes the problems of motivation, the issuance of directives, instructions, assignments, and orders, as well as the guidance and overseeing of employees.

Moreover, the manager should consider his influencing function as a means not only for getting the work done and motivating, but also for developing his employees. The most effective way to achieve such development of employees is diligent coaching and teaching by their immediate superior. Thus, influencing is more than just a matter of giving orders or supervising the employees to make certain that they follow directives. Influencing means building an effective work force and inspiring each member of it to perform at his best. Influencing is the function of getting the employee to work in a large enterprise as effectively as possible and with the same amount of enthusiasm that he would display if he were working for himself, either in his own enterprise or at a hobby. Only by appropriately influencing and supervising the employee will the manager be able to instill in him this motivation to work energetically on his job and at the same time to find personal satisfaction.

Of course, influencing is the job of every manager whether he is the administrator of a health care facility, or the supervisor of one of its departments; whether he is the president of a company, or a regional sales manager. Every manager performs the influencing function regardless of his position. However, the amount of time and effort a manager spends in this function will vary, depending upon his level, the number of employees he has, and the other duties he is expected to perform. It is a fact that the supervisor of a department will spend most of his time influencing and supervising. He will spend much more time at this than the administrator of the hospital. Indeed, influencing is an ever present, continuous function of the supervisor that covers the day-to-day activities within his department.

Naturally, the supervisor's influencing function is interconnected with his other managerial functions. It is obvious that influencing is largely affected by the kind of employee whom the supervisor has selected while performing his staffing function. It is obvious that the plans that the supervisor had made and the organization which he has drawn up also have a bearing on how he performs his influencing function. The controlling function is likewise affected by influencing inasmuch as control often involves human problems. Clearly, influencing is a crucial function, the one which deals most intimately with the human being. Thus, in order to understand this function we must understand something about what makes the human being tick, what motivates him, and more basically what underlies his motivations.

THE NATURE OF HUMAN MOTIVATION

Every action of man is motivated by unsatisfied needs. These unsatisfied needs cause man to behave in a certain manner and to try to achieve certain goals in hopes of reducing the tensions which arise from needs that are unmet. A person eats because hunger creates the need for food. Someone else has a strong need for achievement and he strives for advancement within his field of work. In other words, there is a reason for everything that people do. People are always striving to attain something that has meaning to them in terms of their own particular needs. It is often observed that man never seems satisfied. He is continuously fulfilling needs. After the successful fulfillment of one need, he will start on another round of pursuits. Indeed, we can say that life is a process in which needs constantly arise and demand satisfaction.

The Hierarchy of Needs

However, we should not think that all needs are of the same order of importance. There are many different kinds of needs and some produce stronger motivation or demand more immediate satisfaction than others. This observation has been expressed by the noted psychologist Abraham Maslow in the form of a theory which has gained broad acceptance. Maslow has suggested an explanation of motivation based on a hierarchy of needs.* (See Figure 16-1.)

FIGURE 16-1

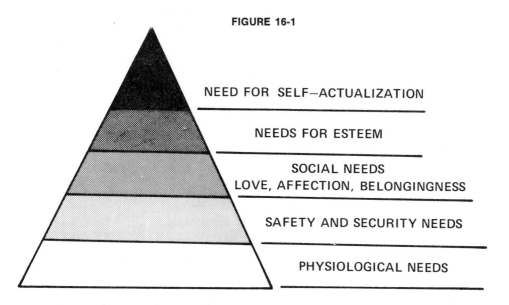

NEED FOR SELF—ACTUALIZATION

NEEDS FOR ESTEEM

SOCIAL NEEDS
LOVE, AFFECTION, BELONGINGNESS

SAFETY AND SECURITY NEEDS

PHYSIOLOGICAL NEEDS

Maslow's model contains five levels of needs which can be visualized as forming a pyramid. The lowest order of needs are the so-called *physiological needs*. These are the needs of a biological nature which everyone has for food, shelter, rest, recreation, and so on. Normally, the paycheck enables an individual to obtain the necessities

*Abraham H. Maslow, *Motivation and Personality,* 2nd ed. (New York: Harper & Row, 1970), Chapter 4.

and comforts of life that are vital to fulfilling these physiological needs.

When the physiological needs are reasonably satisfied, needs at the next higher level begin to dominate and motivate man. These are usually called *safety needs*. They are the needs we have for protection against danger and threat. Such needs are natural reactions which all of us have to insecurity. We all desire more control and protection over the uncertainties of life. In a work environment, these uncertainties would produce safety needs caused by fear of arbitrary management action, of loss of job, of favoritism, of discrimination, of unpredictable administration of policy, and so on. Most enterprises today offer various programs which are designed to satisfy and fulfill these safety or security needs. For example, most enterprises have medical and insurance plans, provisions for retirement benefits, provisions for unemployment compensation, seniority, etc.

Once man's physiological and safety or security needs are satisfied, his *social needs* become important motivators of his behavior. Social needs consist of the need for belonging, for association, for acceptance by fellow men, and for giving and receiving friendship and love. These social needs are often identical with the needs people have for a feeling of group identity, for being part of a group, for being accepted and respected by their peers. A supervisor must be aware of the existence of these needs and hopefully he will allow them to be fulfilled by the organization's informal groups. As we know, tightly knit, cohesive work groups will generally enable employees to gain greater on-the-job satisfaction and will produce a better climate for motivation. This is why the supervisor should look at the positive aspects and the strengths of informal groups. Often supervisors — incorrectly — go to great trouble in order to control and interfere with the natural "grouping" tendency of human beings. This is ill-advised. When man's social needs are thwarted and frustrated, he will behave in ways which are likely to hurt organizational objectives. The manager should always realize that these social needs are fulfilled to a large extent by informal groups and informal organization.

Above the social needs are man's egotistical needs for *esteem*, both self-esteem and esteem from others. Self-esteem includes the need for self-confidence, for independence, for achievement, for competence, for knowledge. These needs are often fulfilled by mastery over part of the environment — for instance, by knowing inside yourself that you can accomplish a certain task. But man also needs the esteem and recognition of others for his accomplishments. These needs relate to one's reputation, one's need for status, for recognition, for appreciation, for the deserved respect of one's colleagues. Many jobs in industrial settings offer very little opportunity for satisfaction of such needs. However, most positions in the health care field are more conducive to the achievement of these needs. Of course, it is desirable that both aspects of the need for esteem are fulfilled. Frequently, however, the esteem of self comes before esteem from others.

The highest level of needs is the need for *self-actualization, self-fulfillment,* or *self-realization.* These are the needs for realizing one's own potentialities, for continued self-development, for being creative in the broadest sense of the term. It has often been said that this is the need "to become what one is capable of becoming." Unlike the other four needs which probably will be satisfied, self-actualization is only seldom fully achieved. Conditions of modern life give very little opportunity to fulfill this need. Most employees are continuously struggling to satisfy the lower needs; they must divert most of their energy to satisfy them. Therefore, the need for self-fulfillment frequently remains dormant and unfulfilled.

The Relationship to Age

It is interesting to note that there seems to be a relation between the hierarchy of needs and age. Physiological and safety needs are paramount in the life of an infant. As a child grows up, love needs become important to him. When he reaches young adulthood needs for esteem seem to dominate the field. If he is successful in life, then he may move on to self-actualization later in life. However, such a step does not necessarily follow because pressing circumstances may arrest his progress at the esteem level or at lower levels. And, as we shall see later, this situation is often the basis of conflict betwen organizational and individual goals.

Levels of Aspiration

A person's level of aspiration is closely related to the hierarchy of needs. An individual's level of aspiration causes his goals to shift as various needs are satisfied. That is, once the needs on one level are satisfied there is a tendency for the individual to aspire to higher levels. Suppose an individual is highly motivated by his need for achievement and his attitudes and personality cause him to look for satisfaction of this need by working in a health care center. Such a person will not be satisfied for any length of time by a low level supervisory position. Once this position has been attained, he will strive for the next higher position, for instance, director of nursing services. After achieving the top position within this service, he may shift his objectives to higher positions within the over-all administration of the hospital, for instance, he may seek to become an associate administrator or even the chief administrator. Or he may shift his objectives to something outside the hospital, for instance, to governmental activities which present possibilities for the satisfaction of his achievement needs. This endless search for alternatives to satisfy increasing aspirations is an important aspect of human motivation. If an organization can provide an individual with a wider range of need satisfactions, his commitment to this organization will be greater.

Attitudes

As we have said, all human behavior is motivated by unsatisfied needs. These needs spring from causes which are deep within the person and which, together with other motives, attitudes, and behaviors, form the configuration usually called the personality. From this point of view, motivations that contribute to personality can be defined as a potential to act in order to satisfy those needs which are not met. The term *potential to act* implies that some motives are stronger than others and hence more likely to produce action. The strength of motivation is determined by the strength of a particular need, the probability that the act required to satisfy that need will be successful, and the rewards forthcoming. Obviously, an individual is more likely to act if the motive is stronger and if the probability for success is high and the reward is significant.

But another factor is also involved in producing human behavior or action. Motives do not stand alone. Closely related to them and significantly affecting their strength are *attitudes*. An attitude is the way an individual tends to interpret, understand, or define a situation or his relationship with others. Attitudes constitute one's feelings about something, an individual's likes and dislikes directed toward persons, things, situations, or a combination of all three. Attitudes are more than casual opinions since they are heavily charged with emotional overtones. Attitudes may include feelings as well as intellectual elements. They also include evaluations and value judgments. Attitudes differ in kind, they differ in strength, and in the extent to which they are open or hidden. Basically, they are revealed in two ways: either by the individual's expressed statements or by his behavior. An individual may say that he dislikes the hospital he works for or he may merely demonstrate this attitude by being absent an excessive amount.

Factors Determining Attitudes

There are in infinite number of factors which determine and influence an individual's attitudes. A major influence is a person's *biological* or *physiological makeup*. Such factors as sex, age, height, race, weight and physique are very important in determining the attitudes which contribute to over-all personality structure. In addition to this, many psychologists feel that the very early years of a person's life are crucial to his attitudinal development. Freudian psychologists, in particular, believe that early childhood is the most critical period of all in what a person actually becomes. This theory is often referred to as *childhood determinism*; it maintains that such factors as feeding patterns, training patterns, and home conditions in early childhood are the primary determinants of personality structure.

Another area which influences a person's attitudes and personality is his immediate *environment*. Factors such as education, employment, income, and many other experiences which confront an individual as he goes through life will influence what he is and what he eventually becomes. Furthermore, one should never forget that the *broader culture* of our society also influences a person's attitudes. In this country, we believe in such things as competition, reward for accomplishment, equal opportunities, and other values which are part of our democratic, capitalistic society. Individuals learn from their early years to strive for achievement, to think for themselves, to work hard, and that these are roads for success. All such cultural influences affect a person's attitudes and thus his behavior. Of course, there are an infinite number of other factors which also influence attitudes and personality. We have only touched on the more obvious ones.

Attitudes and Behavior

No matter what factors have caused their development, however, attitudes become deep seated attributes of the individual's makeup. They are learned and acquired through all life's experiences. As stated above, they do not have to be rational or logical. Attitudes tend to last for a long time. We hold firmly to our attitudes and resist forces which attempt to interfere with them. Attitudes can change, but they change very slowly. Attitudes do not exist only within individuals, but as we brought out in our discussion of informal organization, attitudes are also generated within groups. At that time, we pointed out that often individuals gladly accept as their own the attitudes of the group to which they belong.

As stated above, needs and motives do not stand alone as determinants of behavior. They are influenced by the underlying attitudes of a person. This is shown in Figure 16-2. Indeed, we can say that *attitudes will determine the individual route which the person takes for the satisfaction of his needs*. Although basically the same needs appear in every person, an individual's attitudes will vary greatly and will affect his own unique responses to his needs. In other words, attitudes help determine what motivates a person to take a certain action in order to fulfill a certain need. For example, many people may have a strong need for achievement. But differing attitudes will motivate one individual to seek fulfillment of need by working in a hospital, another by working in government, another by working in industry, and a fourth person may seek the fulfillment by teaching in a university.

FIGURE 16-2

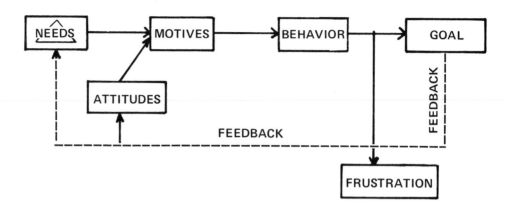

Motivation Versus Frustration

If the individual's chosen route results in goal accomplishment, he will find his need satisfied and his attitudes reinforced. In other words, accomplishment of the goal works as "feedback" to the individual to let him know that his needs are satisfied and his attitudes are reinforced. What happens, however, if the chosen course of action does not result in goal accomplishment? What happens when we cannot achieve what we would like to? What happens when we knock our heads against a wall which seems to hold us back?

Generally speaking, actions that do not succeed in obtaining goals result in blocked satisfactions and frustration. As shown in Figure 16-2, this would mean that feedback notifies the individual that his needs are not being fulfilled. In other words, there is conflict and frustration instead of need satisfaction. Basically, there are five ways in which people commonly resolve the problems of conflict and frustration. The best way would be problem-solving behavior, but there are also other methods such as resignation, detour behavior, retreat, or aggression.

Problem-solving behavior is usually the most desirable way of meeting frustration. It is advantageous if a person can look at his own personal problems objectively and base his decisions upon reasoned analysis of the situation. Unfortunately, many people are not capable of doing this and it is the supervisor's duty to help his employees learn problem-solving behavior. Suppose, for instance, that an LPN is eager to advance to a better position. However, all better positions demand the RN degree as a prerequisite to the job. Of course, the LPN is frustrated because she is beating her head against a wall. In this instance, reasoned analysis of the situation and a thorough discussion with her supervisor could encourage the LPN to go on to school and to obtain the RN degree which will enable her to move up within the hierarchy of nursing services. Such a decision would constitute intelligent problem-solving behavior.

Another way to solve a conflict situation is by *resignation*. Suppose the same LPN were to say to herself, "What else can I do? I have to stick it out." She seems resigned to her lot. She will keep on working for the hospital but may no longer consider herself a part of it. Once an employee has given up in the face of obstacles, it is difficult to build up her morale to the point where hospital and departmental goals are really important to her. Some employees simply stay on the job listlessly until they are able to retire. Such employees who have resigned themselves to their lot are usually passive and resistant to change. They are difficult for the supervisor to deal with because new ideas do not excite or stimulate them. Hopefully, the supervisor can help such subordinates use problem-solving methods of reasoned analysis and objective evaluation. If, however, the supervisor does not succeed in this respect, he may try to restimulate the employee to strive either for her old goals or toward some new and desirable goals. The supervisor knows that the result of resignation is usually inferior performance on the job, lowering of morale, and a climate which is not conducive to the best performance of the department.

A third way to solve a frustrating situation is to resort to *detour behavior*. Since the direct way of reaching the goal is barred, the employee will try to find another way to get there. Such detours, however, are often obscure and sometimes devious. For example, one kind of detour behavior is self-induced illness. Children learn early in life that being sick gives them an acceptable excuse for getting out of doing an unpleasant task. Similarly, employees will often have painful and real physical disorders in order to evade a conflict situation. Of course, some people can stand conflict and frustration better than others. But sooner or later the strain begins to tell and some sort of conflict resolution is necessary.

Leaving the field (retreat) is a fourth way to meet the problems of conflict and frustration. Most people at one time or another have looked at their jobs and have wished that they could quit right there and then. They may feel that they are not getting the satisfaction which they thought the position would bring, that no one realizes the difficulties involved in the job, that their supervisor does not appreciate all the things they are doing, and so on. Certainly, in most people's lives there are occasions when feelings of this sort are prevalent. And in many instances, an employee does quit his job and take another position, possibly even in another town. Whether this reaction to frustration is good or bad, however, will depend upon the major source of the conflict and frustration. If the major source is in the employee's personality and the conflict does not stem from the working situation, then, of course, leaving the field would not be the right answer. In other words, if the frustration is due to the person's own peculiar psychological makeup, then such a change in all likelihood will not bring about the desired result. If, however, the conflict is due to an unfavorable work situation in which the employee finds himself, then leaving the field, quitting, or even leaving the city may represent a real solution to the problem. Often it is difficult for the individual to determine whether or not this is the case. Of course, it is not always necessary to quit the job or move to another city in order to "leave the field." Leaving the field may show itself simply by "daydreaming," by spending a lot of time in the washroom, by a high rate of absenteeism, or by some other form of symbolic escape. Obviously, all of these forms of leaving the field will cause the supervisor additional problems.

Aggression is the fifth way in which people may meet the problem of conflict and frustration. By aggression we mean not only hostile behavior aimed at harming other people or things, but also merely the tendency to commit acts of aggression. This tendency may manifest itself in thoughts or words or even in feelings which have not as yet been put into words. The supervisor should always remember that frustration and aggression are closely tied together and that all aggressions stem from some kind of frustration. Of course, as we have said, some individuals can stand a larger amount of frustration than others and are not as easily moved into aggressive behavior. Moreover, many minor frustrations which could lead to aggressive behavior do not because we hold back and inhibit them. Obviously, the job of the supervisor is to see to it that frustration is minimized. He should try to anticipate the sources of frustration and attempt to eliminate them. If, however, he is not successful in doing this, then the best he can do is to see to it that the causes of frustration are not aggravated. Often patient listening will help to ease employee tensions and it may enable the subordinate to seek the real source of his frustration. Or a good counseling interview may also alleviate a frustrating situation.

Conflicts Between Individual and Organizational Goals

Although there are many causes of the frustration of which we have been speaking, a major cause arises from the fact that individual needs and goals often conflict rather than coincide with those of the organization, or to be more specific, with those of the department. Much has been written about the conflict between the individual who seeks activity and independence and the bureaucratic formalized organization which keeps the individual in a climate that stifles his natural desire for freedom and self-determination. The consequences of such a climate manifest themselves in high turnover, waste, lower productivity, slowdown, lack of innovative and creative behavior, non-acceptance of leadership, and so on. The most serious consequence of a bureaucratic organization, however, is that it blocks the individual from attaining satisfaction of his needs. In this day and age, administrators are becoming more aware of these consequences and of the necessity for an organization to provide a climate which will enable those who work within it to find personal satisfaction. As a matter of fact, the need for an appropriate organizational climate is increasing due to the rising expectations of employees. This is especially true in the health care field where we are confronted with an ever advancing and more sophisticated area of activity, with highly skilled and educated employees, to a large degree with professionals, who expect to fulfill a multitude of their needs right on the job. Since such employees tend to take high wages and appropriate fringe benefits for granted, it should be apparent that the key to long term motivation for them rests in the satisfaction of the higher level needs, that is, their social, esteem, and self-fulfillment needs. It is management's duty to develop an organizational climate which will produce effective motivation and satisfaction of these needs, thereby helping to resolve the conflict between individual and organizationl goals.

MOTIVATION STUDIES: SATISFIERS AND DISSATISFIERS

Extensive research has been carried on in order to demonstrate that many factors which management and supervisors have traditionally believed would motivate people serve primarily to satisfy or dissatisfy, rather than to really motivate them. For this reason, we should not always assume that motivation and satisfaction are one and the same. As stated again and again, each employee, whether he is a supervisor or merely a subordinate, hopes to satisfy his needs and reinforce his attitudes on the job. More specifically, it has been pointed out that these needs and attitudes give rise to expectations and the extent to which expectations are met on the job determine personal satisfaction and morale. It is therefore essential to examine the conditions that underly the realization or satisfaction of employee expectations and to compare these with the conditions that produce motivation.

Frederick Herzberg, a psychologist, has done a great deal of research on job satisfaction and has developed a number of conditions upon which satisfaction is based.* He measures satisfiers and dissatisfiers in terms of the frequency with which they appear and in terms of the duration of the period during which they produce either a marked improvement or a marked reduction in job satisfaction. The factors most frequently involved in events causing job dissatisfaction (*"dissatisfiers"*) are company policy and administration, supervision,

*Frederick Herzberg, "New Approaches in Management Organization and Job Design" *Industrial Medicine and Surgery* 45 (November, 1962): 477-481.

interpersonal relations, and working conditions. Where these kinds of factors are negative or lacking, they are considered to be dissatisfiers. But even when they are positive and appropriate, these factors do not tend to motivate people; rather they merely satisfy. When positive, they are "*satisfiers.*" This, however, does not mean that these factors are unimportant. They are essential but they are only a start in achieving a good organizational climate.

Herzberg's study further indicates that the most frequently mentioned factors in improved job satisfaction are achievement, recognition, work itself, responsibility, and advancement. These are the factors which, if present, truly motivate people. Hence, he calls them "*motivators.*" It is the opportunity for advancement, greater responsibility, the possibility of promotion, growth, achievement, and interesting work — which make a job challenging, meaningful, and really motivating to subordinates. Such factors are obviously associated with the higher level needs of people.

Herzberg's findings have important implications for the supervisor. Although management strives for good organizational "hygiene" through sound wage administration, enlightened supervison, pleasant working conditions, appropriate fringe benefits, and so forth, these factors may not produce a strong motivational climate. If properly fulfilled, such factors are merely satisfiers, but they are not motivators. What is actually required, therefore, is a two-way effort which is directed first at the hygiene and then at the development of motivation. That is, in addition to the need to avoid unpleasantness which comes from largely dissatisfying conditions, the supervisor has to see to it that positive motivation is produced through a more sophisticated set of factors which is closely related to the concept of self-actualization discussed previously.

SUMMARY

Influencing is that managerial function in which the supervisor creates a climate that enables his subordinates to find as much satisfaction as possible while they are getting their jobs done. Influencing is that function which is particularly concerned with behavioral responses and interpersonal relations. Only by appropriately influencing will the supervisor instill in his subordinates the motivation to go about their jobs with enthusiasm and also to find personal fulfillment of their needs.

All human behavior is caused by unsatisfied needs. These needs eventually stimulate the formation of goals which motivate people to take certain actions. Motivation, however, is caused not only by unmet needs but it is also largely influenced by an individual's attitudes and entire personality.

An individual's attitudes are formed from early childhood on. They affect and are affected by an infinite number of factors in the person's life. Attitudes will determine the individual route which a person takes for the satisfaction of his needs. Although they vary in strength, most needs are basically the same in all people. Thus, we can speak of a hierarchy of needs, starting with physiological needs at the bottom, moving up to safety and security needs on the second level, further up to the third level of social needs or the needs for belonging and association. The fourth level needs are often called egotistical needs or the needs for esteem. They lead to the highest level needs, namely self-actualization and self-fulfillment. A person's level of aspiration is closely related to this hierarchy of needs.

If a person is able to understand his needs and attitudes fairly well, he will be able to choose courses of action which result in achievement of his goals. Goal accomplishment serves as a feedback to the individual: his need is satisfied and his underlying attitudes are confirmed. If a goal is not attained, however, conflict often sets in This is because action that does not succeed results in blocked satisfaction and frustration. By and large most people react to conflict and frustration in one of five following ways: problem-solving behavior, resignation, detour behavior, retreat, or aggression.

It is the supervisor's duty to minimize frustrating situations in which the subordinate often finds himself, especially if these result from a conflict between individual and organizational goals. One way to minimize such conflict situations is to realize that in the work environment there are a number of different kinds of factors which influence the realization of an employee's expectations. Some of these factors are merely satisfiers and dissatisfiers, whereas others are real motivators and are able to fulfill the higher level needs and goals of people. These motivations would include the opportunity for advancement, greater responsibility, chance for promotion, growth and achievement, and an interesting and challenging job. A supervisor in his desire to create a good organizational climate must see to it that in addition to satisfying conditions as many of these motivators as possible are at work.

CHAPTER 17

Leadership

A very important component of the organizational climate is leadership, a term which we have mentioned on numerous occasions throughout this text, but merely in passing. Ultimately, management leadership is responsible for establishing the kind of climate which facilitates motivation and the successful performance of the influencing function.

We can define leadership as a process by which subordinates are imaginatively directed, guided, and influenced in choosing and attaining goals. In any organized activity, a leader mediates between organizational and individual goals so that the degree of satisfaction to both is maximized. A manager, of course, also plays this mediating role but he does not necessarily do it in the same manner that a leader does. Although the terms manager and leader are often used interchangeably, leadership is not synonymous with managerial ability. A manager can do a reasonably good job of managing without being a leader. However, since the manager's job is getting things done through people it is obvious that he will be a much more effective manager if he is also the leader of his employees. But, we may ask, what enables him to be their leader, what qualities does he have to possess in order to be a leader as well as a manager?

LEADERSHIP THEORIES

Much has been written and said about leadership ever since the days of antiquity when emphasis was focused on the leader himself to the exclusion of everything else. Many theories have been formulated as to what constitutes a good leader and what enables some people to be a leader and others not. We shall look at a few of these theories briefly.

The Early Genetic Theory

For hundreds of years observers recognized leadership as the ability to influence people in such a manner that they willingly strove toward an objective. It was believed that this ability was something apart from official position. It was held that certain people were born to be leaders, having inherited a set of unique traits or characteristics which could not be acquired in any other way than through heredity. Leadership was thought to be inherited simply because it emerged frequently within the same prominent families. In reality, however, strong class barriers made it impossible for anyone outside these families to acquire the skills and knowledge required to become a leader.

The Trait Theory

As the social and economic class barriers were broken down and as leaders began to emerge from the so-called "lower classes" of society, the early genetic theory was modified. This modification was largely due to the fact that beginning in the middle 1930's behavioral scientists began to contribute to the literature on leadership. The first contribution was made by writers who, rather than considering leadership only a function of inherited characteristics, held that it could also be *acquired* through experience, education, and training. These writers tried to focus upon all the *traits*, whether inherited or acquired, which were found in men regarded as leaders. Lists of qualities which recognized leaders had in common were compiled. The traits found on these lists frequently included physical and nervous energy, a sense of purpose and direction, enthusiasm, friendliness and affection, integrity, technical mastery, decisiveness, intelligence, teaching skill, faith, and so on.

The inadequacy of this approach soon became obvious, however. Seldom, if ever, did any two lists agree on the essential leadership characteristics. Furthermore, the lists were confusing because they used different terminology and had different numbers of characteristics. Nevertheless, the trait approach was widely accepted for a long time. It was extremely plausible because studies of various successful leaders almost always indicated many similar personality and character traits. However, the intensity and the degree of the traits varied. Moreover, no satisfactory answer could be reached about which traits were most essential for leadership, or whether a man could be a leader if he was lacking some but possessed others. Nor was there any suggestion of how to isolate and identify all the specific traits common to leaders. A further weakness of the trait approach was that it did not distinguish between those characteristics which were needed for acquiring leadership and those which were necessary for maintaining it.

Although the trait approach is partially discredited today, there is a considerable body of research showing that leaders *do* have in common certain very general characteristics. Some of these are intelligence, communication ability, and sensitivity to group needs. Such traits are found interwoven in the personality of the leader, but they are always considered relative to the group. For example, the most intelligent person in the group will not necessarily emerge as the leader. Instead the leader is more likely to be the person with the optimal combination of these traits for the particular situation in which the group finds itself.

The Situational Approach

This leads us to another major weakness of the trait approach, namely, that it does not consider the influence of situational factors on the leadership process. In their search for the "universal traits" of leaders, behavioral scientists discovered the importance of situational factors which make it easier for certain persons to acquire positions of leadership. The proponents of the situational approach do not deny that the characteristics of individuals play an important part in leadership, but they point out that leadership is also the product of situations in particular groups. They point out that leadership in one group will differ from leadership in another group, that in one situation a certain person might evolve as the leader whereas in a different situation someone else would emerge as the leader. For example, on a sinking boat a person with strong swimming ability may emerge as the leader, but in a political meeting someone with good speaking ability may rise to the top. In other words, who becomes the leader of a group engaging in a particular activity and what leadership characteristics are needed are a function of the specific situation in which the group finds itself.

In their desire to deemphasize the traits approach, however, some behavioral scientists may have gone overboard in emphasizing the situation. In so doing, they may have ruled out the possibility that at least some characteristics *predispose* their possessors to attain leadership positions or at least increase their chances of becoming leaders. The fact is that *both* characteristics and the situation are involved in the concept of leadership.

The Follower Approach

A more sophisticated theory of leadership incorporates the follower's personality and needs into the leadership concept. This approach maintains that the follower must also be studied because in the last analysis it is the follower as an individual who perceives the leader, who perceives the situation, and who accepts or rejects leadership. Proponents of this approach further maintain that it is the follower's persistent motives, his point of view, and his frame of reference which will determine what he perceives and how he reacts to it. The follower approach does not neglect the importance of the group situationist at a particular point in time, nor does it fail to take into consideration the fact that certain characteristics will help one person to emerge as the leader rather than another person. However, the satisfaction of the follower's needs is a very important aspect.

More specifically, the follower approach stresses the idea that the leadership function must be analyzed and understood in terms of a dynamic relationship between the leader and his followers. The leader appears to the latter as the best means available for the satisfaction of their needs. The group members will follow the leader because they see in him the means for personal fulfillment. For a group to act as a unit a leader is essential. The members look at him as their leader not only because he possesses certain characteristics such as intelligence, skill, drive, and ambition, but also because of his functional relationship to the members of the group. "The functional relationship which is leadership exists when a leader is perceived by a group as controlling means for the satisfaction of their needs. Following him may be seen either as a means to increased need satisfaction or as a means to prevent decreased need satisfaction."*

Of course, a leader may also arise in the reverse fashion. Instead of him answering group needs, his own personal need satisfaction may cause him to seek out the leadership of the group. That is, he may want to accomplish an objective which can only be attained if he can direct the activities of other people. The latter situation is more typical of a manager formally appointed to a managerial position within an organization.

Conclusions

This leads to the conclusion that a leader is an individual perceived in harmony with the needs of the group and responsive to the group situation. But because leaders must always be recognized as such by group consensus and because *managers* who are appointed do not necessarily reflect subordinate group choice, they are not generally regarded as leaders at the outset. They may *become* true leaders of the group but they do not start out as such. Obviously, it is desirable from an influencing standpoint that subordinates quickly accept the manager as a leader and not merely as the head of their department.

LEADERSHIP STYLE

This is where leadership style comes in since it is so important in winning subordinate acceptance of managers. Generally speaking, leadership styles can be classified in three broad categories: autocratic, democratic, and free rein.

---

*Irving Knickerbocker, "Leadership: A Conception and Some Implications," *The Journal of Social Issues,* Vol. IV, No. 3 (Summer, 1948), 33.

Autocratic Leadership

This type of leadership usually reflects tight supervision, a high degree of centralization, and a narrow span of supervision. The autocratic style is repressive and normally withholds communication other than that which is absolutely necessary for doing the job. Autocratic management makes decisions unilaterally and does not consult with the members of the department. Therefore, the autocratic style of leadership minimizes the degree of involvement by the subordinates.

In more specific terms, autocratic leadership is described by Douglas McGregor's Theory X.* According to McGregor, a manager who fits into "Theory X" leans toward an organizational climate of close control, centralized authority, authoritarian practices, and minimum participation of the subordinates in the decision-making process. As we already know, the reason why a Theory X manager accepts this combination is that he makes certain assumptions about human behavior. Theory X assumptions, according to McGregor, are that:

1) the average man dislikes work and will avoid it to the extent he can;
2) stemming from the above, most people have to be forced or threatened by punishment to get them to make the effort necessary to accomplish organizational goals;
3) the average individual is basically passive and therefore prefers to be directed, rather than to take any risk or responsibility. Above all else he prefers security.

Democratic Leadership

The democratic style emphasizes a looser kind of supervision and greater individual participation in the decision-making process. Authority is delegated as far down as possible and a wide span of management is advocated. A free flow of communication is encouraged among all members of the department so that a climate of trust and confidence can be established.

In McGregor's terms, the democratic style is represented by Theory Y. The "Theory Y" manager operates with a completely different set of assumptions regarding human motivation. He maintains that an effective organizational climate utilizes more general supervision, greater decentralization of authority, little reliance on coercion and control, democratic techniques, and consultation with subordinates on departmental decisions. The assumptions upon which this type of organizational climate is based include the following:

1) that work is as natural to man as play or rest and, therefore, it is not avoided;

---

*Douglas McGregor, *The Human Side of Enterprise* (New York: McGraw-Hill Book Co., 1960), Chapters 3 and 4.

2) that self-motivation and inherent satisfaction in work will be forthcoming in situations where the individual is committed to organizational goals; therefore, coercion is not the only form of influence that can be used to motivate;

3) that commitment is a crucial factor in motivation, and it is a function of the rewards coming from it;

4) that the average individual learns to accept and even seek responsibility given the proper environment;

5) that the ability to be creative and innovative in the solution of organization problems is widely, not narrowly, distributed in the population;

6) that in modern businesses and organizations the intellectual potentialities of employees are just partially utilized.

McGregor underscores the notion that Theories X and Y are beliefs held by management about the nature of man. As such, they constitute the foundation upon which the organizational climate is built. The supervisor who follows Theory X has a basically limited view of people and their capabilities. He feels that individuals must be controlled, closely supervised, and motivated on the bases of money, discipline, and authority. Thus, he feels that the key to motivation is in the proper implementation of approaches designed to satisfy the lower level needs of people.

The Theory Y supervisor, however, has a much different opinion of the capabilities and possibilities of people. He feels that if the proper approach and conditions can be presented, people will exercise self-direction and self-control toward the accomplishment of objectives. He recognizes that the supervisor's activities must fit into the scheme of each employee's own particular set of needs. He also believes that the higher level needs of people are more important in terms of personality and self-development.* Thus, he uses his supervisory skills to try to enable his employees to achieve at least partial satisfaction on the job of their needs for esteem and self-actualization.

Of course, this confronts the supervisor with the question as to which management philosophy and organizational climate will produce the best results. On the surface one is inclined to say that Theory Y would be more desirable than Theory X because on the surface it is humanistic and less harsh. Also it is more optimistic about human motives at work.

Free-Rein Leadership

The free-rein style goes beyond democratic leadership and Theory Y. It is often called *laissez-faire* leadership because the climate of the

---

*For those who would like to read more about theories of changing organization climates: Rensis Likert, *The Human Organization* (New York: McGraw-Hill Book Company, 1967), pp. 14-24 and 120-121; also see Robert R. Blake and Jane Scryglie Mouton, *The Managerial Grid* (Houston, Texas: Gulf Publishing Company, 1964.)

organization is such that people are left almost entirely alone to do their jobs. On the assumption that individuals are self-motivated, an absolute minimum of supervision is imposed. Although the manager is available as a consultant to help out if need be, he leaves the individual with enough authority to provide his own solutions.

Making a Choice

A good manager knows when to use one or the other style of leadership. Obviously, each of these three styles has a place in the practice of management. Free-rein is probably the most useful in an organization of professional people who desire and have shown the capacity for independent work. This would apply, for instance, to research scientists, professors, and so on. The democratic style seems to be appropriate in those situations where a relatively unfettered environment is necessary under which skilled and educated people seem to thrive. This would probably include most activities performed in any health care center. It would be wrong to state, however, that a democratic leadership style is beneficial for all organizations regardless of the nature of their activities and the skill levels of their employees. In some situations, even the autocratic leadership style will produce good results, especially among unskilled subordinates who are poorly prepared to participate in decision-making and who might be uncomfortable if urged to do so.

Therefore, in concluding it is proper to state that leadership style must be adapted to each specific situation. However, it seems that in general a more democratic, more open style achieves greater leader acceptance than an autocratic one. Such a style is more humanistic and more optimistic which also makes it more acceptable to most employees. In addition, much of the research evidence indicates that the Theory Y, democratic approach is more likely to achieve better results. Nevertheless, it is a sign of a good manager and a good leader to be able to utilize any one of these three techniques whenever the need or occasion arises.

LEADERSHIP ROLES

No matter which leadership style is chosen, it will require the manager to assume definite leadership roles. Most of us have had the occasion to observe individuals and the different roles they play in groups. One person may organize the group to achieve goals, whereas another plays the "devil's advocate" raising a stream of objections, and yet someone else is a "synthesizer" who puts together the ideas of all group members. These roles and many others are essential for group life. They fulfill the needs of the individual members of the group and are vital to the group's accomplishment. Of course, the group's leader is not expected to assume all of these roles, but he is expected to fulfill some of them. Generally speaking, leadership roles fall into two broad classifications — task leadership roles, and emotive leadership roles.

Task roles are those that the leader plays in organizing and influencing the group to achieve specified objectives. Usually in an organized activity these objectives are imposed on the group from above. However, in groups which arise spontaneously objectives are generated from within the group itself. In both instances, the leader must facilitate the accomplishment of the group's goals. That is, he plays the role of getting the group to fulfill its tasks.

Emotive roles are just as important as task roles. They provide satisfaction for the individual needs of the group's members. The emotional needs of people are of a social and psychological nature. The leader playing the emotive role helps the members of the group to gain satisfaction of these needs and at the same time he prepares the way for task performance.

Frequently, the ideal leader is one who plays both roles effectively. But the leadership of a group can be shared without diminishing the group's performance or morale. In such a case, one person plays the task role and another takes the emotive role. This would not be an unusual situation in a large institution. The formal organization of such an institution often forces a supervisor to be primarily concerned with getting the job done. He must concentrate largely on task leadership. However, under these conditions the group will probably select another individual, the informal leader, who will function in the emotive role. The supervisor, of course, should not object to the informal leader's role. Rather, he must realize that it is a necessary part of the leadership process, one which fulfills important human needs and which is an essential component of high employee morale, the subject of our next influencing chapter.

SUMMARY

Leadership is a process by which subordinates are imaginatively directed, guided, and influenced in choosing and attaining goals. One cannot equate the term leadership with that of management; a person does not have to be an outstanding leader in order to be an adequate manager, but to a certain extent the characteristics of both overlap.

This can be seen in the earlier genetic theories about leadership which maintained that it was a function of specific characteristics with which a leader was born. Later the genetic approach was altered to state that leadership was a function of numerous personal traits which could be acquired as well as inherited. More recent studies point out that the particular situation at hand also has a significant bearing upon who emerges as a leader. The follower approach adds to the concept of leadership the importance of the perception of the followers and the group which they constitute. By and large, a person must be accepted by his group as a leader before he can actually function as one. Thus, it is important for each manager to adopt a leadership style which facilitates such acceptance.

There exist three broad categories of leadership style, namely autocratic (Theory X), democratic (Theory Y), and free-rein styles. Managers will use these styles in their efforts to be regarded as a leader. A manager who is appointed to a position of organizational authority is not generally perceived as a leader at the outset. Hopefully, however, he will emerge eventually as the leader of his subordinates, thus becoming a much more effective manager as well.

Hopefully also, in his leadership function, the manager will be able to fulfill both the task role of influencing the group to achieve its goals and the emotive role of satisfying the emotional needs of group members. If, however, it is impossible for him to fulfill the latter role, he should not object if an informal leader is chosen by the group to substitute for him.

CHAPTER 18

Morale

The interpersonal skills of the supervisor have a great bearing on the morale of his subordinates. Writers sometimes distinguish between morale and satisfaction; they connect satisfaction with an *individual's* needs and attitudes whereas morale pertains to the spirit of a *group*. However, this distinction is largely academic since the factors used in measuring group morale are usually the same as those used in measuring an individual's satisfaction.

THE MEANING OF MORALE

Although there are many definitions for morale, a particularly useful one is to describe it as a state of mind and emotion affecting the attitudes, feelings, and sentiments of individuals and groups toward their work, environment, administration, and colleagues. Morale is not a single feeling, however. It is a composite of feelings, sentiments, and attitudes which, when it is high, makes the employees strive hard to accomplish the objectives of the enterprise; and conversely, when it is low, prevents or deters them from doing this.

The Range of Morale

Supervisors often make the mistake of speaking of morale as something which is either present or absent among their employees. But morale is always present and by itself has neither favorable nor unfavorable meaning. Morale can range from excellent and positive through a large number of intermediate degrees to poor and completely negative. If the attitude of the subordinates is very poor, then the morale is also poor; but if the subordinates' state of mind and emotion affecting their willingness and dedication to strive hard for the best possible patient care is high, then we speak of high morale. An employee with high morale finds satisfaction in his position in the enterprise, has confidence in his own and his associates' ability, and shows enthusiasm and a strong desire for voluntary cooperation in achieving the hospital's objectives to the fullest extent of his ability.

But high morale of this type cannot be ordered. It can only be created by introducing certain conditions into the work situation which are favorable to its development. High morale is not the cause of good human relations, rather it is the result. It is the result of good motivation, respect and dignity of the individual, realization of individual differences, good leadership, effective communication, participation, counseling, and many other human relations practices. In other words, the state of morale will reflect how appropriately and effectively the administration practices good human relations.

Morale — Everybody's Concern

Every manager, from the top administrator down to the supervisor, should be concerned with the level of morale in the organization. A good supervisor is aware that it is his function to elicit and to maintain the morale of his subordinates at as high a level as possible. It is the immediate supervisor who, in his day-to-day contact with his employees, influences and determines the level of morale more than anyone else. Raising morale to a high level and maintaining it there is a long-run project and cannot be achieved solely on the basis of short-run devices such as pep talks or contests. And the supervisor will also find that although good morale is slow to develop and difficult to maintain, it can change very quickly from good to bad with many shadings in between. Indeed, the level of morale varies considerably from day to day and is far more changeable than the weather. Morale, moreover, is contagious. The higher the degree of individual satisfaction of group members, the higher the morale of the entire group. This, in turn, tends to raise the over-all level of morale even higher since individuals get personal satisfaction from being in a high morale group. But although favorable attitudes spread, it is true that unfavorable attitudes among employees spread even more quickly. It seems to be human nature to quickly forget the good and to remember the bad.

Of course, management is not alone in their desire for a satisfactory level of morale. Each employee of the institution is likewise concerned since bad morale is simply not as satisfying to them as good morale. A state of bad morale creates an unpleasant environment for the employees of the hospital and they have as much at stake as the administration. Good morale, on the other hand, will make the employee's day at work a pleasurable and satisfying experience and not a misery. The employee will find satisfaction in working with his supervisors and associates. High morale is also of importance to the patient in the hospital and his family. They will quickly sense whether the employees of the institution are operating on a high or a low level of morale, and they will respond accordingly. But what, we may ask, determines the level of morale?

FACTORS INFLUENCING MORALE

Almost anything can influence the morale of the employees up-ward or downward. Some of these factors are within the control of the supervisor, whereas others are not. Although there are an infinite number of morale determinants, they can generally be classified into two broad groups: those factors which have their primary source in situations which are external to the institution; and those factors whose source lies mostly within the daily supervisory practices.

External Factors

The first broad source of factors affecting morale, namely, those factors which are connected with events and influences outside the institution, are generally beyond the scope of the supervisor to con-trol. Although they are external in origin, these factors nevertheless concern the supervisor since everyone takes his problems right to his station of work and does not leave them in the car or on the parking lot. Examples of external factors are marital problems, associations with friends, a breakdown of the car, sickness in the family, hobbies, and so forth. Obviously, what happens away from the job may change the employee's feelings very quickly; an argument before leaving home may set the emotional tone for the rest of the day. The head-lines in the morning paper may be depressing or they may be con-ducive to high morale.

This outside-of-the-hospital source of morale factors can gene-rally be dealt with only indirectly. Nevertheless, the supervisor should try to sense such factors because they are reflected in the work atti-tudes of his subordinates. If something has happened to lower an em-ployee's morale and if the supervisor is familiar with the cause, he should try to get the employee to forget the incident as quickly as possible by supplying an antidote. One of the best ways to erase the effects of an occurrence that depresses morale is to encourage the employee to talk about it freely. In so doing, the supervisor will find out what is happening and why, and he may be able to devise effective means of action to raise the morale. But aside from this sort of counseling interview, for which the supervisor may not have time or to which the employee may not wish to submit, there is little a super-visor can do to cope with these outside factors affecting morale. The supervisor must remember that he or the institution is not always the cause of shifts in the level of morale.

Internal Factors

However, there are a large number of important factors affect-ing the morale of employees which are within the realm of the super-visor's activities. These include appropriate incentives, good working conditions, and above all, the quality of supervision. When considering incentives, the first thing that comes to mind is pay. Of course, wages are exceedingly important, but aside from wages and fringe benefits there are many other things which are essential to the employee. Considerations such as job security, interesting work, good working conditions, appreciation of a job well done, chance for advancement, recognition, prompt and fair treatment of grievances, etc., are all necessary components of a high morale environment (see Chapter 16). None of these will take the place of appropriate compensation in dollars and cents. But assuming that the pay is at the going rate, the additional factors mentioned above play a significant role. For example, although reasonable monetary incentives may be provided and the quality of supervision is high, morale can still sink quickly if, for example, working conditions are neglected. The important factor is that an honest attempt is made to improve working conditions whenever possible. There are many cases where employees work under undesirable conditions and still maintain high morale as long as the supervisor has made a serious effort to correct the conditions.

The Supervisor's Attitude

Aside from these on-the-job factors influencing the morale of employees, the most significant influence is exercised by the supervisor himself in his immediate, day-to-day relationship with them. The boss's over-all manner of supervision, directing, leadership, his interpersonal skills, and general attitude will, more than anything else, make for good or bad morale. The employees will put forth their best efforts when they are given an opportunity to obtain their need satisfactions through work which they enjoy and which at the same time achieves the department's objectives. Such job satisfaction will raise and keep morale at a high level. It can only be maintained if the supervisor lets his employees know how significantly they contribute to the over-all goals of the hospital and how their work fits into the over-all effort, if he gives them a feeling of accomplishment in their work and allows them to be their own boss as far as possible. The supervisor who practices democratic supervision, as discussed in the previous chapter, is likely to reduce the undesirable features of a job and to create an environment in which his employees derive genuine satisfaction from the work they do every day. In addition to this, the supervisor should not forget the importance of social satisfactions on the job. He should provide his employees with an opportunity to develop friendships and to work as a team. In other words, he must not forget the positive contributions that informal groups and informal organization make.

The supervisor should bear in mind that his employees' morale is affected not only by what he does, but also by how he does it. There is little doubt that if the supervisor's behavior indicates that he feels superior to his employees or that he is suspicious of their motives and actions, only a low level of morale can result. The supervisor should not forget how little it takes to make his own spirits rise or fall. A word of appreciation from his own boss or even from the hospital administrator can change the supervisor's outlook toward his whole work situation. He will become more cheerful and so in all likelihood will his employees.

The supervisor also knows that a frown or a quizzical expression on his boss's face can have the opposite effect. He will begin to wonder what he did wrong, his face will drop, and his morale will sink. The supervisor should remember that the employees of his department react the same way to him that he does to his own boss. He should remember that attitudes beget like attitudes. If the supervisor shows that he is worried, his employees tend to follow suit. If he loses his temper, others do the same and become angry. However, when the supervisor appears to be confident in the operation of the department, his employees will react accordingly and feel that things are going well. This does not mean that the supervisor should only see the good side of departmental operations and refuse to acknowledge difficulties and troubles. What it does mean is that he should show his employees that as a leader of his department he has the situation well in hand, and that if anything goes wrong, he will give them an opportunity to correct the situation and to see to it that it does not happen again in the future.

Obviously, the supervisor can never relax his efforts to build and maintain a high degree of morale among his employees. Nor should he be discouraged if, from time to time, the morale drops, since there are so many factors to cause such a change which are beyond his control and out of his reach. The supervisor can be reasonably satisfied when his employees' morale is high most of the time.

THE EFFECTS OF MORALE

The question arises as to how good or poor morale affects other variables such as turnover, absenteeism, the rate of accidents, teamwork and productivity. Much research has been done in this area and some general conclusions can be drawn. Normally, higher morale reduces the rate of turnover and results in lower absenteeism. Probably the same holds true for a lowered rate of accidents although some of them have no relation whatsoever to high or low morale. Let us look at the evidence for these conclusions a bit more carefully.

Morale and Teamwork

The term teamwork is often associated with morale. However, the two do not mean the same thing. Morale applies to the *attitudes* of the employees in the department, whereas teamwork is the smoothly coordinated and synchronized *activity* achieved by a small, closely knit group of employees. Although good morale is usually helpful in achieving teamwork, it is possible that teamwork may be high yet morale low. Such a situation could exist in times when jobs are scarce and when the employees will put up with close and tight supervision for fear of losing their jobs. It is also conceivable that teamwork may be absent when morale is high; in such a case, the employee probably prefers individual effort and finds satisfaction in his own job performance.

Morale and Productivity

It is generally assumed that high morale is automatically accompanied by high productivity. Supervisors feel that as long as the morale of employees is high, their output will be accordingly high. They are aware that the willing cooperation of employees is almost always necessary to get continuous superior performance. Moreover, there is substantial research evidence to back up the contention that employees produce best in an environment of high morale. Every supervisor also knows from his own experience that a highly motivated, self-disciplined group of employees will consistently do a more satisfactory job than a group which is forced to perform at a certain rate. It is therefore obvious that every supervisor will do all in his power to keep the level of morale as high as possible in order to keep the output of his department at a high level.

However, more recent studies show that this general statement does not hold true in all situations. There is proof that the morale-productivity relationship can appear in many forms, namely, low morale and high productivity, high morale and low productivity, as well as high morale and high productivity, and low morale and low productivity. Much depends upon other factors, for example, the economic situation, the job market, and so on. Thus, a supervisor cannot automatically depend upon the positive relationship between morale and productivity.

MEASURING CURRENT MORALE

Much of the foregoing discussion has assumed that the level of morale can be measured, but it should be realized that morale cannot be measured directly. Nevertheless, there are suitable indirect ways and means of determining the prevailing level of morale and its trends. Although some supervisors pride themselves on their ability to intuitively detect low morale, the wise supervisor will do better to approach this problem more systematically in either of two ways. One approach is through observation of activities, events, trends, and changes; and the other approach is to use what is commonly referred to as attitude surveys.

Measurement by Observation

Observation is a tool that involves watching people and their reactions. Although this tool is available to every supervisor, it is not often fully utilized. However, if the supervisor does consciously and systematically observe his employees, he can appraise their level of morale and major changes in it. He will watch his subordinates' behavior and listen to what they have to say; he will observe their actions and notice any changes in their willingness to cooperate. He will probably find it fairly easy to recognize by observation the extremes of high and low morale. Finer means of measurement, however, may be required to differentiate among the intermediate degrees. Of course, personal observation can note such obvious manifestations of morale as a facial expression or a shrug of the shoulder, but often it is very difficult to interpret these. It is also difficult to determine how far from normal the behavior must be in order to indicate a shift in morale. Thus, it takes an extremely sensitive supervisor to correctly conclude from indicators of this sort that a change in morale has taken or is taking place.

Moreover, the supervisor may not be able to make the detailed observations necessary for accurate morale appraisal. Although the closeness of the day-to-day working relationship usually offers much opportunity for supervisors to become aware of morale changes, it often happens that they are so burdened with work that they do not have the time to look or, if they do look, they do not actually see. At times, they may even be afraid to look for fear of what they might find. And although some supervisors may realize that changes are taking place, they are frequently inclined to ignore them and give the matter no further attention. Only later, after the change in the level of morale has taken place to such a degree that it has openly manifested itself, will the supervisor recall these first indications, and only then will he admit that he had noticed them, but had not thought much about them at the time.

In order to avoid situations of this sort, the supervisor must take care not to brush any indicators conveniently aside. He must realize that the most serious shortcoming of observation as a yardstick for measuring current morale is that when the activities and events causing an observable lowering of morale are recognized, the change has probably already occurred. The supervisor, therefore, should be extremely keen in his observation in order to do as much as possible to prevent such changes before they take place or to speedily counteract them if they have already begun. Naturally, the closer the supervisor's relations are with his employees, the more sensitive will he become to these changes and the shorter will be his reaction time.

Morale or Attitude Surveys

Many institutions use morale or attitude surveys as a way of finding out how employees feel about their jobs, their supervisors, the hospital as a whole, specific policies, and so on. Expressions of the opinions of employees are requested in the form of answers to written questionnaires. These questionnaires are prepared with the aid of the personnel department or some outside consulting firm. They may be filled out on the job or at home. Although there are many advantages in filling out questionnaires in the privacy of the home, it is to be expected that a high percentage of those questionnaires which are sent home will never be returned. However, it is better to have more meaningful answers even if the number of replies is smaller. Of course, regardless of whether they are filled out on the job or at home, care must be taken that the questionnaires remain unsigned and that the replies be kept secret.

In a health care center, such attitude surveys cover the entire field of operations. But it is feasible to limit the inquiry to only one department, e.g., the nursing services. This, however, must be cleared with top administration since too many surveys at too frequent intervals would not be advisable. Once a survey is decided upon, the administrator and all other managers must be prepared to have their feelings hurt as many dissatisfactions will probably be expressed. But more important than this is the fact that management must be prepared and willing to act upon the complaints once they are revealed. Up until the time the survey is taken, management could always plead complete ignorance; but now everyone knows that the administration has heard about the problems causing dissatisfaction. Hopefully, many of the complaints can be adjusted; at least a serious and honest effort must now be made. If, however, administration is not prepared to act, it would have been far better not to have had any survey whatsoever.

Taking the Survey and Analyzing Its Results

Questionnaires submitted to employees come in a variety of types (see Figures 18-1 and 18-2). Some questionnaires offer a specific choice of answers; others are not so specific, giving the employee an opportunity to answer freely in his own words. But since many employees have difficulty in stating their opinions in complete sentences or even in completing a started sentence, the best results are usually obtained by a form that enables the employee to check the box which seems to provide the most appropriate answer for him.

Once the forms have been filled out, the results must be tabulated and analyzed. This is usually done by the personnel department or by an outside consultant. The analysis must be thorough and instead of simple straight run answers, it should produce more meaningful interpretations. For instance, instead of simply stating that 65 percent of the subordinates have frequent communication with their boss whereas 35 percent do not, or that 75 percent of the respondents like their jobs whereas 25 percent do not, it would be better to state that of those 75 percent who like their jobs 85 percent have frequent contact with their boss whereas 15 percent do not. At the same time, we can learn that among those 25 percent who do not care for their jobs, 55 percent claim that they have infrequent communications with their superiors. Crosstabulations of this type show the correlation between good communication and job satisfaction.

After such correlation analysis and interpretation of the survey has been done, the results are presented to the top administrator, if the survey originated there. He, in turn, passes them on to all supervisors. As a matter of fact, in some organizations the results of morale surveys are used as discussion material in supervisory training. But aside from this, attitude surveys provide the administrator and his supervisors with information to guide them in their over-all efforts to improve morale. Occasionally, the surveys will reveal certain deficiencies and the supervisor can do something very specific about them. Frequently, however, the results of initial surveys are not so clear. They raise a lot of questions, and sometimes additional surveys are required to probe deeper. But survey techniques are becoming more and more sophisticated and with their help management should be able to arrive at a solution to almost any morale problem which arises.

SUMMARY

Morale is a state of mind and emotion affecting the attitudes, feelings, and sentiments of individuals and groups of employees toward their work environment, colleagues, supervision, and the enterprise as a whole. It is a composite and not a single feeling. Morale is always present, and it can range all the way from high to low. The level of morale varies considerably from day to day. It is contagious; that is, favorable attitudes spread, but unfavorable attitudes spread even more quickly. High morale is not only the concern of the supervisor — the employees are just as interested in a satisfactory level of morale. Moreover, not only do insiders feel the effect of high or low morale, it is also recognizable to outsiders such as patients and visitors coming in contact with the institution.

Morale can be influenced by a multitude of factors which can be classified in two broad groups, namely, those factors affecting the employee's activities outside of the enterprise and those factors pertaining to on-the-job situations. There is relatively little the boss can do to directly change the effects of outside factors on his subordinates' morale, but there are many internal factors such as incentives, working conditions, and his own attitudes which are within the supervisor's power to control. These factors can be used to significantly raise the level of subordinates' morale. If the supervisor succeeds in maintaining high morale, it is likely that good teamwork and increased productivity will result. However, recent research indicates that this is not always the case.

FIGURE 18-1

Opinion Survey*

St. X Y Z Health Center

Dept. . . . .
Unit . . . .

    Each question may be answered in several ways, any one of which will give us the information we need. Check only *one* answer that most closely expresses your true feelings. DO NOT sign the form. Seal your questionnaire in the accompanying envelope and drop it in a box in the Personnel Department tomorrow or any day on or before July 15.

1. How would you rate the hospital as a place to work?
☐ Poor place ☐ Not so good ☐ Better than most ☐ Good place
2. Are you kept informed on the policies of the hospital and changes in them?
☐ Never ☐ Sometimes ☐ Usually ☐ Always
3. Do you feel that the policies of the hospital are fair to you?
☐ Never ☐ Sometimes ☐ Usually ☐ Always
4. Are you kept informed about what is going on at the hospital?
☐ Never ☐ Sometimes ☐ Usually ☐ Always
5. Where do you get most of your information about what is going on?
☐ Grapevine ☐ Local newspapers ☐ Bulletin boards ☐ Supervisor
6. Were you given a satisfactory introduction and explanation of your new job before you started to work?
☐ No explanation ☐ Very little ☐ Fair amount ☐ Sufficient
7. Were you made to feel at home and at ease by your supervisor and fellow worker?
☐ Never ☐ Sometimes ☐ Usually ☐ Always
8. Do you like your job?
☐ Not at all ☐ Neither like it or dislike it ☐ Fairly well ☐ Very much
9. How well do you feel your experience and abilities are used in your job?
☐ Poorly ☐ Not so well ☐ Fairly well ☐ Very well
10. What do you think of your department head and supervisor?
Department Head
☐Poor ☐ Below average ☐ Above average ☐ Very good Why?

Immediate Supervisor
☐Poor ☐ Below average ☐ Above average ☐ Very good Why?

11. Are your duties and responsibilites clear to you?
☐ Never ☐ Sometimes ☐ Usually ☐ Always
12. Can you depend on your department head's and supervisor's promises?
☐ Never ☐ Sometimes ☐ Usually ☐ Always
13. Does your supervisor and department head give you full credit for suggestions you make about your job or department?
☐ Does not ☐ Seldom does ☐ Almost always does ☐ Always does
14. Do you get conflicting orders because of too many "supervisors"?
☐ Never ☐ Sometimes ☐ Usually ☐ Always
15. When your department head and supervisor criticizes you or your work, is it done in a friendly and helpful way?
Department Head
☐ Never ☐ Sometimes ☐ Usually ☐ Always
Supervisor
☐ Never ☐ Sometimes ☐ Usually ☐ Always
16. Does your department head and supervisor give clear, exact and easily understood instructions about your work?
Department Head
☐ Never ☐ Sometimes ☐ Usually ☐ Always
Supervisor
☐ Never ☐ Sometimes ☐ Usually ☐ Always

17. Does your department head or supervisor have a tendency to show favoritism?
Department Head
   ☐ Does ☐ Usually does ☐ Seldom does ☐ Never does
Supervisor
   ☐ Does ☐ Usually does ☐ Seldom does ☐ Never does

18. When changes are made in your work, are you usually given a reason for them?
   ☐ Never ☐ Sometimes ☐ Usually ☐ Always

19. Does your department head or supervisor take an understanding attitude toward your difficulties?
Department Head
   ☐ Never does ☐ Seldom does ☐ Usually does ☐ Does
Supervisor
   ☐ Never does ☐ Seldom does ☐ Usually does ☐ Does

20. If you were in trouble whether it is your fault or not, what are your chances of a fair hearing and getting a "square deal"?
   ☐ No chance ☐ Very little chance ☐ Fair chance ☐ Good chance
Why?

21. Do you feel that you can appeal to a higher authority if your immediate supervisor decides a point against you?
   ☐ I do not ☐ Reasonably so ☐ Almost always ☐ Always can
If not, why?

22. Is your job and future secure if you do good work?
   ☐ No ☐ Fairly secure ☐ To a large extent ☐ Very secure

23. Are your associations with your fellow workers and superiors as pleasant as they should be?
   ☐ Not pleasant ☐ Fairly pleasant ☐ Almost always pleasant ☐ Most pleasant
If not, why?

24. Do you feel that your fellow workers in your department are doing their fair share of the work?
   ☐ Very few ☐ About half of them ☐ Most of them ☐ All or almost all
Please list by number (1-10) items in the order of importance to you.
   ☐ Physical working conditions ☐ Doing something worthwhile
   ☐ Opportunity for advancement ☐ Liking of job ☐ Job security
   ☐ Satisfactory relations with co-workers ☐ Wages ☐ Knowing what is going on
   ☐ Fair supervision ☐ Credit for work done
What do you like best about your job?
What do you like least about your job?
Length of service at St. X Y Z Health Center (check one)
   ☐ One month or less ☐ 1 - 3 months ☐ 3 - 6 months ☐ 6 - 12 months
   ☐ 1 - 5 years ☐ 5 - 10 years ☐ 11 years or more
Age (check one)
   ☐ 16 - 20 years ☐ 21 - 25 years ☐ 26 - 34 years ☐ 35 - 45 years
   ☐ 46 - 50 years ☐ 51 - 70 years
Marital status (check one)
   ☐ Single   ☐ Married
Employed   ☐ Part-time   ☐ Full-time
   Please add any additional information that you feel would make the hospital a better place in which to work.

*This example is for illustrative purposes only and should not necessarily be considered a recommended form.

FIGURE 18-2

Employee Opinionnaire*

Column headers (left group): Agree | Don't Know | Disagree

Column headers (right group, "Importance of this item to me"): Very Important | Important | Not So Important

1. My relationship with my immediate supervisor is clearly spelled out.
2. The deductions from pay check are adequately explained.
3. I am in favor of a no smoking area in the cafeteria.
4. The employees lockers are conveniently located and easy to use.
5. The doctors on SMHC's staff are pleasant to work with.
6. My supervisor knows whether or not I am doing a good job.
7. I would be willing to rotate shifts more often.
8. I will accept the first chance to leave my job.
9. The hallways and stairways are spacious and clean.
10. My co-workers are usually friendly and courteous to other employees.
11. Compared to other cafeterias SMHC's meal costs are reasonable.
12. As long as I do a good job I will have a job at SMHC.
13. Do you think the employee who "yells the loudest" gets the "better pay."
14. I find the in-service training and education sufficient.
15. My work area is too small.
16. The pay at SMHC is competitive with other places for which I could work.
17. I consider the fringe benefits at SMHC to be good.
18. Considering the job I do, my pay is good.
19. The personnel policies have been clearly explained to me.
20. I know what responsibility I have should there be a disaster or fire.
21. My supervisor could have been more helpful in orienting me to my job.
22. I get a salary increase only when my supervisor feels like it.
23. There are many employees who abuse the sick leave policy.
24. More often than not I am criticized for the job I do rather than given credit for a job well done.
25. My job orientation was adequate.
26. I feel that administration is concerned about me and my fellow employees.
27. I find it more convenient to go to the canteen or bring my lunch rather than go to the cafeteria.
28. My work area is the cleanest in which I have ever worked.
29. Whenever a complaint is filed it takes too long to get it settled.
30. The patients at SMHC are getting the best care available.
31. My supervisor encourages and assists me in improving my skills so I may have the opportunity to advance.
32. Many of my co-workers love to gossip.
33. The people I work with help each other get the job done.
34. My job is a challenge.
35. The cafeteria has a wide selection of food from which to choose.

	Agree	Don't Know	Disagree	Very Important	Important	Not So Important

36. My supervisor is vague on instructions given me. ☐ ☐ ☐ ☐ ☐ ☐
37. I think the Personnel Department is doing a good job. ☐ ☐ ☐ ☐ ☐ ☐
38. My supervisor really tries to explain new policy changes or new ideas. ☐ ☐ ☐ ☐ ☐ ☐
39. Visitors are treated courteously. ☐ ☐ ☐ ☐ ☐ ☐
40. The parking lots are secure. ☐ ☐ ☐ ☐ ☐ ☐
41. I find that the noise in my work area is distracting. ☐ ☐ ☐ ☐ ☐ ☐
42. My supervisor is an asset to SMHC and knows his/her job well. ☐ ☐ ☐ ☐ ☐ ☐
43. My work area is well lighted and ventilated. ☐ ☐ ☐ ☐ ☐ ☐
44. I am interested in extracurricular activities such as team sports, social outings, baseball and football games, etc. ☐ ☐ ☐ ☐ ☐ ☐
45. My job description clearly spells out the work I am doing. ☐ ☐ ☐ ☐ ☐ ☐
46. I would recommend SMHC to my friends and relatives if hospitalization is needed. ☐ ☐ ☐ ☐ ☐ ☐
47. There exist some jealousy between my co-workers. ☐ ☐ ☐ ☐ ☐ ☐
48. My work is tiring — I am exhausted at day's end. ☐ ☐ ☐ ☐ ☐ ☐
49. If an emyloyee is dismissed at SMHC there is always just cause. ☐ ☐ ☐ ☐ ☐ ☐
50. My supervisor treats me with respect and listens to my suggestions. ☐ ☐ ☐ ☐ ☐ ☐
51. I would rather "time in" and "time out" with a time clock rather than with a time sheet. ☐ ☐ ☐ ☐ ☐ ☐
52. No one ever has a chance for promotion from within the ranks. ☐ ☐ ☐ ☐ ☐ ☐
53. My supervisor doesn't have enough time to spend with me when I have a problem. ☐ ☐ ☐ ☐ ☐ ☐
54. Safety is stressed in my work area. ☐ ☐ ☐ ☐ ☐ ☐
55. My work group always has all the supplies it needs to get the job done. ☐ ☐ ☐ ☐ ☐ ☐
56. Parking facilities at SMHC are adequate. ☐ ☐ ☐ ☐ ☐ ☐
57. My supervisor is fair in any disciplinary action that is taken. ☐ ☐ ☐ ☐ ☐ ☐
58. Most news reaches me through the grapevine and not through the regular channels. ☐ ☐ ☐ ☐ ☐ ☐

59. *Do not sign* the opinionnaire. However, please check one of the following boxes so that the results of this opinion survey will be more meaningful.

I am a member of the:

Nursing Services ☐

Professional Care Division
(Pharmacy, clinical labs, medical records, dietary, rehabilitation, therapy, radiology, nuclear medicine, social service, central supplies) ☐

Administrative Services
(Executive offices, data processing, general clerical, admitting, public relations, purchasing, switchboard, volunteer services, accounting, personnel, etc.) ☐

Plant Operation and Maintenance Services
(Engineering, maintenance, housekeeping, laundry, dispatch, security, grounds, etc.) ☐

60. I have been employed by SMHC

for less than one year	From one to three years	from three to five years	from five to ten years	for more than ten years
☐	☐	☐	☐	☐

Please return in one week. Please do not sign.

*Much of this is taken from a questionnaire used at St. Mary's Health Center, St. Louis, Mo. Reprinted with special permission.

An astute supervisor can sense changes in the level of morale by keen observation of his subordinates. But often supervisors do not realize that a change has taken place until it is too late. In addition to observation, there is another way for the supervisor to become familiar with the level of morale. He can perform an attitude survey with the help of the personnel department. This is done primarily by questionnaires submitted to employees. Once a morale survey has been performed, it is absolutely necessary that management do something about those points which appear to contribute to a lowering of morale. In conclusion, good management as advocated throughout this text will be able to raise low morale to high morale.

CHAPTER 19

Giving Directives

Now that we know something about the influencing function in psychological terms, in terms of motivation, leadership, and morale, we are ready to deal with it in more concrete terms, in terms of issuing directives and exercising positive discipline. Discipline will be discussed in the next chapter after we have had a chance to explore the essence of the influencing function, namely, the art of giving directives.

In order to get the job done, every supervisor spends a great deal of his time and efforts in giving directives to his subordinates. In this connection, it is advisable to recall the principle of *unity of command* to which reference was made earlier. Unity of command, as we know, means that in each department there is only one person who has the authority to make decisions appropriate to his station. It means that each employee has a single immediate supervisor, who is in turn responsible to his immediate supervisor, and so on up and down the chain of command. It also means that a subordinate is responsible to only one supervisor. The principle of unity of command further states that the supervisor is the only one who can give directives to his employees. All directives can come only from the immediate supervisor, and there should be no interference in the guiding and overseeing of his employees by anyone else. In other words, there is a direct line of authority from the supervisor to his subordinate, just as there is one from the administrator to the director of a service and from there to the supervisor of a department. The administrator's line, however, extends only to the directors of services and not to the supervisors and the employees under particular supervisors. Thus, all supervision of the employees of a department rests with the supervisor of that department and must not be exercised by anyone else — emergencies excepted. Otherwise, the principle of unity of command is violated; no man can serve two bosses.

THE IMPORTANCE OF ORDER GIVING

Because issuing directives is such a basic and integral part of the supervisor's daily routine, it has often been taken for granted that every supervisor knows how to give orders. It is frequently assumed that anybody can give orders. This is probably not true. But even if it were true, there is general agreement that some ways of issuing directives are much more effective than others. The experienced supervisor knows that faulty or bad order giving can easily upset even the best laid plans, and instead of coordination of efforts, a general state of chaos is created.

To the uninitiated outsider, it may seem that some supervisors can get excellent results even though they appear to break every rule in the book. Other supervisors may use all the best techniques of order giving and phrase their requests in the most courteous ways and still only get grudging compliance. The question of what is the most appropriate method of order giving depends upon the employee concerned, the particular situation, the supervisor, the way he views his job, his attitude toward people, and many other factors. There are definite techniques for giving orders, however, and since the supervisor's own success depends largely on how his subordinates carry out the orders he gives, it is essential for him to possess the knowledge and the skill for good directing. In other words, since directing is the fundamental tool employed by supervisors to start activities, to stop them, or to modify them, it is necessary for every supervisor to become familiar with the basic characteristics which distinguish good and accomplishable directives from those which are not.

CHARACTERISTICS OF A GOOD DIRECTIVE

It Should Be Reasonable

The first essential characteristic of a good directive is that it must be reasonable, i.e. that compliance can reasonably be expected by the supervisor. Unreasonable orders will not only undermine morale, but they will aso make controlling impossible. This requirement of reasonableness immediately excludes orders pertaining to activities which physically cannot be done. In judging whether or not a directive can reasonably be accomplished, the supervisor should not only appraise it from his own point of view, but he should also try to place himself in the position of the employee. The supervisor should not issue a directive if the capacity or experience of the employee receiving the instruction is not sufficient to comply with the order. This becomes particularly important in the case of recent graduates of various programs who may have had an excellent education in many areas, but certainly lack experience and even some of the knowledge required. The supervisor should not forget the value of his own on-the-job training.

It can still easily happen that a supervisor issues unreasonable instructions. For instance, in order to please the director, a supervisor promises the completion of a job at a particular time and then issues such an order without considering whether the employee who is to carry out the order can actually do so. In this type of case, the supervisor should make it clear to his boss that he will do the best he can to get the job done in time; but he should not put unreasonable pressure on his subordinate. The supervisor should place himself in the position of the subordinate, and ask himself if compliance can reasonably be expected. His decision will depend upon all the conditions prevailing at the time. There are some borderline cases where the directive may actually be intended to stretch the subordinate's capabilities a little bit beyond what had previously been requested. Then the question of reasonableness becomes a question of degree. But generally speaking, a prime requirement of a good directive is that it can be accomplished by the employee to whom it is assigned without undue difficulty.

It Should Be Intelligible

Another requirement is that a good directive should be intelligible to the employee — he should be able to understand it. The subordinate cannot be expected to carry out an order which he does not understand. For example, a directive in a language not intelligible to the subordinate cannot be considered an order. But the same also applies if both speak the English language, and the supervisor uses words that the employee does not comprehend. This, then, becomes a matter of communication. (See Chapter 5.) The supervisor must make certain that the employee understands him, and it is the supervisor's duty to communicate in words and forms which the employee actually understands, and not merely should understand. Instructions must be clear but not necessarily lengthy. What is clear and complete to the supervisor, however, is not always clear and complete to the employee. And sometimes the supervisor himself has not made up his mind as to exactly what it is that he wants done. Here, too, it is advisable for the supervisor to project himself into the position of the employee. A supervisor simply cannot expect his subordinates to carry out his directives if he has not made them clear and intelligible.

It Should Be Worded Appropriately

Every good supervisor knows that the tone and words used in issuing directives significantly affect the subordinates' acceptance and performance of them. A considerate tone is likely to stimulate willing and enthusiastic acceptance, which, of course, is preferable to routine or grudging acceptance or outright resignation. Those in the health care field who are closely involved with the care of the patient will use the term "order" without unpleasant connotations. But most other supervisors should refrain from using the term "order" as much as possible and instead use such terms as directives, assignments, instructions, suggestions, and requests.

Requests

Phrasing orders more as requests does not reduce their character as a directive, but there is a big difference in the reaction a request will inspire as compared to a command. With the majority of subordinates, a request is all that is commonly needed and used. It is a pleasant and easy way of asking an employee to get the job done, particularly with those employees who have been working for the supervisor for some time and who are familiar with the personality of the supervisor, and vice versa. A request works best with this kind of employee, and it usually does not rub him the wrong way.

Suggestions

In other instances, it might be advisable to place the directive in the form of a suggestion which is a still milder form than a request. For example, the supervisor might say, "Mary, we are supposed to get all of this work done today and we seem to be a bit behind. Do you think we can make up for it?" Suggestions of this type will accomplish a great deal for the supervisor as they will be understood and accepted by his responsible and ambitious employees. Such employees like the feeling of not being ordered around and of being left on their own to get the job accomplished. However, this suggestive type of order would not be advisable where the supervisor is dealing with new employees. The new employees simply do not have the background of the department and have not been around long enough to have received sufficient training and familiarity with its activities. Nor is the form of suggestion the proper way of giving orders to those employees who are less competent and less dependable.

Moreover, some subordinates must be told what to do simply because a request or a suggestion might invite an argument as to why they should not do it. Sometimes the command type of order is the only way to get things done. Everyone remembers commands from parents and schoolteachers as a part of the process of growing up. Most people, however, feel that once they are adults commands are no longer necessary. Thus, the best rule for a supervisor is to avoid the command form of giving an order whenever possible but to remember to use it on those occasions when it is needed.

Compatible With Objectives

A good directive must be compatible with the purposes and objectives of the organization. If the instructions are not in conformance with the objectives of the enterprise, the chances are that the subordinate may not execute them adequately, or may not execute them at all. It is therefore necessary that the supervisor, when issuing directives which appear to be in conflict with the main organizational objectives, explain to the employee why such action is necessary; or explain that the directive merely appears to be in conflict, but actually it is not contrary to the objectives of the enterprise. Instructions must also be consistent; they must not be in opposition to orders or directives previously given unless there is a good reason for the discrepancy.

Time Element

An additional characteristic of a good directive is that it specify the time within which the instructions should be carried out and completed. The supervisor should allow a reasonable amount of time, and if this is not feasible, he must realize that the quality of the performance can only be as good as can be produced under the time limit. In many directives, the time factor is not clearly stated, although it is probably implied that the assignment should be carried out within a reasonable length of time. What is a reasonable length of time will, of course, depend upon the circumstances of the situation.

The above are some of the major characteristics which should be incorporated in a good directive. Because the performance of the employee depends to a great extent on the quality of directives given by the supervisor, the latter should make certain that his directing fulfills these most essential characteristics.

MAJOR TECHNIQUES OF DIRECTING

On several occasions, we have discussed various theories describing the supervisor's underlying managerial attitudes such as Theories X and Y, autocratic and democratic leadership, participation in decision-making, broad or narrow delegation of authority, and so forth. The following is a more detailed discussion of how these managerial attitudes manifest themselves in the daily working environment where the supervisor depends upon his subordinates to actually get the job done.

Generally speaking, the supervisor may choose from two basic techniques of direction: autocratic, close supervision on the one hand, or democratic, consultative, general supervision on the other. In our discussion, we can clearly distinguish between these two extremes. But in practice, the supervisor usually combines and blends these techniques. It is conceivable, for example, that he might use one or another of these techniques at different times. It is also possible that for some of his employees he might consider it more advisable to use one method and for other employees another. No one form of supervision is equally good in all situations. Whether it is better to apply a more autocratic or a more democratic type of supervision will depend upon many factors: the kind of work, the situation at hand, the attitude of the employee toward the supervisor, the personality and the ability of the employee, and the personality, experience, and ability of the supervisor. A good supervisor is sensitive to all of these factors and to the needs of each situation, and he will adjust his style of supervision accordingly.

Autocratic Close Supervision

When the supervisor employs the autocratic technique of directing — close supervision — he gives direct, clear, and precise orders to his subordinates with detailed instructions as to exactly how and in what sequence he wants things done. This, as we know, allows little room for the initiative of the subordinate. The supervisor who normally uses the autocratic technique of supervision is the kind of person who will delegate as little authority as possible, and who believes that in all probability he can do the job better than any of his subordinates. He relies on command and detailed instructions followed by close supervision. He is the kind of supervisor who feels that his subordinates are "not paid to think," that they are expected to follow instructions, that he alone is to do the planning and decision-making and that this is what he is trained and paid for. The autocratic supervisor does not necessarily distrust the subordinate, but he feels that without minute instruction from him the subordinate could not properly carry out the directive. He believes that only he can specify the best method and that there is only one way — namely, his way — to get the job done. In other words, he practices Theory X management.

With most people the consequences of this type of supervision can be fatal. Employees lose interest and initiative; they stop thinking for themselves because there is no need or occasion for independent thought. They are obedient but silent and lack initiative, sparkle, and ingenuity. It becomes difficult to remain loyal to the organization and to the supervisor; the subordinate secretly rejoices when his boss makes a mistake. This kind of supervision tends to make the employee somewhat like an automaton. His freedom is curtailed and it is difficult for him to learn even by making mistakes; he justly concludes that he is not expected to do any thinking about his job, and although he perfunctorily performs his duties he finds little involvement in his work. He certainly is not motivated.

These shortcomings of the autocratic technique of close supervision are obvious. Generally speaking, young men and women who have been brought up in a democratic and permissive society from their earliest days resent autocratic order giving. It is contrary to our traditional democratic way of life in America. No ambitious employee will remain in a position where the supervisor is not willing to delegate some degree of freedom and authority. Any subordinate who is eager to learn and to progress will resent being constantly given detailed instructions that leave no room for his own thinking and initiative. He will be stifled, and sooner or later he will leave the enterprise. This method of supervision does not produce good employees and will only chase away those who have the potential.

On the other hand, it must not be forgotten that under certain circumstances and with certain people a degree of close supervision may be necessary. But this is the exception, not the rule. Suppose, for example, that the subordinate is the kind of person who does not want to think for himself and who prefers to receive clear orders. Firm guidance gives him reassurance, whereas loose and general supervision may be frustrating to him. There are some employees who lack ambition and imagination, and who do not want to become at all involved in their daily job. There are also employees who have been brought up in an authoritarian manner by their families here or in a foreign country, and whose previous work experience leads them to believe that general supervision is no supervision at all. Moreover, there are occasions when a work situation is so chaotic that only autocratic techniques can bring order. Aside from these rather unusual situations, however, it can generally be assumed that autocratic, close supervision is the least desirable and least effective method.

It should be noted, moreover, that the autocratic supervisor usually makes the basic Theory X assumption that the average employee does not want to do the job, that close supervision and threats of loss of job are needed in order to get people to work. Such a supervisor feels that if he were not on the job and "breathing down their necks," all his subordinates would stop working. And under these conditions, they very likely would. On the other hand, the supervisor who follows Theory Y and believes in general supervision assumes that the average employee is eager to do a good job, that he wants to do the right thing, and that he must have motivation to perform at his best. Obviously, autocratic, close supervision is not conducive to motivating employees to perform at their best; general supervision, however, will.

The Consultative Technique and General Supervision

The opposite of autocratic, close supervision is what is commonly known as the consultative, participative, democratic, or permissive way of directing. This is similar to the concept of general supervision to which we referred earlier. Its basic assumption is that employees are eager to do a good job and are capable of doing so. The supervisor behaves toward them with this basic assumption in mind, and the employees, in turn, tend to react in a manner that justifies the expectations that their supervisors have.

This democratic, permissive approach to the directing function manifests itself in the practice of general supervision when it comes to routine assignments within the department. When new jobs have to be performed and new assignments made, this democratic method of supervising will manifest itself in what we shall call the *consultative* or *participative* technique of directing. Both, of course, have the underlying assumption that employees will be more motivated if they are left to themselves as much as possible. We shall first discuss the types of situations which require consultation and, then, the meaning of general supervision for routine assignments.

Consultation

The essential characteristic of this method is that the supervisor consults with his employees concerning the extent, nature, and alternative solution to a problem before he makes a decision and issues a directive. When the supervisor uses the consultative or participative approach before issuing directives, he is earnestly seeking help and ideas from the employees, and he approaches the subject with an open mind. More important than the procedure is the attitude of the supervisor. A subordinate will easily sense superficiality and he is quick to perceive whether or not his boss genuinely intends to consult with him on the problem or whether he intends only to give the impression of so doing.

There is a danger that some supervisors are inclined to use such *pseudoconsultation* merely to give employees the feeling that they have been consulted. In many instances, supervisors ask for participation only after they have already decided on the directive. Here the supervisor is using the consultative technique as a trick, as a device for manipulating people to do what he wants them to do. The subordinate will quickly realize that he is not being taken seriously and that his participation is not real. The results achieved will be much worse than if the superior had used the most autocratic method. If a supervisor really wants to practice consultative management when it comes to the issuing of new directives and new assignments, he must be ready to take it seriously and he must be willing to be swayed by the employee's opinion and suggestions. If he is not sincere, it would be better for him not to apply this technique in the first place.

If the subject matter concerns only the supervisor and one employee, the consultative or participative method can be carried out in a *most informal* manner. There are numerous occasions during the day to hold such private consultations. Of course, there is a danger that if the supervisor uses this approach all the time, his subordinates may begin to doubt whether or not he has any opinions of his own and whether he is able to make any decisions. In some instances, it is probably correct that the supervisor is incapable of making a decision. But in most cases, the supervisor has probably just gone too far in utilizing this philosophy of direction. Somehow, while implementing the technique of participation he has not been able to retain the atmosphere of managing.

To reinstate the atmosphere it should be recalled that consultative direction does not lessen or weaken the supervisor's formal authority because the *right to decide* still remains with him. Moreover, the supervisor using this approach is just as much concerned with getting the job done economically and expeditiously as the manager who uses another kind of approach. But the supervisor must not dominate the situation to the point that it excludes any participation by the employee. This is not to say that the supervisor cannot express his opinions. He must, however, express them in a manner which indicates to the employee that even the supervisor's opinions are subject to critical appraisal. Similarly, participative consultation does not mean that the suggestions of the employee cannot also be criticized or even rejected. True consultation implies a sharing of information between the supervisor and the employee and a thorough and impartial discussion of alternate solutions regardless of who originated them. Only then can it be said that the manager really consulted the subordinate.

In order for such consultative practices to be successful, moreover, it is not only necessary that the supervisor be in favor of them, but the employee must also want them. If he is the kind of subordinate who believes that "the boss knows best" and that making decisions and giving directives is none of his concern, then there is little likelihood that the opportunity to participate will induce better motivation or better morale. In this connection, it must also be kept in mind that an employee should be consulted only in those areas in which he is capable of expressing himself and in which he can draw on a certain fund of knowledge. The problems involved must be consistent with the subordinate's ability. Asking participation in areas which are outside his scope of experience will make the employee feel inadequate and frustrated instead of motivating him.

In using consultation there is the danger that at the end of an extended discussion the employee may not have a clear, crisp idea of the solution which was arrived at. It is therefore desirable and even necessary that the supervisor or the subordinate summarize the conclusions in order to avoid such a pitfall. This is even more essential if several employees participated in the consultation.

One of the obvious advantages of summarizing the results of the consultation is that the directive emerging therefrom does not appear to the employee as an order, but rather as a solution which came directly from him or in which he participated. This assures the subordinate's best cooperation and enthusiasm in carrying the directive out. It gives him a feeling of importance since it is evident that his ideas were desired and valued. Active participation also provides an outlet for reasoning power and imagination and an opportunity for the employee to make a worthwhile contribution to the organization. Since there is a considerable degree of talent among employees, their ideas often prove of real value in improving the quality of directives. An additional advantage of this technique is that it will bring the employee closer to the supervisor which will make for better communication and understanding between them. Looking at these impressive advantages of consultation, it becomes apparent that it is by far the best method to use whenever the supervisor has to issue new assignments, new directives, and new instructions.

General or Loose Supervision

This democratic, participative approach to directing subordinates leads to what we have already referred to as general or loose supervision when it comes to *routine assignments* and to carrying out the daily chores involved in each employee's job. General supervision, as we know, means to let the subordinate work out the details of his job, to let him make the decisions of how best to do it. Through this process, the worker will gain great satisfaction from being on his own and from having a chance to express himself and to make decisions himself. Instead of having a specific, detailed list of orders to comply with, his supervisor will just generally indicate to him what needs to be done and might make a few suggestions as to how to go about it. In so doing, the supervisor assumes that given the proper opportunity the average employee wants to do a good job. The supervisor is primarily interested in the results and once he tells his subordinate what he wants accomplished, establishes the goals, and fixes the limits within which he can work, he leaves him on his own. Obviously, this kind of thinking and supervision can only lead to higher motivation, higher morale, and ultimately to a better job. It gives the employee the opportunity to satisfy his need for self-expression and being his own boss.

Explaining Why. The supervisor who practices general supervision creates an atmosphere of understanding and mutual confidence in which the employee will always feel free to call on his boss whenever the need arises without fear that this would indicate incompetence. By the same token, the supervisor takes great pains to explain to his workers the reasons for his general directives and why certain things have to be done. By explaining the purpose behind the directives, the employee will be able to understand the environment of his activities. This will make him better informed and the better informed the subordinate is, the better he will be able to perform his job.

Indeed, it is a common complaint in many enterprises that subordinates are kept in the dark most of the time and that supervisors hoard knowledge and information which they ought to pass on. In most instances, it is exceedingly difficult to issue directives so completely as to cover all particulars. However, if the person who receives the directive knows the purpose behind it, he is in a better position to carry it out than one who does not know. This will enable him to put the environment in total perspective and to make sense out of it so that he can take firm and secure action. Without such knowledge, the employee might find himself in an anxiety-producing situation. He may run into unforeseen circumstances, and if he knows why the directive was given he will probably be able to use his own good judgment and carry it out in a manner that will bring about proper results. He could not possibly do this if he were not well informed.

There is an often-told story illustrating the importance of explaining why. A foreman had a crew of workers dig holes at random in the factory yard. Each time two men had dug a hole four feet deep, the foreman was called over to inspect the hole, after which he ordered the men to fill it up again. After the lunch break, the work crew refused to do the job because they thought it completely useless. At that point, the foreman explained the purpose, telling them that the blueprints for an old water main line had been lost and that they were searching for the water main. With this explanation the workers were happy to return to their job. It is obvious that the supervisor could have saved himself some trouble had he explained the reason for the job in the beginning. As each hole was dug, the workers could have searched for the water main themselves and the supervisor could have avoided the inspection of these holes.

However, this story should not blind us to the fact that sometimes a supervisor in his desire to explain can overdo a good thing and instead of clarifying he offers so much information that ultimately the subordinate is utterly confused. Explanations should include only enough to give the subordinate background without confusing him. If the directive involves a very minor activity and if not much time is available, the explanation will probably be very brief. The supervisor, of course, must use his own judgment in deciding how far he will go in explaining the reasons why. He will take into consideration such factors as the capacity of the subordinate to understand, the training he has had, the content of the directive, his own underlying managerial attitude, as well as the time available. After evaluating these factors, he will be in a better position to decide what constitutes an adequate explanation.

General or Loose Supervision Does Not Mean "No Supervision." It should be recalled that general supervision is not the same as no supervision at all. General supervision requires that the employee be given a definite assignment. But this assignment is definite only to the extent that the employee understands the results expected of him. It is not definite regarding the specific instructions which tell him precisely how the results are to be achieved. General supervision does not mean that the subordinate can set his own standards. Rather, the supervisor will set the standards, but he will make them realistic, high enough so that they represent a challenge, yet not higher than can possibly be achieved. Although general supervision excludes direct pressure, employees know that their efforts are being measured against these standards and this thought alone should lead them to work harder. By setting the standards reasonably high, the general supervisor does apply a degree of pressure. But this kind of pressure is quite different from the pressure exerted by "breathing down some-one's neck."

General supervision requires a continuous effort on the supervisor's part to develop the potential of his employees. Everyone knows that active learning is more effective than passive learning. Employees learn more easily when they work out a solution for themselves, than if they are given the solution. It is a known fact that employees learn best from their own mistakes. In general supervision, the supervisor spends considerable time teaching his employees how to solve problems and how to make decisions as problems arise in their work situation. Continuous training of employees is an absolute necessity in general supervision. The better trained the employees become in basic problem-solving methods, the less need there will be for supervision. In fact, one way to judge the effectiveness of a supervisor is to see how the employees in his department function when he is away from the job.

General supervision, however, is a way of life which must be practiced over a period of time and the supervisor cannot expect instantaneous results if he introduces general supervision into a situation where the employees have been accustomed to close supervision. It will take time before the results can be seen. The general supervisor is just as much interested in results as any other kind of supervisor. But he is also interested in the individual development of his employees which differentiates him from the autocratic and close supervisor.

Although the supervisor may be a firm believer in general supervision and will practice it wherever he can, this does not mean that from time to time under certain conditions he must not show his firmness, fortitude, and decisiveness. There may be occasions and there may be certain employees who just do not seem to thrive under this kind of loose, general supervision and who are in need of a closer type of supervision. This, however, should be the exception and not the rule. Although general supervision is *not a cure-all* for every problem, all research studies seem to indicate that it is more effective than close supervision in terms of productivity, morale, and achievements. General supervision permits the employee to acquire pride in his work and in the results which he has achieved. It helps develop his talent and capability. It permits the supervisor to spend less time with his employees and more time on the over-all management of the department. General supervision provides the motivation for the employee to work on his job with enthusiasm and energy, thus deriving full satisfaction from his work.

INFLUENCING AND THE INTRODUCTION OF CHANGE

The supervisor's influencing function is extremely important whenever he is faced with the introduction of a change. Since every enterprise operates in a larger context and since the environment is of a dynamic nature, change is to be expected as a part of everyday life. As a matter of fact, the growth of most undertakings depends largely upon the concept of change.

We all know that the speed with which changes are occuring has increased greatly in the last few decades, particularly in the field of health care services. And there is little doubt that most of these changes have been very beneficial. Hospital floors are filled with patients benefiting from one new technique or another. Indeed, the health care center as a social system produces an ever shifting equilibrium of forces due to the amazing advances in medical sciences and technologies. The supervisor's own department is a small social subsystem, interdependent with the larger system of the health care center. Any change imposed from without is likely to shift the equilibrium of forces within each individual department as well as within the organization as a whole.

Moreover, it is the departmental supervisor who finds himself in the forefront of change as he is the one who in the daily working situation has to facilitate its introduction in order to make it a reality. The supervisor must "sell" the idea of change to his subordinates. Most of the time he has had little to do with the decision to make the change or with its timing. It originated higher up in the administration. Hopefully, however, the supervisor understands and accepts the change as it is now his role and duty to introduce it, to explain it to his subordinates, and to feed back their reactions to his superiors. Of course, the supervisor will encounter reactions from his employees which range all the way from ready acceptance to outright rejection and hostility with varying degrees of everything in between.

Most people pride themselves on being modern and up-to-date, and most gladly accept and welcome changes in material things, whether it be a new automobile, new design of homes, clothing, or any kind of gadgets. But when it comes to changes in jobs and interpersonal relations, there is a tendency to resist them. This is unfortunate because if an enterprise is to survive, it must be able to react to the prevailing conditions by changing itself and by issuing directives which will incorporate and realize the necessary changes. However, since resistance to change is a common phenomenon, it is essential for the supervisor to learn about the causes for this resistance and what he can do to help his employees accept necessary changes.

He must not fail to realize that even a trifling change may cause deep reactions within some of the employees of his department.

Reasons for Resistance to Change

One reason for resisting change is that change disturbs the equilibrium of the current state of affairs. The assumption is that prior to the change the employee exists within an environment in which his *need satisfaction* has reached a high degree of stability, and the change may prevent or decrease the satisfaction of his needs. Therefore, it is natural that he does whatever he can to thwart the introduction of the change.

A second reason for resisting change is that any change is seen as a potential threat to the employee's *security*. He is to give up the known, familiar routine which he has mastered for something new and unpredictable. For example, new apparatus in the lab could make some of a technologist's previous skills superfluous. This could undermine his sense of occupational identity. The change may require him to upgrade his skills and he is not sure that he can master these new responsibilities. At the outset, any new ideas and methods almost always represent a threat to the security of the individuals involved in the change. Usually people fear change because they cannot assess or predict what it will bring in terms of their own position, activity, and future. It makes no difference whether the change is actually threatening or not. What matters is that the subordinate believes or assumes this.

A third reason for resistance to change is that the change may threaten the employee's *status* within the organization. He may fear that his status will be lowered and someone else's raised. Such fears have, for example, caused many new computer installations to be used less effectively than anticipated or to be slowed down in their effects on the over-all organization. This was because the "accounting boys" started to gain a different status in the organization once the computer became their domain. Its introduction caused what appeared to be threatening changes in the reporting relationships and status of numerous employees.

Often threats of an *economic* nature provide an additional reason for resistance to change. The subordinate may fear that the change will affect his job economically. Hundreds of years ago, hand weavers in the Low Countries of Europe tried to destroy mechanic looms by throwing their wooden clogs (sabots) into the machinery (sabotage) because they feared that the machines would destroy their jobs and income. The same fears still prevail today when it comes to the size of the pay check.

In general, we may say that changes affect different people in different ways. A change that causes great disturbance to one person may create little disequilibrium for another. The type and severity of reaction which occurs in a particular situation will depend upon the nature of the change and the person concerned. The important thing for the supervisor to recognize is that changes do disturb the equilibrium of the employee, and that when individuals become threatened they develop ways of behavior that serve as barriers to the thing that threatens. Therefore, it is the supervisor's duty to facilitate the inevitable process of adjustment when changes are necessary. Let us see how this can be done.

How to Facilitate Change

The supervisor should always remember that employees seldom resist change just to be stubborn. From the foregoing discussion, we learned that there are valid reasons for resistance. Subordinates resist because the change affects their equilibrium socially, psychologically, and possibly economically. However, with the proper attitude and the right techniques the supervisor can facilitate the introduction of change to a great extent.

One of the factors which is particularly important in gaining acceptance of change is the relationship that exists between the supervisor who is trying to introduce the change and the employee who is subject to the change. If a relationship of mutual confidence and trust exists between the two, the employee is much more likely to go along with the change than otherwise.

The supervisor should assume that a considerable amount of time is necessary to implement a change, that a rigid time table for change is unrealistic. The change must be planned far in advance and its impact on each position and job should be anticipated. Even if the change is well thought out and carefully planned, however, some ramifications will in all likelihood be overlooked. The supervisor must leave room to discuss and accommodate them.

Explanation

Of course, the most important aspect in facilitating the introduction of change is the supervisor's duty to *explain* the change to his employees in advance. This should begin long before the change is to be initiated. There should be ample time prior to the changeover to familiarize the employees with the idea, to allow them to think through the implications and ramifications, and by all means to ask questions for more clarification. In other words, there must be sufficient time for feedback and additional communication.

In *explaining* the change, the supervisor should put himself into his subordinates' position and discuss its *pros and cons* from their point of view. This discussion should explain what will happen and why. It should clarify the way in which the change will affect the employee and what it means to him. It should show how the change will leave him no worse off or even improve his present situation. All of this information should be communicated to the entire department, to those employees who are directly involved as well as to those who are indirectly involved. Overstatements are, however, ill-advised and it is essential to be absolutely truthful. The supervisor cannot afford a credability gap.

The supervisor must also try to *communicate* and explain to his employees all those things which the latter consciously and subconsciously wants and needs to know in order to resolve his fears. Only then can the employee assess and understand what the change would mean in terms of his own position and activity. The supervisor must help the subordinate understand the need for the change. This will be easier if the supervisor has always been concerned with setting the proper stage and giving the proper background information for all of his directives. In such a case, the employee is thoroughly acquainted with the underlying factors and he is more likely to view the change as a necessary adjustment in a dynamic environment. He might ask a few additional questions about it, but he then can quickly adapt to it and resume his previous behavior. When the subordinate has been informed of the reasons for change, he knows what to expect and why. Instead of blind resistance, there will be intelligent adaptation to the instructions, and instead of insecurity, there will be a feeling of security. In the final analysis, it is not the change itself which leads to so much misunderstanding, it is more the *manner* in which the supervisor *introduces the change*. In other words, resistance to change that comes from fear of the unknown can be minimized by supplying appropriate information.

Participation

Another effective way of reducing the resistance to change is to permit the individual or individuals involved to participate in the planning of the change. No doubt those who are affected by the change may have something to contribute since they are close to the situation and could see some aspects that management might overlook. Furthermore, playing a part in planning the change will remove most of the fears and threats which normally would be the causes for resistance.

This participation may be in the form of *consultation* whereby criticism and suggestions are sincerely solicited from the employees in connection with the comtemplated change. In face-to-face conversations, the supervisor discusses with his employees the problems, asks questions, and tries to get their ideas and reactions. Hopefully, management will then incorporate as much of this into the change as possible and the employees will consider themselves a partner in the change.

A more advanced stage of participation occurs when the supervisor lets his employees *make the decision themselves*. He defines the problem and sets the limits. But he lets his subordinates develop the alternatives and choose between them. If several employees are involved, this group decision-making is an effective means for overcoming resistance to change. Such an approach recognizes the fact that if the employees who are threatened by a change have the opportunity to work through the new ideas and methods from the beginning and can assure themselves that their needs will be satisfied in the future, they will accept the new ideas and methods as something of their own making and will give them their support. Group decision-making also makes it easier for each member of the group to carry out the decision once it is agreed upon, and the group will put strong pressure on those who have reservations or who do not want to go along.

Both kinds of participation should be encouraged as they help to facilitate the introduction of change. Of course, in trying to implement change in his department the supervisor will make use of all means available to him — persuasion, discussion, participation, and group decision-making.

SUMMARY

The influencing function of the manager is that function which forms the connecting link between planning, organizing, and staffing on one side, and controlling on the other. Issuing directives is perhaps the most important part of the influencing function because without them, nothing or at best very little would be achieved. In order to be properly carried out, there are certain prerequisites which each good directive should possess. A good directive must encompass the formula of who, what, where, when, how, and why. The directive should be accomplishable, intelligible, properly phrased, and compatible with the objectives of the enterprise. In addition to this a reasonable amount of time should be permitted for its completion.

In issuing directives, the supervisor may employ two major techniques: the autocratic technique which brings about close supervision, or the participative, democratic, permissive kind of technique usually called consultative or general supervision. There are certain occasions, certain employees, and certain conditions under which the autocratic technique is probably the more effective one; but for most situations it is far better for a supervisor to apply consultative, participative techniques in order to produce the highest motivation and morale among the employees. This means that in the case of new assignments the supervisor will consult with his employees as to how the job should best be done. He will elicit their contributions to the decision. In those directives which are primarily concerned with routine assignments and the daily performance of the job, the supervisor will employ a form of general supervision instead of close supervision.

In so doing, he gives his employees the freedom to make decisions themselves on how the job is to be done, after he has set the goals and standards which they are to achieve. This also gives employees the freedom to use their own ingenuity and judgment, and experiences of this type offer continuous ground for further training and improvement. In addition, it motivates the employees to the extent that they find satisfaction in their jobs. All indications are that general supervision produces better results than close supervision.

Since the health care field is of a dynamic nature necessitating continuous and often substantial changes, the supervisor is confronted with the problem of how to introduce change. In order to successfully cope with the average employees' normal resistance to change, the supervisor must know the social, psychological, and economic reasons for this resistance. Then he can explain and interpret the change in a manner which will seek to overcome his subordinates' fear of it. He can also allow his subordinates to participate in planning for the change. In the final analysis, the supervisor is in the front line and it is up to him to accommodate change and to make it become reality.

CHAPTER 20

Positive Discipline

Good influencing and maintaining positive discipline go hand in hand. The word discipline is used in many connections and understood in several different ways. When one hears the word discipline, one is often inclined to think immediately of the use of authority or force. To many, discipline carries the disagreeable connotation of the need for punishment. However, there is another way of considering the matter of discipline, a way which is far more in keeping with what we have been saying about good management practices.

THE NATURE OF ORGANIZATIONAL DISCIPLINE

For our purposes, discipline can be thought of as a state of affairs — as a condition in an enterprise in which there is orderliness, in which the members of the enterprise behave themselves sensibly and conduct themselves according to the standards of acceptable behavior as expressed by the needs of the organization. Discipline is said to be good when the employees willingly practice self-discipline, willingly follow the rules of the enterprise. Discipline is said to be bad when subordinates either do this reluctantly or actually disobey regulations and violate the standards of acceptable behavior.

Discipline and Morale

Discipline is not the same as morale. Morale, as discussed before, is an attitude, a state of mind, whereas discipline is a state of affairs. But the level of morale significantly influences the problems of discipline. Normally, it can be expected that there will be fewer problems of discipline whenever the morale is high. By the same token, low morale brings about increased problems of discipline. Yet it is also conceivable that there could be a high degree of discipline in spite of a low level of morale. Under these conditions, discipline would probably be controlled by fear and sheer force. On the other hand, however, it is usually not possible to maintain a high level of morale unless there is also a high degree of discipline.

Self-Discipline

The best discipline, as we said, is self-discipline. By this we mean the normal human tendency to do what needs to be done and to do one's share, to do the right thing, and to subordinate some of one's own needs and desires to the standards of acceptable behavior set for the enterprise as a whole. Experience shows that most employees want to do the right thing. Even before they start to work, most mature persons accept the idea that following instructions and fair rules of conduct is a normal responsibility which goes with any job. Thus, most employees can be counted on to exercise a considerable degree of self-discipline. They believe in coming to work on time, in following the supervisor's instructions, in signing the time sheet, in refraining from fights, drinking at work, or stealing, and so on. In other words, such self-imposed discipline involves conformity with the rules, regulations, and orders which are necessary for the proper conduct of the institution.

Once the employees know what is expected of them and feel that the rules by which they are governed are reasonable, they usually will observe them without problems. Of course, from time to time the supervisor must ask himself whether some of these rules and regulations are still reasonable. Times are changing and certain rules that were once reasonable are no longer considered to be so. For example, the dress codes and codes of general appearance have most certainly undergone changes in the past decade. It would be unreasonable to request subordinates to comply with a dress and appearance code set up years ago.

When new rules are introduced, however, the supervisor must make it his business to show their current reasonableness and need to the employees. For instance, women's fashion may dictate a style such as miniskirts which is not conducive to a nurse's appearance on the job. But instead of simply outlawing miniskirts, a rule giving nurses their choice between wearing a certain length of hemline, wearing culottes, or wearing uniforms with long pants might be considered a more reasonable dress code. Or let us take another example, that of the operating room supervisor faced with the new trend toward long hair and facial hair. Realizing that hair is known to be a danger to asepsis, this supervisor together with possibly the chief of surgery, the infection committee, and the director of nursing might work out a rule which will make a hood or helmet-type covering mandatory for operating room personnel. Heretofore, there was no need for such a device, but old rules do not provide the necessary protection any longer. In other words, the supervisor must be alert to changing styles and mores and he must make certain that the rules and regulations truly respect them; otherwise, he will have a great many disciplinary problems which need not arise.

Of course, a strong sense of self-imposed discipline on the employees' part will exert group pressure on any possible wrongdoer, thus further reducing the need for disciplinary action on the supervisor's part. The employee knows that he will have the unqualified support of his supervisor as long as he stays within the ordinary rules of conduct and as long as his activities are consistent with what is expected of him. Proper discipline makes it necessary for the supervisor to give positive support to the right action, and also criticize and punish the wrong action. The subordinate must know that failure to live up to what is expected of him will result in "punishment."

However, the administration cannot expect its employees to practice self-discipline unless self-discipline starts at the top. Similar restrictions must be imposed upon all managerial personnel to remain within the acceptable patterns of behavior. For example, supervisors cannot expect their workers to impose self-discipline if they themselves do not show it. Proper conduct with respect to the needs of the organization requires the supervisor also to comply with the necessity to be on time, to observe "no smoking" and "no drinking" rules, and to dress and to behave in a manner commensurate with his activities.

Maintaining Positive Discipline

Although the vast majority of employees will exercise a considerable degree of self-discipline, there are unfortunately a few employees in every large organization who for some reason or other occasionally fail to observe established rules and standards even after having been informed of them. There are some employees who simply will not accept the responsibility of self-discipline. Since the job must go on, however, the supervisor cannot afford to let those few "get away with" violations. Firm action is called for to correct the situation. Unless such action is taken, the morale of the other employees in the work group will be seriously weakened. This is the time when the supervisor has to rely on the authority inherent in his position even though he may dislike doing so. On such an occasion, the supervisor must clearly realize the fact that he is in charge of the department, that he is responsible for discipline within it. If the supervisor does not correct the situation, it may encourage some individuals who are merely on the borderline of being undisciplined to follow the bad example. When a defect in discipline becomes apparent, it is the supervisor's responsibility to take proper action firmly and, of course, wisely.

The Purpose of Discipline

Discipline is not for the purpose of "getting even" with an employee. Rather, its purpose is improvement of the employee's future behavior. It corrects the subordinate's breach of the rules and tells him there would be more serious consequences in the future. Discipline, of course, also serves to warn the other people in the department. It reminds the disciplined individual's co-workers that rules exist and that violating them does not go unnoticed or without any action from the supervisor. Moreover, discipline reassures all those employees who respect the rules out of their desire to do the right thing. Its primary purpose most certainly is not punishment or retribution.

Indeed, the supervisor should administer discipline so that it motivates rather than demotivates. In other words, he must exercise positive discipline. This is not an easy task, however, since inherently the act of punishing a subordinate for violating a rule always presupposes that he was caught violating it. Yet there are many others who may have done the same thing but who go free, so to speak, because the supervisor did not catch them. This invariably injects a note of unfairness into the disciplinary process. Another reason that it is difficult to administer positive discipline is because any discipline is normally resented and it may damage the relationship between the supervisor and his subordinate. Sometimes all it does is make the subordinate double his efforts not to be caught again. Nevertheless, positive discipline can generally be successful if the supervisor follows a few simple rules when taking disciplinary action.

TAKING DISCIPLINARY ACTION

Do Not Shirk Responsibility

Normally, a good supervisor will not have too much occasion to take disciplinary action. But whenever it becomes necessary, it is the supervisor's job to do so.* The supervisor is best qualified to know the employee, the alleged violations, and the circumstances. Since he is the manager in charge of the department, he has the authority and responsibility to take appropriate action. Although it may be expedient for the moment to let the personnel director handle unpleasant problems of this type, the supervisor would be shirking his responsibility and abdicating and undermining his own position if he allowed this.

The same thing would happen if the supervisor were to ignore or to conveniently overlook for any length of time a subordinate's failure to meet the prescribed standards of conduct. If he condones such breaches, the supervisor is merely communicating to the rest of the employees the fact that he does not intend to enforce the rules and regulations. Thus, he must not procrastinate in administering discipline. On the other hand, the supervisor must caution himself against

---

*In all of our discussions it is assumed that the employees of the department do not belong to a union, and therefore no contractual obligations restrict the supervisor's authority in the realm of disciplinary action.

haste or unwarranted action. Before he does anything, it is necessary for him to investigate what has happened and why. In addition, he should check the employee's past record and all other pertinent information he can easily obtain before he takes any action.

Do Not Lose Temper

Whenever taking disciplinary action, the supervisor must also continuously caution himself not to lose his temper. Regardless of the severity of the violation the supervisor must not permit himself to lose control of the situation, thus running the risk of losing the respect of his employees. This does not mean that he should face the situation half-heartedly or haphazardly. But if the supervisor should feel that he is in danger of losing control of his emotions he should, by all means, avoid action until he has cooled down. Even if the violation is significant, the supervisor cannot afford to lose his temper. Moreover, the supervisor should follow the general rule of never laying a hand on an employee in any way. Except for emergencies where an employee has been injured or becomes ill, or where he needs to separate employees who are fighting, such a gesture could easily make matters worse.

Discipline in Private

The supervisor must make certain that all disciplinary action takes place between himself and the employee involved as a private matter. It most certainly should never be done in public. A public reprimand builds up resentment in the employee being reprimanded, and it may permit unrelated factors to enter the situation. For instance, if in the opinion of the other workers, a disciplinary action is too severe for the violation, the disciplined employee would appear as a martyr to the rest of them. If the supervisor is disciplining in public, he is bound to have his performance judged by every other employee in the department. It is possible that the employees may not agree with the facts on which the supervisor is basing his disciplinary action. Before he knows it he will be arguing with the other employees over what happened, and it is likely that varying eyewitness reports will only confuse the situation. In addition to this, of course, public discipline would humiliate the disciplined employee in the eyes of his co-workers and would cause considerable damage to the entire department. Therefore, privacy in taking disciplinary action must be the rule.

TYPES OF DISCIPLINARY ACTION

The question of the type of disciplinary action is answered differently in different enterprises. But in recent years many enterprises have accepted the idea of a progressive discipline which provides for an increase in the penalty with each "offense." Unless a serious wrong has been committed, the employee would rarely be discharged for the first offense. Rather, a series of progressive steps of disciplinary action would be taken. The steps presented below are merely suggested; they are not the only means of disciplinary action nor are they necessarily in their proper order. But many enterprises have found the majority of these steps to be quite workable: 1) informal talk; 2) oral warning or reprimand; 3) written or official warning; 4) disciplinary layoff; 5) demotional downgrading or transfer; 6) discharge.

The Informal Talk

If the incident is of a minor nature and if the employee is one whose record has no previous marks of disciplinary action, an informal, friendly talk will clear up the situation in many cases. In such a talk, the supervisor will discuss with the employee his behavior in relation to the standards which prevail within the enterprise. He will try to get to the underlying reason for the undesirable behavior. At the same time, he will try to reaffirm the employee's sense of responsibility and re-establish his previous cooperative relationship within the department. It may also be advisable to repeat once more why the action of the employee is undesirable and what it may possibly lead to. If the supervisor later finds that this friendly talk was not sufficient to bring about the desired results, then it will become necessary for him to take the next step, namely, that of an oral warning.

Oral Warning or Reprimand

In this interview between the employee and the supervisor, it should again be pointed out how undesirable the subordinate's violation is and how it could ultimately lead to more severe disciplinary action. Naturally, such an interview will have emotional overtones since the subordinate is likely to be resentful for having been caught again and the supervisor may also be angry. The violation should be discussed in a straightforward statement of fact, however, and the supervisor should not begin with a recital of how the fine reputation of the employee has now been "tarnished." Neither should the supervisor be apolegetic, but he should state his case in specific terms and then give the subordinate a chance to tell his side of the story.

The supervisor should also stress the preventive purpose of discipline by his manner and words but, nevertheless, he must put the employee on notice that such conduct cannot be tolerated. In some enterprises, a record is made on the employee's papers that this oral warning has taken place. Of course, the purpose of the warning is to help the employee correct his behavior and to prevent the need for further disciplinary action. The warning should leave the employee with a confident feeling that he can do better and will improve in the future. Some supervisors may feel that such an oral reprimand is not very effective. However, if it is carried out skillfully, many employees will be straightened out at this stage.

Written or Official Warning

A written warning is of a formal nature insofar as it becomes a part of the employee's record. Written warnings are particularly necessary in unionized situations so that the document can serve as evidence in case of grievance procedures. The written warning, of which the employee receives a duplicate, must contain a statement of the violation and the potential consequences. Another duplicate of the warning is also sent to the personnel department so that it can be inserted in the permanent record.

Disciplinary Layoffs

This penalty would be next in line in cases where the employee has continued his offense and where all previous steps were of no avail. Under such conditions, the supervisor must determine what length of penalty would be appropriate. This, of course, will depend on how serious the offense is and how many times it has been repeated. Usually, disciplinary layoffs extend over several days or weeks. Seldom are they more than a few weeks, however.

Some employees may not be very impressed with oral or written warnings, but they will find such a disciplinary layoff without pay a rude awakening and they will be convinced that the institution is really serious. A disciplinary layoff may bring back a sense of compliance with rules and regulations. There are, however, a number of disadvantages to invoking a disciplinary layoff, and some enterprises do not apply this measure at all. They reason that they are hurting their own productivity by laying off one of their trained employees, especially in times of labor shortages when they will not be able to replace him with someone who is just as skilled. It is also felt that the employee might return from his layoff in a much more unpleasant frame of mind than when he left. Therefore, quite a few institutions are no longer using disciplinary layoffs; instead they move on to discharge.

Demotional Downgrading

This is another disciplinary measure the usefulness of which is seriously questioned. To demote for disciplinary reasons to a lesser paying job is likely to bring about dissatisfaction and discouragement. As a matter of fact, to lose pay over an extended period of time is a form of constant punishment. The dissatisfaction which results may easily spread to other employees in the department. For this reason, many enterprises avoid downgrading as a disciplinary measure just as they avoid layoffs. If so, they will have to use termination of employment as the ultimate penalty in serious cases.

Discharge

Discharge is the most drastic form of disciplinary action, and it should be reserved exclusively for the most serious offenses. Supervisors should resort to it infrequently and only after some of the preliminary steps have been taken. Of course, when a very serious wrong has been committed, discharge should be invoked at once. For instance, when a nurse is caught stealing narcotics immediate discharge is in order and necessary. Even for lesser offenses, there are hospitals where the supervisor goes through the steps of friendly and more formal oral and written reprimands, and then points out that the next measure would be discharge without any further discussion. There is no intermediate penalty such as a three-day disciplinary layoff which could hurt the superior-subordinate relationship. Discharge is the only step left in this scheme.

For the employee, discharge eliminates all the seniority standing he may have had and makes it difficult for him to obtain new employment. As far as the enterprise is concerned, discharges involve serious losses and waste, including the expense of training a new employee and the expense of the disruption caused by changing the makeup of the work team. Discharge may also cause damage to the morale of the group. Because of these serious consequences of discharge, some enterprises, especially those in unionized settings, have reserved the right of discharge for higher management and have taken it away from the supervisor. In unionized situations, management is concerned with possible prolonged arbitration procedures, knowing full well that arbitrators have become increasingly unwilling to permit discharge except for the most severe violations. Of course, there may be cases where there is no other answer but to fire the employee for "just cause." But these cases will be the exception and not the rule.

Time Element

In all of the disciplinary steps that we have just discussed, the time element is of significance. In other words, it is important to decide how long the breaking of a rule should be held against an employee. Current practice is inclined to disregard offenses which have been committed more than a year ago. Therefore, an employee with a poor record on account of tardiness would start a new life if he maintained a good record for one year or maybe even for six months. This time element, of course, will vary depending upon the nature of the violation. If an employee should be brandishing a loaded gun in a heated argument during work, there is no need to worry about any time element or previous offenses. This is enough to warrant immediate discharge!

THE SUPERVISOR'S QUANDARY

In spite of all the restraint and wisdom with which the supervisor takes disciplinary action, it still puts him in a sensitive position. It is very difficult to impose discipline without generating resentment because disciplinary action is by nature an unpleasant experience. The question therefore arises as to how the supervisor can apply the necessary disciplinary action so that it will be the least resented.

The "Hot Stove" Approach

To help answer this question, Douglas McGregor refers to what he calls "the hot stove rule" and draws a comparison between touching a hot stove and experiencing discipline.* When one touches a hot stove, the resulting discipline has four characteristics: it is immediate, with warning, consistent, and impersonal. First, the burn was immediate, and there was no question of the cause and effect. Second, there was a warning. Everyone knows what happens if he touches a hot stove, especially if the stove is red hot. Third, the discipline is consistent. Every time one touches a hot stove, one is burned. Fourth, the discipline is impersonal. Whoever touches the hot stove is burned. He is burned because of what he does, because he touched the hot stove, not because of who he is.

This comparison illustrates the fact that the act and the discipline are almost one. The discipline takes place because the person did something, because he committed a particular act. The discipline is directed against the act and not against the person. Following the four basic rules expressed in this "hot stove" approach will help the supervisor take the sting out of many disciplinary actions. It enables him to achieve positive discipline while at the same time to generate in the employee the least amount of resentment toward punishment.

Immediacy

The supervisor must not procrastinate in administering discipline. A prompt beginning of the disciplinary process is necessary as soon as possible after the supervisor notices the violation. The sooner the discipline is invoked, the more automatic it will seem and the closer the connection with the offensive act. Of course, as we have already said the supervisor should refrain from taking hasty action, and enough time should elapse for tempers to cool and for the assembling of all necessary facts.

There are instances when it is apparent that the employee is guilty of a violation although the full circumstances may not be known. Here the need for disciplinary action is unquestionable, but there is some doubt as to the amount of penalty. In such cases, the

*As cited in George Strauss and Leonard R. Sayles, *Personnel, The Human Problems of Management,* 2nd ed., (Englewood Cliffs, New Jersey: Prentice-Hall, Inc., 1967), pp. 311-320.

supervisor should tell the employee that he realizes what went on, but that he will need some time to reach his conclusions. There are other cases, however, when the nature of the incident makes it necessary to get the offender off the premises quickly. Some immediate action is required even if there is not yet enough evidence to make a final decision in the case.

Temporary Suspension. To solve this dilemma, many enterprises invoke what is called "temporary suspension": the employee is suspended pending final decision in the case. This device of suspension protects management as well as the employee. It gives management a chance to make the necessary investigation and it provides an opportunity for tempers to cool off. In cases of temporary suspension, the employee is told that he is "suspended" and that he will be informed as soon as possible of the disciplinary action that will be taken. The suspension, in itself, is not a punishment. If the investigation shows that there is no cause for disciplinary action, the employee has no grievance since he is recalled and he will not have suffered any loss of pay. If, on the other hand, a penalty is decided upon and if this penalty should be a disciplinary layoff, then the time during which the employee was suspended will constitute part of whatever layoff is assessed. The obvious advantage of this device of suspension is that the supervisor can act promptly without any prejudice to the employee. Nevertheless, the suspension method of disciplinary action should not be used indiscriminately.

Advance Warning

In order to have good discipline and to have the employees accept disciplinary action as fair, it is absolutely essential that all employees be clearly informed in advance as to what is expected of them and what the rules are. There must be warning that a certain offense will lead to disciplinary action. Some enterprises rely upon bulletin board announcements to make such warnings. But these cannot be as effective as a section in the employee handbook which every new employee receives whenever he starts working for the institution. Along with the written statements in the handbook, it is advisable to include oral clarification of the rules. During the induction process shortly after a new employee is hired, he should be orally informed of what is expected of him and of the consequences of not living up to behavioral expectations.

In addition to the forewarning about general rules, it is essential to let the employees know in advance about the kind of disciplinary action that will be taken. It is necessary to clarify the various steps of disciplinary action to which employees would become subject *before* they could possibly become involved in an offense. There are considerable doubts, however, as to whether or not a standard penalty should be provided and stated for each offense. In other words, should there be, for example, a clear statement that falsifying attendance records will carry a one week disciplinary layoff? Those in favor of such a list suggest that it would be an effective warning device and that it would provide greater disciplinary consistency. But such a list would not permit management to take into consideration the various degrees of guilt and the circumstances. In general, it is probably best not to provide a list with standard penalties for specific violations, but merely to state the progressive steps of disciplinary action which will be taken in an orderly sequence. It should be clearly understood that continued violations will bring about more severe penalties. There are some enterprises which do specify that certain offenses such as drinking liquor on the premises or fighting will bring the penalty of immediate discharge. But for most violations it is unwise to spell out a rigid set of disciplinary measures.

The practice of forewarning before taking disciplinary measures also applies to rules which have not been enforced lately. If the supervisor has not disciplined anyone who violated them for a long time, the employees do not expect these rules to be enforced in the future. Suddenly the supervisor may decide that in order to make a rule valid he is going to make "an example of one of the employees" and take disciplinary action. Of course, he should not do it in this manner. The fact that a certain rule has not been enforced in the past does not mean that it cannot ever be enforced. What it does mean is that the supervisor must take certain steps before he can begin to enforce such a rule. Instead of acting tough suddenly, he should give his employees some warning that this rule, enforcement of which has heretofore been lax, will be strictly enforced in the future. In such cases, it is not enough to put the enforcement notice on the bulletin board. It is essential that in addition to a clear written warning, supplemental oral communication be given. The supervisor must explain to his subordinates, perhaps in a departmental meeting, that from the present time on he intends to enforce this rule.

Consistency

A further requirement of good discipline is that it must be consistent. The supervisor must be consistent in the enforcement of discipline and in the type of disciplinary action he takes. By being consistent, he sets the limit for acceptable behavior, and every individual wants to know what the limits are. To be inconsistent, on the other hand, is one of the fastest ways for a supervisor to lower the morale of his employees and to lose their respect. If the supervisor is inconsistent, then the employee finds himself in an environment in which he cannot feel secure. Inconsistency will only lead to anxiety, creating doubts in the employee's mind as to what he can and cannot do. At times, the supervisor may feel inclined to be lenient and to overlook an infringement. In reality, however, he is not doing the employee any favor. He is only making it harder for him and for the others.

Mason Haire, a well known psychologist, compares this situation to the relations between a motorist and a traffic policeman.* He says that whenever we are exceeding the speed limit on the highway, we must feel some sort of anxiety since we are breaking the rule. On the other hand, the rule is often not enforced. We think that perhaps this is a place where the police department does not take the rule seriously and we can speed a little. But there is always the lurking insecurity because the motorist knows that at any time the policeman decides to enforce the rule, he can do so. Most motorists probably feel that it would be easier to operate in an environment where the police would at least be consistent one way or the other. The same holds true for most employees who have to work in an environment where the supervisor is not consistent in his disciplinary activities.

Of course, at times extenuating circumstances may make it very difficult for the supervisor to exercise consistent discipline. There are occasions when the department is particularly rushed with a large amount of work, and the supervisor may be induced to overlook infringements because he does not want to upset the work force or he is afraid that if he has to suspend someone he will lose a valuable employee at a critical time. The same kind of consideration may apply whenever it is difficult to get an employee with a certain skill and the offending employee possesses that skill.

In addition to this, the supervisor faces another problem in trying to be consistent. On the one hand, he has been continuously cautioned to treat all of his employees alike and to avoid favoritism, while on the other hand he has been told again and again to treat people as individuals in accordance with their special needs and situations. On the surface, these two requirements appear to contradict each other and to make it impossible to always apply consistent discipline. But the supervisor must realize that treating people fairly does not mean treating everyone in exactly the same manner. What it does mean is that when an exception is made, it must be considered as a valid exception by the other members of the department. The rest of the employees will regard an exception as fair if they know why it was made and if they consider the reason to be justified. Moreover, the rest of the employees must be confident that if any other employee were in the same situation he would receive the same treatment. If these conditions are fulfilled, the supervisor has been able to exercise fair play, to be consistent in his discipline, and still treat people as individuals.

The extent to which a supervisor can be consistent and yet consider the individual's situation is illustrated as follows: Assume that

*Mason Haire, *Psychology in Management,* 2nd ed. (New York: McGraw-Hill Book Company, 1964), p. 74.

three employees were engaged in some kind of horseplay. It could very well be that the supervisor will merely have a friendly, informal talk with one of the employees since he just started work a few days ago. The second employee may receive a formal or written warning since he had been warned about horseplay before. And it is conceivable that the third employee would receive a three-day disciplinary layoff since he had been involved in many previous cases of horseplay. Each case must be considered on its own merit and each employee must be judged according to his background, personal history, length of service, and other factors of this type. Of course, if two of the employees had been in the same situation with the same amount of previous warnings, then their penalty would also have to be identical. In this respect, then, consistency must prevail.

Being Impersonal

Another way that a supervisor can reduce the amount of resentment and keep the damage to his future relations with his subordinates at a minimum is to take disciplinary action on as impersonal a basis as possible. In recalling the "hot stove" rule, it is worth repeating that whoever touches the stove is burned regardless of who he is. The penalty is connected with the act and not with the person. Looking at disciplinary action in this way reduces the danger to the personal relationship between the supervisor and his employee. It is the specific act which brings about the disciplinary measure, not the personality.

Keeping this in mind, the supervisor will be able to discuss the violation in an objective manner, excluding the personal element as far as possible. The supervisor should take disciplinary action without being apologetic about the rule or what he has to do to enforce it and without a sign of anger. Once the disciplinary action has been taken, the supervisor must let bygones be bygones. He must treat the employee as he always has treated him before and he must try to forget about what happened. However, the supervisor and the employee may feel like avoiding each other for a few days afterwards. Such feelings are understandable, but it would be far more advisable for the boss to lean over backward to find some opportunity to show his old friendly feelings toward the disciplined employee as a person. This, of course, is easier said than done. Only the mature person can handle discipline without hostility or guilt. But, as we have said, these feelings can be minimized by following the "hot stove" approach and by practicing positive discipline.

AVENUES OF APPEAL

In every human organization, it is always possible that an individual in a position of authority might treat a subordinate unjustly. Thus, there must be a system to right such wrongs, there must be a system of corrective justice in every enterprise which is concerned with maintaining a healthy organizational climate. There must be a system for grievances which will enable employees to obtain satisfaction for unjust treatment.

Everyone is familiar with the various steps of the grievance procedure to which each employee has access if he belongs to a union. But this right of appeal should also exist in an enterprise which does not have a union. It must be possible for any employee to appeal his supervisor's decision in regard to disciplinary action. Following the chain of command, the immediate supervisor's boss would be the one to whom such an appeal would be directed. Many health care centers have provided for just this type of appeal procedure.

But great care must be taken that the right of appeal is a real right and not merely a formality. There are supervisors who will gladly tell their subordinates that they can go to the next higher boss, but who will never forgive them if they do. Statements and thinking of this type merely indicate the supervisor's own insecurity in his managerial position. As a superior, he must permit the employee to take an appeal to his boss without any resentment. It is management's obligation to provide such an appeal procedure, and the supervisor must not feel slighted in his role as manager or as leader of his department when it is used. Indeed, it is very likely that management's failure to provide an appeal procedure is one of the chief reasons why employees take recourse to unionization.

There is no doubt, however, that it requires a mature supervisor not to see some threat to his position from appeals which go over his head. Such a situation should be handled very tactfully by the supervisor's boss. It is possible that in the course of an appeal the disciplinary penalty imposed by the supervisor may be reduced or completely removed. It is understandable that under these circumstances the supervisor may become discouraged since his boss has not backed him up. This usually happens in situations where there remains doubt as to the actual events and where the boss cannot get two stories to coincide. In such cases, the "guilty" employee normally goes free. Although this is unfortunate, it is preferable that in a few instances a guilty employee go free instead of an innocent employee being punished.

Another reason for the reversal of a decision by higher level management is that the supervisor may have been inconsistent in his exercise of discipline or he may not have obtained all the necessary facts before he imposed a disciplinary action. In order to avoid such an unpleasant situation, it is necessary for the supervisor to adhere closely to all that has been said in this chapter about the exercise of positive discipline. If a supervisor is a wise disciplinarian, he will normally find his verdict upheld by his boss. And even if it should be reversed, this is still not too high a price to pay in order to guarantee justice to every employee.Without justice, of course, a good organizational climate cannot exist and the influencing function cannot be performed satisfactorily.

SUMMARY

Discipline is a state of affairs. It is likely that if morale is high, discipline will be good and less need will exist for the supervisor to take disciplinary action. A supervisor is entitled to assume that most of his employees want to do the right thing and that much of the discipline will be self-imposed — imposed by the employees upon themselves. However, if the occasion should arise, it is essential for the supervisor to know how to take disciplinary action himself. There is usually a progressive list of disciplinary measures leading all the way from an informal talk or an oral warning to "capital punishment," namely discharge. The supervisor should bear in mind that the purpose of such disciplinary measures is not retribution or humiliation of employees. Rather, the goal of disciplinary action is the improvement of the future behavior of the subordinate in question and of the other members of the organization. The idea is to avoid similar violations in the future. Nevertheless, taking disciplinary action is a painful experience not only for the employee but also for the supervisor. In order to do the best possible job, the supervisor must see to it that all disciplinary action fulfills the requirement of immediacy, forewarning, consistency, and it must be impersonal in nature. Moreover, the need for a good organizational climate makes it mandatory that a system of corrective justice exist whereby a subordinate can appeal any disciplinary action which he feels is unfair.

PART SEVEN

Controlling

CHAPTER 21

Basic Control Requirements

Controlling is the process which checks performance against standards. It makes sure that the organizational and departmental goals and objectives are achieved. The controlling function is closely related to the other four managerial functions, but it is most closely related to the planning function. When the manager plans goals, objectives, policies and so on are set and become standards against which performance is checked and appraised. If deviations are found, the manager has to take corrective action and such action may very well entail new plans and new standards. This is how planning decisions affect controls and how control decisions affect plans. This again illustrates the circular nature of the entire management process.

THE NATURE OF CONTROLLING

Control and the Other Managerial Functions

The fact that our discussion of controlling comes last in this book — just as in all other textbooks — leads many readers to believe that controlling is something that the manager does only *after* he has done everything else. In other words, it conveys the general impression that controlling is concerned *only* with events *after the fact*. This impression is reinforced by practical considerations, for example, faulty workmanship in a product is usually not discovered until after the mistake was made. In spite of such considerations, however, it is much more appropriate to look at controlling as something that goes on *simultaneously* with the other functions. Although the relationship between planning and controlling is particularly close, controlling is interwoven with *all* managerial functions. The better the manager plans, organizes, staffs, and influences, the better can he perform his controlling function and vice versa. As we have said, there is a circular relationship among all of these functions and their interrelatedness does not permanently place any one function first or last.

Of course, a supervisor cannot expect to have good control over his department unless he follows sound managerial principles in persuing his other duties. Well made plans, workable policies and procedures, a properly planned organization, appropriate delegation of authority, continuous training of employees, good instructions, and good supervision all play a significant role in the department's results. Naturally, the better these requirements are fulfilled, the easier will be the supervisor's function of controlling and the less the need for taking corrective action.

Control is Forward-Looking

To a large degree, controlling is a forward-looking function; it has *anticipatory* aspects. That is, management is concerned with controls which anticipate potential sources of deviation from standards. Past experience and the study of past events tell the supervisor what has taken place, where, when and why certain standards were not met. This enables management to make provisions so that future activities will not lead to these deviations. For example, the procedures and methods prescribed for giving medication consist of steps to prevent mistakes. There should be requirements that only one nurse gives all medications on a particular nursing unit, that she check and double check with the patient's file, that she check as to the label on the bottle, the patient's name, room, and bed number, and the time and amount of medication. She should check all of these things at least twice before she finally gives the medication. In this sense, then, controls are anticipatory. Unfortunately, the anticipatory aspect of controls is not always sufficiently stressed and much of the time we are primarily concerned with their *corrective* and *reactive* aspects. Deviations from standards are detected after they have occurred and are corrected at the point of performance, rather than anticipated.

Even if this is the case, however, the corrections will have an effect on the future. There is normally precious little the supervisor can do about the past. If, for instance, the work assigned to a subordinate for the day has not been accomplished, the controlling process cannot correct that. There are some supervisors who are inclined to scold the person responsible and assume that he was negligent and deliberate because something went wrong. But there is no use "crying over spilled milk." The wise supervisor will look forward rather than backward. However, the supervisor must study the past in order to learn what has taken place and why. This will enable him to take the proper steps to assure corrective and hopefully preventive action for the future.

Since control is forward-looking, it is essential that deviations from the established standards are discovered by the supervisor as quickly as possible. Therefore, it is the supervisor's duty to minimize the time lag between results and corrective action. For example, instead of waiting until the day is over, it would probably be more advisable for a housekeeping supervisor to check at mid-day to see whether or not the job is progressing satisfactorily. Even then, that particular morning is already past and nothing can be done about it any longer. Although this is a painful thought to the supervisor, he cannot alter the fact that sometimes effective control must take place after the event has occurred. Indeed, such control is often unavoidable. But minimizing the time lag between results and doing something about them will enable the supervisor to institute corrective action before the damage has gone too far.

The Closeness of Control

Knowing how closely to control or to follow-up the work of a subordinate is a real test of any supervisor's talents. The closeness of follow-up is based on such factors as the experience, initiative, dependability, and resourcefulness of the employee who is given the assignment. Giving an employee an assignment and allowing him to do the job is part of the process of delegation. This does not mean, however, that the supervisor should leave him completely alone until it is time to inspect the final results. Nor does it mean that the supervisor should be "breathing down his subordinate's neck" and watching every detail. Rather, the supervisor must be familiar enough with the ability of his subordinate so that he can accurately determine how much leeway to give him, how close he has to follow through with his control measures.

The Human Aspects of Controls

There is another important aspect of control and that is the *response of people* to it. In previous chapters, we had a great deal to say about work and human satisfaction; we spoke about tight versus loose supervision, delegation of authority, and on-the-job freedom in connection with motivation. Although controls are an absolute requirement in any organized activity, it must be kept in mind that in behavioral terms control means placing constraints on behavior so that what people do in organizations is more or less predictable. The amount of control will determine how much freedom of action an individual has in performing his job. Complete absence of control, however, does not maximize an individual's perception of freedom. As a matter of fact, some controls are needed to maximize human perception of freedom. The reason for this is that controls not only restrict one's own behavior, but also the behavior of others toward him.

A certain amount of control, therefore, is essential for any organizational freedom. But, neither the extreme of tight control nor complete lack of control will bring about organizational effectiveness. What is needed is a mix between these two extremes. This mixture will take into consideration the amount of decentralization in the organization, management styles, motivational factors, the situation, the professional competence of the employees, etc. In other words, in order to arrive at the most desirable mix of freedom and control, the manager must try to balance the goals of organizational effectiveness and individual satisfaction. These goals must be kept in mind whenever a manager is determining the degree of controls.

The Supervisor and Control

Control is the process of checking to determine whether or not plans and standards are being adhered to, whether or not proper progress is being made toward objectives, and acting, if necessary, to correct any deviations. The essence of control for a supervisor is mainly that action which adjusts performance to predetermined standards, if deviations from these standards occur. The supervisor is responsible for the results of his department. He must make certain that all functions within his department adhere to the established standards, and, if not, that corrective action is taken. At times, the supervisor may enlist the aid of experts within the organization for assistance in obtaining control information data, and counsel. But it would be out of order for the supervisor to expect anyone else to perform the controlling function for him.

As we have said, planning, organizing, staffing, and influencing are the preparatory steps for getting the work done. Controlling is concerned with making certain that the work is properly executed. Without controlling, the supervisor is not doing a complete job of managing. Control remains necessary whenever a supervisor assigns duties to a subordinate because the supervisor cannot shift the responsibility he has accepted from his own superior. He can and must assign tasks and delegate authority, but, as stated on many occasions, he does not delegate his responsibility. Rather, he must exercise control to see that his responsibility is properly carried out.

The supervisor knows that the eventual success of his department depends upon the degree of difference between what should be done and what is done. Having set up the standards of performance, the supervisor must keep himself informed of the actual performance through observation, reports, discussion, control charts, and other devices. It is the supervisor's job to use these tools to evaluate the difference between what should be done and what is accomplished. Only then can he prescribe the corrections necessary to bring about full compliance between the standards and the actual performance.

REQUIREMENTS OF A CONTROL SYSTEM

In order for any control system to be workable and effective it must fulfill certain basic requirements. It is necessary that the controls be understandable, that they register deviations quickly and are timely, that the system provide for appropriate, adequate, and economic control, that it is flexible to a degree, and that it point to where corrective action should be applied. These requirements are applicable to all activities in a hospital and to all levels within the management hierarchy. However, we will discuss them only in a general sense since it would be impossible to spell out the specific characteristics of controls used in each department or unit of a health care center.

Controls Must Be Understandable

The first requirement of a workable control system is that the controls must be understandable. Both the manager and the subordinates must understand what kind of control is to be exercised. This is necessary on all managerial levels. Of course, the further down in the hierarchy the system is to be applied the less complicated it must be. Thus, the top administrator may use a very complicated system of controls based on mathematical formulae and statistical charts, whereas the control system for the lower supervisory level will have to be much less sophisticated. It must be designed so that whoever is to use it will be able to understand it. If the control system given to a supervisor is too complicated, he will frequently have to devise his own more effective control system which, for all practical purposes, will fulfill the same need.

Controls Must Register Deviations Rapidly

In order to have a workable control system, controls must indicate deviations without delay. As pointed out above, controls are forward-looking and the supervisor cannot control the past. However, the sooner the supervisor is aware of such deviations, the sooner can he take corrective action. It is more desirable to have deviations reported quickly, even if substantiated only by partial information, approximate figures, and estimates. In other words, it is far better for the supervisor to have such approximate information that is prompt than to have highly accurate information that is too late to be of much value. This does not mean that the supervisor should jump to conclusions or take corrective action hastily. The supervisor's familiarity with the job to be done, his knowledge, and past experience, will come in handy in sensing quickly when something is not progressing the way it should be. For most supervisors, it is not necessary to wait until the day is over or the week is past to know whether the job will be or has been accomplished properly. His proximity to his employees should make it possible for him to observe deviations much more rapidly.

Controls Must Be Appropriate and Adequate

Controls must always be appropriate for the activity which they are to monitor. The control tools that are suitable for the dietary department are different from those used in nursing. Even within nursing the tools used by the Director of Nursing Services are different from those that the head nurse uses on the floor. The latter's controls have to be more specific and precise, whereas the former's have to be more far reaching. It is obvious that an elaborate control system which is necessary in a large undertaking would not be needed in a small department. Nevertheless, the need for control exists just the same, only the magnitude of the control system will be different. Whatever controls are applied, it is essential that they be appropriate for the job involved. Any system of control should not require more than is absolutely necessary.

Controls Must Be Economical

Controls must be worth the expenses involved; that is, they must be economical. At times, however, it may be difficult for management to ascertain how much a particular control system is worth and how much it really costs. One of the important criteria might be the consequences that would follow if the controls did not exist. Thus, the control of narcotics is very stringent and exact whereas no one is too concerned with close control of bandaids or aspirin tablets.

Controls Must Be Flexible

Since all undertakings work in a dynamic situation, unforeseen circumstances and happenings could play havoc even with the best laid plans and standards. The control system must be built so that it will remain flexible. It must be designed to keep pace with the continuously changing pattern of a dynamic setting. It must permit change as soon as the change is required or else the control system is bound to fail. If the employee seems to run into unexpected conditions early in his assignment, it is necessary for the supervisor to recognize this and to adjust the plans and standards accordingly. In other words, the supervisor must adjust the criteria by which he will check the employee's job.

Controls Must Point to Corrective Action

A final requirement of effective controls is that they must point the way to corrective action. It is not enough to show deviations as they have occurred. The system must also indicate *who* is responsible for them and *where* they have occurred. The supervisor must make it his business to know precisely where the standards were not met and who is responsible for not coming up to the standard. If successive operations are involved, then it may be necessary for the supervisor to check the performance after each and every step has been accomplished and before the work is passed on to the next employee or to another department.

SUMMARY

Controlling is that managerial function in which the manager checks performance against standards and takes corrective action if there are deviations. Control is most closely related to the planning function, but it is interwoven with all the other managerial functions as well. Control is essential in every organized activity, although in behavioral terms control means placing constraints on people. However, a good control system must be designed so that it will bring about organizational effectiveness without infringing upon individual satisfaction.

Since control is forward-looking a control system should be designed so that it reports deviations as quickly as possible. The supervisor must make sure that his subordinates fully understand the controls and that the controls he establishes are appropriate for the situation. Controls must also be worth the expense involved; in other words, they must be worth the effort put forth. It is likewise imperative that a good control system provide for sufficient flexibility in order to cope with new situations and circumstances in a dynamic setting. Last, but not least, a viable control system must clearly indicate where and why deviations have occurred so that the supervisor can take appropriate corrective action at the proper place.

CHAPTER 22

Steps in the Controlling Process

In performing his controlling function, the supervisor should follow three basic steps: first, it is necessary for the supervisor to set standards. Next, the supervisor must check performance and appraise it on the basis of these standards. In so doing, he will learn whether the performance meets the expected standards or not. If not, the supervisor must take corrective action which is the third step in the controlling process (see Figure 22-1). This sequence of steps is necessary for effective control. As a matter of fact, the supervisor cannot check and report on deviations without having set the standards in advance, and he cannot take corrective action unless he has discovered that there are deviations from these standards.

FIGURE 22-1

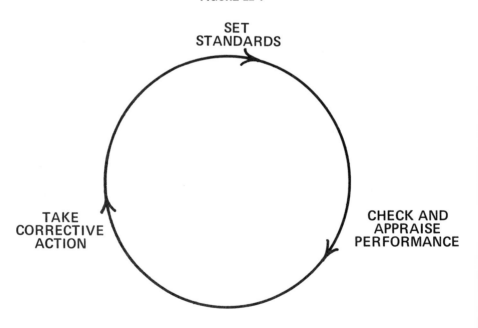

SET
STANDARDS

TAKE
CORRECTIVE
ACTION

CHECK AND
APPRAISE
PERFORMANCE

SETTING STANDARDS

Standards are criteria against which to judge results. They are closely related to, though more specific than, goals and objectives. In planning, as we know, the chief administrator sets the over-all objectives and goals that the health care center hopes to achieve. These over-all objectives are then broken down into narrower objectives for the individual departments. From these the supervisor establishes even more specific goals which relate to quality, costs, time standards, quotas, schedules, budgets, and many other measurements of detailed operations. These goals become the criteria, the standards for exercising control. Of course, those that we have just mentioned are of a tangible nature; however, there are also standards which are intangible. Although the latter are much more difficult to work with, a health care institution has to apply many intangible standards especially when it comes to patient care. Let us look at both kinds of standards in more detail.

Tangible Standards

The most common tangible standards are physical standards which pertain to the actual operation of a department where goods are produced (for instance, in the dietary department), or where services are rendered (for example, in nursing, in the laboratories, in the laundry, and so on). These standards are quantitative and qualitative. Not only do they define, for example, how much money can be spent per patient on food, supplies, and materials for three meals a day, but they also state what quality these meals are to be as far as nutritional values, taste and aesthetic appeal are concerned. Likewise, there are standards on how much one pound of laundry should cost and how many pounds are to be produced in what amount of time, taking into consideration the state of mechanization and automation of the laundry. Furthermore, the laundry will have qualitative standards as to sanitation and sterilization, standards as to "cleanliness" of the linens, as to "color," absence of "stains," and so forth. Or to take another example, there are standards which specify the number of nursing personnel on a floor in relation to the number of patients to be cared for. Such standards vary depending upon the time of the day, the particular nursing unit in question (e.g., an intensive care unit versus regular floor nursing), and many other factors. There are also standards as to the comfort of the patient, his safety, meeting his physical needs, cleanliness and orderliness of the room, and so on.

In setting all these types of standards, the supervisor is aided by his experience and by his knowledge of the various jobs to be done within his department. A supervisor has a general idea of how much time it takes to perform a certain job, how much material it requires, what constitutes a good quality of performance, and what is a poor job. Such job knowledge and experience will be one of the resources which the supervisor uses to help him establish the standards against which he judges the performance of his department.

However, there are also better, more scientific and systematic ways of establishing objective standards. In some departments, the supervisor can call on industrial engineers who will use work measurement techniques to help him determine the exact amount of work an employee should turn out within a given time period. There are many tasks in the housekeeping department, in the laundry, in the laboratories, in dispatch, in the dietary department, and even possibly in nursing where this approach is worth the effort and the cost. Standards arrived at through work measurement techniques help the supervisor distribute the work evenly and judge fairly whether an employee is performing satisfactorily. They also make it possible for the supervisor to predict the number of employees required and the probable cost of the job to be done. In many activities outside the health care field standards of this type serve as a basis for incentive plans.

The supervisor rarely conducts these work measurement techniques himself, however. As we have said, they are usually assigned to an industrial engineer or perhaps to an outside consultant trained in doing motion and time studies. Motion study involves an analysis of how the job is currently performed with a view to eliminating or combining certain steps, and devising a method which will be quicker and easier. Often flow charts are drawn up which analyze the steps taken in performing the jobs. After a thorough analysis of the motions and the work flow arrangements, the engineer will come up with what is considered the "best method" for doing the job in question. Once the "best method" has been designed, time studies are performed in order to find out the standard time required to do the job using this method.

All of this is done in a rather scientific and systematic manner by selecting an employee for observation, by measuring the times used for the various elements of the job, by applying correction factors, and by making allowances for fatigue, personal time, unavoidable delays, and so on. The combined result then leads to a standard time necessary to perform the job. Although this method sounds rather scientific, it must be kept in mind that considerable judgment and many approximations will be used to arrive at the standard time. There is still the need for decisions involving judgment and discretion. However, standard times are a sound basis on which to determine objective standards.

If the supervisor should not have the assistance of industrial engineers, he can perform some of this work himself by simply observing and timing the various operations and by making the necessary adjustments for fatigue, delay, and so on. If the job to be performed in the department has never been done there before, the supervisor should try to base his tentative standards on similar operations. If the new job has no similarity to any previous function, then the best the supervisor can do — unless he can call on the help of industrial engineers — is to observe the operation while it is being performed for the first few times. He will have to make approximate time and motion studies himself in order to arrive at a standard for the new function. Sometimes, of course, the manufacturer of a new piece of equipment can be helpful to the supervisor in providing standard data, for example, how long it will take the machine to perform a certain task, etc.

It should be kept in mind that although they may not be as scientific, the standards are more likely to be effective if they are set with the participation of the supervisor and the subordinate instead of being handed down by a staff engineer, a top manager, or an outside consultant. The purpose of any standard is to establish a specific goal for the employee to strive toward and, just as with directives, the employee is likely to be more motivated to achieve those standards which he and his boss have had some part in determining.

Intangible Standards

In addition to the tangible standards which can be expressed in physical terms, there are also standards of an intangible nature. In a hospital or related health care facility, some of the intangible standards consist of the institution's reputation in the community, the excellence of patient care or the degree of "tender loving care," including attention to the patients' psychological needs, the high morale of the employees, and so on. It is exceedingly difficult, if not impossible, to express the criteria for such intangible standards in precise and numerical terms. It is much simpler to measure performance against tangible standards, e.g., the number of nursing personnel in relation to number of patients. Nevertheless, a supervisor should not overlook the intangible achievements even if it is difficult to set standards for them and just as difficult to measure their performance. Tools for appraising some of these intangible standards are being developed in the form of attitude surveys, questionnaires, and interviews. Although these tools are not exact, they should be helpful in determining to what extent certain intangibles are being achieved.

How to Select Standards

Strategic Standards

Obviously, the number of standards which can be used to ascertain the quality of performance within a department is very large and increases rapidly as the department expands. As the operations within the department become more complex and as the functions of the departments increase, it will become more and more difficult for the supervisor to check against all the possible standards. Therefore, he will need to concentrate on certain standards by selecting some of them as the strategic ones. For example, a head nurse making the rounds knows which are the strategic points that should be checked first. She probably checks with the cardex file and makes certain that the tests and treatments are being done on time, that the physical set-up of the room is in order, that the patient is comfortable, and that he understands what is being done for him on that day. She also observes where the other nursing personnel are and what they are doing. Each of these areas constitutes a strategic point of control for the head nurse.

Unfortunately, there are no specific guides on how to select these strategic control points. The peculiarities of each departmental function and the makeup of the supervisor and the employees will be different in each situation. Thus, only very general guides can be suggested for selecting strategic standards.

Guidelines for Selection

One of the first considerations in choosing one standard as more strategic than another is *timeliness*. Since time is essential in control and since controls look to the future, as stated before, the earlier the deviation can be discovered the better. Keeping this in mind, the supervisor can determine at what point in time and process the work should be checked. For example, in the maintenance department, the strategic control point may be the time after a crack has been repaired, but before it has been repainted. In other words, timeliness may tell the supervisor to choose one standard as a stragetic control point before additional processing and performance costs are incurred.

Another consideration in choosing strategic control points is that they should permit *economic observations*. In the previous chapter, it was pointed out that any control system must be worth the expense involved, that it must be economical. Naturally, the same applies to the strategic control points which make up the system. A further consideration is that the strategic standards should provide for *comprehensive and balanced control*. The supervisor must be aware of the fact that the selection of one strategic control point might have an adverse effect on another. Excessive control on the quantity of achievements often has an adverse effect on the quality. On the other hand, if expenses are selected as a strategic control point, the quality or the quantity of the output may suffer. For instance, the laundry supervisor must not sacrifice the quality standards which have been designed to prevent infections in order to achieve his goal of so much cost per pound. All of these decisions will naturally depend upon the nature of the work within the department and what serves well as a strategic control point in one department will not necessarily apply in another.

Standards and Individual Responsibility

In order for control to have an effective influence on performance, the supervisor must make certain that the goals and standards are known to all the employees within the department. He must make it clear with whom the responsibility lies for the achievement of these standards so that he knows whom to blame for deviations if the results do not come up to standard and whom to praise if they do. After all, the supervisor is interested in having the standards and objectives reached. Only if each employee knows exactly what is expected of him as far as his own work is concerned can he try to achieve it. This is why it is necessary to tie the standards in with the individual responsibilities of each employee.

CHECKING ON PERFORMANCE

The second step in the process of control is to check on performance. Once the standards have been set, it is the supervisor's job to compare the actual performance with these standards. Work is observed, output is measured, and reports are compiled. Such checking activities are usually carried on by the supervisor *after* the subordinate has done his function. Since the supervisor does not shift his responsibility when he assigns a duty to a subordinate and when he delegates authority to him, he must make certain that enough controls are available to take corrective action in case the performance does not come up to standards.

There are several ways for a supervisor to check on performance. He can do this either by directly observing the work, by personally checking on his employees, or by studying various summaries of reports and figures which are submitted to him. He compares the information thus obtained with existing standards. Such comparisons are a continuous function of the supervisor which he has to perform daily, weekly, and monthly.

Reports

Written reports — with or without oral presentation — are an especially good means of checking on performance if a department operates twenty-four hours a day and seven days a week, or if it is very large, or if it operates in different locations. When a department operates around the clock and one supervisor is responsible for it twenty-four hours each day, he depends very much on reports to cover those shifts during which he is normally absent. Even with such reports, it is wise for the supervisor to get to work a little earlier and stay a little later in the day, so that he overlaps a bit with the night supervisor in the morning and can have a few words with the afternoon supervisor when he comes to work. This gives these supervisors a chance to add some oral explanations to their reports. Of course, the reports should be clear, complete, concise, and correct. They must be brief, but still include all important aspects.

As the departmental supervisor checks these reports, he will in all likelihood find many activities which have been performed up to standard and he can pass over those quickly. He should concentrate on the *exceptions,* namely on those areas where the performance significantly deviates from the standard. Only they require the supervisor's attention. As a matter of fact, if the supervisor depends on reports from the different shifts, he may even request his subordinates not to send any data on those activities which have reached the pre-established standards but to merely report on those items which do not meet the standards or which exceed them. In this way, the supervisor can concentrate all of his efforts on the problem areas. However, in such situations it is essential that a climate of trust exist between the supervisor and his subordinate so that the latter can freely report the deviations. The subordinate should know that his boss has full confidence in the rest of his activities even though he doesn't report on them.

If the supervisor does depend on reports for his information, he must review them immediately after they are received and take action without delay wherever action is needed. He should request only those reports which are of significance; it is demoralizing to send reports to a supervisor who does not even read them.

Direct Observation

A second means for checking on performance is direct observation. Indeed, there is no better way to check than by personally observing what is accomplished. Unfortunately, personal observation is time-consuming, but *every* manager should spend a certain part of each day away from his desk inspecting the performance of his employees. For example, regular rounds are not only necessary for the head nurse; they are just as important for the director of nursing. In the latter case, they will be less frequent, but even the director should make some personal observations on the results of the department.

For the supervisor, such direct observations are the most effective way of maintaining close contact with his employees as a part of their continuous training and development for more efficiency in their jobs. Indeed, this opportunity for close personal observation is one of the great advantages of the supervisor's job; it is something which the top administrator cannot do to any great extent. The further removed a manager is from the firing line, the less will he be able to personally observe and the more will he have to depend upon summary reports, with or without oral presentation.

Of course, whenever the supervisor observes his employees at work he must assume a questioning attitude and not necessarily a fault-finding one. The supervisor should not ignore mistakes, but the manner in which he questions is very essential. He should ask himself whether or not there is any way in which he could help his employees do the job more easily, more safely, or more efficiently; whether there is anything in the way the employee is going about his job that should be particularly noticed, whether it is good or bad. Such observations can check specific areas, for instance, inadequate patient care, lack of orderliness, not meeting the physical needs of the patient, sloppy work, poorly performed jobs, etc. At times it may be difficult to convince an employee that "his work is unsatisfactory"; but if reference can be made to concrete cases it is not easy for the subordinate to deny that they exist. Indeed, it is essential for the supervisor to observe specifically because without being specific he cannot realistically appraise performance and take appropriate corrective action.

TAKING CORRECTIVE ACTION

The third stage in the process of control is taking corrective action. Of course, if there are no deviations of performance from the established standards, then the supervisor's process of controlling is fulfilled by the first two steps. But if there is a discrepancy or a variation, then his controlling function is not fulfilled until and unless he has taken the third step, namely, the step of corrective action. Of course, data must be examined as quickly as possible after the observations are made, so that immediate corrective action can be taken in order to curb undesirable results and to bring performance back into line.

In case of such deviations, it is necessary for the supervisor to first make a careful analysis of the facts and to look for the reasons behind the deviations. He must do this before he can prescribe any specific corrective action. The supervisor must bear in mind that the performance standards were based on certain prerequisites, forecasts, and assumptions, and that some of these may not have materialized. A check on the discrepancy may also point out that the trouble was not caused by the employee in whose work it showed up, but in some preceding operation. For instance, a patient's infection might not be caused by floor-nursing activities, but rather by conditions or actions in the recovery room or in the surgical suite. In such a case, of course, the corrective action must be directed toward the real source of the discrepancy. In this instance, the corrective action would emanate right from the Nursing Director's office, assuming that the latter is the common line superior to all the departments concerned.

The supervisor might also discover that a deviation may be caused by an employee who is not qualified or who has not been given the proper directions and instructions. If the employee is not qualified, additional training and supervision might help, but then again there might be cases where a replacement would be in order. If there is a situation where directions have not been given properly and the employee was not well enough informed of what was expected of him, it is the supervisor's duty to again explain the standards which he is required to maintain. It might also be helpful if the subordinate's motivation could be made stronger.

Only after a thorough analysis of such reasons for a deviation has been made will the supervisor be in a position to take corrective action. It should be stated again that it is not sufficient to merely find the deviation, rather controlling means to correct the situation. The supervisor must decide what remedial action and what modifications for the future are necessary in order to secure improved results. This corrective action may consist of revising the standards, of replacing certain employees, or of devising better work methods. Of course, the supervisor must study the effect each corrective action has on his total control system and he must be certain to check again after he has instituted the corrective action to make sure that it brings about the desired results.

SUMMARY

In performing the controlling function, the manager should follow three basic steps. First he must set standards, then he must check performance, and third, he must take corrective action. In setting standards the supervisor must be aware of both intangible and tangible standards. Many of the latter group can be established with the help of motion and time studies. It is much more difficult, however, to establish standards for intangible aspects of performance. Moreover, since the number of both types of standards is so large, the supervisor must select certain control points as strategic ones. In each and every department, the supervisor alone can best determine which these are. After establishing the strategic standards, it is the supervisor's function to check and appraise performance against them. In some instances, he will have to depend upon reports, but in most cases direct personal observation and inspection is the best means for appraising performance. If discrepancies from standards are revealed, the supervisor must take corrective action in order to bring matters back into line.

CHAPTER 23

Budgets and Cost Controls

Of all available control devices, the budget is probably the one with which the supervisor is most familiar and with which he has been coping for the longest time. The budget is the most widely used control device not only in health care centers, but also in all other kinds of organized activities. Such is the case because budgetary control is an extremely effective managerial tool for any manager, whether he is the executive director of a hospital or the supervisor of a department. For this reason it is essential that every manager learn how to work out budgets, how to live within their boundaries, and how to use them properly for control purposes.

As we have pointed out earlier in the text,* budget making is a planning function, but its administration is part of the controlling function. Budgets are pre-established standards to which operations are compared and, if need be, adjusted by the exercise of control. In other words, a budget is a means of control insofar as it reflects the progress of the actual performance against the plan and in so doing provides information which enables the supervisor to take action, if necessary, to make results conform with the plan.

THE NATURE OF BUDGETING AND BUDGETARY CONTROL

The term *budgeting* usually refers to the preparation of a plan which covers all operations for a definite period in the future. Budgetary plans generally include an over-all budget for the organization as a whole and many sub-budgets for the various divisions and departments. Whereas the over-all budget is of great concern to the top administrator and the Board of Directors, the supervisor is mainly involved with his own departmental budget although over-all budget considerations do have their effects on every sub-budget. The term *budgetary control* refers to the use of budgets to control the actual daily operations of the department so that they will be in conformance with the goals and standards set by the budget. Budgetary

*See the discussion on budgets in Chapter 6.

control goes beyond merely evaluating actual results in relation to established goals. It also means taking corrective action where and when needed.

Numerical Terms

The budget states the anticipated results in specific numerical terms. Although the terms are usually of a monetary nature, not all budgets are expressed in dollars and cents to begin with. There are many budgets which are stated in non-financial numerical terms such as man hours, nursing hours, quantities of supplies, raw materials, and so forth. There are also personnel budgets which indicate the number of workers needed for each type of skill required, the number of man hours allocated to perform certain activities, etc. Although budgets may start out with numerical terms other than monetary values, ultimately however every non-financial budget must be translated into dollars and cents. This is the common denominator for all activities of an organization and this is why one normally thinks of a budget as a plan expressed in monetary terms.

Improved Planning

The making of a budget, whether it is financial or otherwise, leads to improved planning. For budgetary purposes, it is not sufficient just to make a general statement. It is necessary to quantify, date, and state specific plans in a budget. There is a considerable difference between making a general forecast on one hand and attaching numerical values to specific plans on the other. The figures which are put into the budget are the actual plan which will become the standard of achievement. The plans are then no longer merely predictions. Rather they are the basis for daily operations and they are looked upon as standards to be met.

THE MAKING OF THE BUDGET

A complete budgetary program requires that all levels of management are involved in it, giving it serious and honest consideration. This kind of rigorous budgetary thinking is bound to improve the quality of organizational planning. Indeed, real participation by all the managers and supervisors who will be affected by the various budgets is a prerequisite for their successful administration. Again, this is important because it is natural for people to resent arbitrary orders. Thus, it is imperative that all budget allowances and objectives are determined with the full cooperation of those who are responsible for executing them.

Participation in Budgeting

As stated above, the supervisor responsible for living up to his budget should play a significant role in preparing it. He should submit his own budget and participate in what is commonly known as "grass roots" budgeting. For instance, as the year draws to a close, the operating room supervisor should sit down and gather together those figures which will make up next year's budget. In this endeavor, she will need the help and assistance of her immediate line superior, in this case the Director of Nursing Services. The supervisor must gather all available information as to past performance, how much was spent for salaries of nursing personnel, for other wages, for supplies, for maintenance, and so forth. Then the supervisor should think of new developments, for example, an increase in wages, increased costs of supplies, and all kinds of other inputs, before she can prepare an intelligent and achievable budget.

Of course, the full responsibility for preparing the budget does not lie with the supervisor alone. It is the administrator's and every upper level manager's duty to work on budgets, and they in turn — together with the accounting department — will give the departmental supervisor a great deal of information on past performance and figures. The supervisor will use such information to substantiate his estimates and proposals in a free exchange of opinions with his line superior. After both reach a certain level of agreement, the line boss will carry the over-all departmental budget to top administration. For example, let us assume that the Director of Nursing Services supervises three different areas of activities: the regular floor nursing function, the operating rooms, and the in-service nursing education. After the supervisors of each of these three activities have worked out their departmental budgets and have discussed and substantiated them fully with the Director of Nursing Services, she will come up with a complete budget for all the nursing services and she will then discuss this budget with the top administrator, if he is her immediate line superior. Ultimately, the final budget will be adjusted and set at top administrative levels. Yet its effectiveness is assured since true grass roots participation has taken place.

Such participation does not mean, however, that the suggestions of the supervisor should or will always prevail. A careful and thorough analysis and study of the figures are necessary. There should be a full discussion between the supervisor and the line superior and the former should have ample opportunity to be heard and to substantiate his case. But the budget suggestions of subordinate supervisors will not be accepted if the superior thinks that the figures are unrealistic, incorrect, or inadequate.

Indeed, some subordinates are inclined to suggest budgets at levels which they hope to achieve without too much effort. This is obviously done for self-protection and because the supervisor wants to play it safe. He feels that by setting his estimates of expenses high enough he can be sure to stay within the allocated amount, and that he will be praised if he stays well below his budget. Of course, this is defeating the purpose of grass roots budgeting. The line superior should remind the supervisor that the purpose of budget participation is to arrive at realistic budgets. He should explain to him that favorable as well as unfavorable variances will be carefully scrutinized and that his managerial rating will depend among other factors upon how realistic a budget proposal he submits. Obviously, there will need to be many discussions before the budget is completed and brought to top administration for final approval.

Budget Director and Budget Committee

Although the authority and responsibility for the budget rests with the line officers, and ultimately with the Administrator or Executive Director and the Board of a health care institution, they will be helped in some cases by a staff unit headed by a budget director or the controller. This staff unit will provide the line people with assistance, advice, and data, but it should not attempt to prepare the budgets for them. It will, however, be particularly helpful in putting the various budget estimates together in final form so that the top administrator can submit it to the board.

Some institutions have also established a budget committee to serve in an advisory capacity in coordinating the various budgets. Clearly, such a committee also performs a staff function. It must be distinguished, however, from those budget committees to which the Board has delegated the line function of setting rather than just coordinating the budget. In this situation, it is the budget committee which considers all departmental budget estimates and which makes the final decisions. Such a budget committee has ultimate line authority and responsibility for determining the budget instead of this responsibility belonging to the top Administrator or Executive Director of the hospital. The budget is approved by the committee and nothing can be done without its approval. If, thereafter, budget revisions and changes are requested it is also up to the budget committee to allow or disallow them.

Length of the Budget Period

Although the length of the budget period may vary, most health care centers choose the accounting period of one year. This period is then broken down into quarters and many hospitals will even divide it by months at the time of the original budget preparation. This is what is commonly referred to as periodic budgeting.

Aside from the annual budget or without periodic breakdowns, it is quite common for hospitals to also have budgets extending over a longer term such as three, five, ten, or even more years in advance. These budgets usually cover such items as capital expenditures, research programs, expansion, and so forth. Long-term budgets of this nature are not direct operating budgets and of no direct concern to the supervisor. Rather they are a concern of the chief administrator and the board of directors.

Flexibility of the Budgetary Process

The supervisor should keep in mind the fact that budgets are merely a tool for management and not a substitute for good judgment. Also, care should be taken not to make budgets so detailed that they become cumbersome. Budgets should always allow the supervisor enough freedom to accomplish the best objectives of his department. There must be a reasonable degree of latitude and flexibility. In fact, one of the most serious shortcomings of budgeting is the danger of inflexibility. Although budgets are plans expressed in numerical terms, the supervisor must not be led to believe that these figures are final and unalterable. Realizing that a budget should never become a strait jacket, enlightened management builds into the budgetary program a degree of flexibility and adaptability. This is necessary so that the hospital can cope with changing conditions, new developments, and even possible mistakes in the budget due to human errors and miscalculations. Flexibility should not be interpreted to mean, however, that the budget can be changed with every whim, nor that it should be looked upon lightly.

Nevertheless, if operating conditions have appreciably changed and if there are valid indications that the budget cannot be followed in the future, a revision of the budgetary program is in order. Such circumstances may be caused by unexpected events, unexpected wage increases, or fluctuations in demand. Consider, for instance, the budget of the department of inhalation therapy where activities have and are increasing constantly due to new ideas, technology, applications and so forth. Naturally, the revenues derived from this service are increasing rapidly at the same time. It would be absurd to expect the supervisor of this department to be able to stay within his budgeted figures for salaries and supplies. If he is to respond and supply the increased demand, his budget must be expanded. In such a case, the old budget has become obsolete and unless provisions are available to make the budget flexible it will lose its usefulness altogether.

Budget Review and Budget Revision

Because of situations like the above increasing attention has been given to ways of assuring budget flexibility in order to avoid the danger of rigidity. Most health care centers are achieving this by means of periodic budget reviews and budget revisions. At regular intervals of one, two, or three months the budget is reviewed and if necessary changed. Each time the actual performance will be checked and compared with the budgeted figures in meetings between the departmental supervisor and his line superior. At these meetings, the supervisor will be called upon to explain the causes for any variations or inadequacies that he finds in the budget. A thorough analysis must be made to discover the reasons for the variances from the budgeted amount. This may then lead to budget revisions or to other corrective measures in order to prevent further deviations.

Of course, an unfavorable variation by itself does not necessarily require a budget change. But in the above cited example, the supervisor of the inhalation therapy department will not have any difficulties in showing his superior the need for an upward budget revision. In some organizations, such a revision can be made right on this level, while in other institutions it must be carried up to the chief administrator or even the budget committee. If the deviations are of a sufficient magnitude, then it is advisable to make the necessary revisions no matter how high up they have to go or how much work they may involve. If the variation is minor, however, it may be more expedient to let it go since it is *explainable*, instead of revising the entire budget.

No matter what decision is made in a particular case, regular budget reviews and revisions seem to be the best way of insuring the flexibility of the budgetary process. They prevent the budget from being looked upon as a straitjacket and allow the supervisor to consider it a living document and a valuable tool for control purposes.

BUDGETING AND HUMAN PROBLEMS

Budgets necessarily represent restrictions, and for this reason subordinates generally do not like budgets. It often happens that subordinates have a defensive approach to budgets, an approach which they acquire through painful experience. Many times the subordinates become acquainted with budgets only as a barrier to spending or the budget is blamed for failure to get a raise in salary. Moreover, the term "budget" in the minds of many subordinates has often become associated with penurious and miserly behavior rather than with planning and direction.

It is line management's job to correct this erroneous impression by pointing out that budgeting is a trained and disciplined approach to many problems and that it is necessary to maintain standards of performance. The budget must be presented to the supervisor as a planning tool and not as a pressure device. Most of the problems, of course, arise at the point of budgetary control. In other words, when deviations from the budget occur subordinates are often censored for exceeding the budget. Such budget deviations necessitate explanations, discussions, and decisions. However, the subordinate should always know that enough flexibility is built into the budget system to permit good common-sense departures necessary for the best functioning of the institution.

Avoiding unnecessary pressures over the budget, of course, presupposes that a good working relationship exists between the supervisor and his immediate superior. This in turn rests on clear-cut organizational lines and a thorough understanding that the line managers are responsible for control. Staff people are really excluded from the process of controlling; they cannot take operating personnel to task for deviations of the budget; they can merely report the situation to the administrative officer. In the final analysis, the effective utilization of budgetary procedures will depend upon the administration's attitudes toward the entire budget process, whether they want it to be an effective planning tool or a pressure device. Only in the first instance will a supervisor believe that whatever can be done without a budget can be done so much more effectively with a budget.

COST CONTROLS

Allocation of Costs

Every supervisor must see to it that his department contributes effectively to the operation of the institution. In this context of overall controls we are not referring to the qualitative aspect, but to the financial operation of a department. At times a supervisor is told that he is operating in the red and that his department is losing money each year instead of contributing to a financial surplus. Take, for instance, an operating room supervisor who has been confronted with such a statement. The supervisor may be at a complete loss to understand this. Everyone is working as effectively as possible, the utilization of the operating rooms is very high, there is no surplus of employees, there is no waste of materials or supplies, and she is complying with the expense figures set out in the budget. The charges for the operating room to the patient have been arrived at by the accounting department in conjunction with the administration. But still the over-all figures at the end of the year indicate that the operating rooms are costing the hospital a great deal of money because it ends up as a deficit activity.

The administration must realize, however, that in a health care center some departments are revenue producing departments whereas others are not. Clearly, the operating rooms should produce revenues, and so should nursing services. But these patient care departments could not function without the facilities provided by the non-patient care departments, for instance, laundry, housekeeping, dietary, medical records, and administration. Admitting, credit and collections, executive offices, the personnel department, public relations, purchasing, telephone service, to mention just a few more, are additional services without which no other department in the hospital could function. But these also are not revenue producing departments. Yet their costs must be carried if the hospital is to break even. Indeed, some hospitals allocate such costs to those patient care departments which do produce revenue. However, the question arises as to *how* the costs of the many non-revenue producing departments are *allo-*

cated to the revenue producing departments. It is this portion of a department's expenses over which the supervisor has no control whatsoever which can make the difference between ending up with a surplus or with a deficit.

It would be beyond the confines of this text to go into a detailed discussion of the various methods of cost analysis, contribution margin approach, and other bases for allocations. However, it is a good idea for the supervisor to be informed in a general way of the bases on which his department is being charged for these various expenditures. This is merely for his own information, however, as in reality he is powerless to influence these costs allocated to his department often on an arbitrary or even capricious basis. The supervisor can readily understand the direct expenses such as wages, salaries, supplies, materials as well as some of the indirect expenses such as social security with which his department is charged. He can also understand that his department is charged with housekeeping based on the hours of service provided, with maintenance figured on maintenance work orders, with linen based on pounds of laundry, and so forth. But when it comes to the allocation of many other charges, the supervisor should find out what the basis is. Of course, the hospital will try to select a basis of distribution which is fair to all departments and feasible from an accounting point of view.

Obviously, the over-all financial performance of a department will be greatly affected by how allocations are made for other expenditures, for example, for administrative expenses, for operation of the plant, for depreciation, for intern and resident service cost, for in-service education, for interest expenses, and a host of others. Although all of this is determined higher up in the administrative hierarchy, the supervisor is well advised to obtain some information and explanation on how it is done. Then he can possibly explain why his department is operating in the red in spite of the effective work he and his subordinates are doing.

Other Control Devices

Aside from the budget and cost controls, the supervisor has other control devices at his disposal. These are mainly more scientific tools and statistical data in form of tables, charts, and curves. A discussion of these would also be beyond the scope of this text. But if a supervisor wishes to explore and use some of the more scientific approaches within his controlling function, he would do well to call on someone within the organization who is familiar with mathematics and other statistical procedures.

SUMMARY

Of all control devices, the budget is the one most widely used and hence the one with which most supervisors are familiar. Budget making is planning whereas budget administration falls into the manager's controlling function. Budgets are plans expressed in numerical terms which will ultimately be reduced to dollars and cents since this is the common denominator used in the final analysis. Budgets are also pre-established standards to which the operations of the department are compared and, if need be, adjusted by the exercise of control.

The supervisor responsible for living up to his departmental budget must play a significant role in its preparation. Budget making is a line responsibility to be shared by the supervisor together with his direct line superior. Ultimately all budgets are submitted and approved by top administration, but it is essential that lower level management participate in making their own sub-budgets and have sufficient opportunity to be heard and to substantiate their cases.

In order for a budget to be a live document and not to become a strait jacket, the budgetary process must provide for flexibility. There must be frequent periodic budget reviews within the normal one year budgeting period and provisions for budget revision. Such provisions will lessen the human problems which budgetary controls often cause.

In addition to budgetary controls, the supervisor should be aware of cost controls which will influence the over-all performance of his department. Here he will be concerned mainly with how the expenditures of the non-revenue producing departments in a health care institution are allocated to those departments which do produce revenues. The bases of these allocations can often make the difference between showing a surplus or operating at a loss. There are also a number of other control devices available to the supervisor, many of which are of a sophisticated, mathematical and statistical nature. Some institutions may have staff experts who can apply these devices, thus helping the supervisor considerably in his controlling function.

PART EIGHT

Labor Relations

CHAPTER 24

The Supervisor and the Union

There is little doubt that the introduction of a union into a hospital or related health care facility may be a traumatic experience for the supervisors as well as for the administrator. It may bring a time of tension during which constructive solutions to problems may be difficult. Gradually, however, both sides, namely the union and the administration, must learn to live with each other. Every manager must accept the fact that the trade union is a permanent force in our society. Every manager must realize that the union, just as any other organization, has in it the potential for either advancing or disrupting the common effort of the institution. It is in the self-interest of the administration to create a labor-management climate which directs this potential toward constructive ends. But there is no simple or magic formula for overnight cultivation of a favorable climate which will result in cooperation and mutual understanding between union and management. It takes wisdom and sensitivity from every manager of the organization, from the administrator down to the supervisor, to demonstrate in the day-to-day relationship that the union is accepted as a responsible part of the institution.

However, in this effort to create and maintain a constructive pattern of cooperation between the hospital and the union, we may say that the simple most significant factor is the supervisor of a department. It is the supervisor who in his day-to-day relations with the employees makes the labor agreement a living document for better or for worse. Therefore, the supervisor must be given continuous training in the fundamentals of collective bargaining and in the nature of labor agreements. This is essential for the development of good labor relations. Actually, the supervisor is involved in two distinct phases of labor relations: first, in the phase of negotiations, and second, in the day-to-day administration of the union agreement, which includes the handling of complaints and grievances. Although the supervisor is primarily concerned with the latter aspects of relations with the union, he also plays a role in the former.

THE SUPERVISOR AND LABOR NEGOTIATIONS

On the surface, it might not look as if the supervisor is significantly involved in the negotiations of a labor agreement. As we have said, the period when a union is first entering a department of a hospital is usually filled with tensions. Emotions run high and considerable disturbance can result. Under such conditions, it is understandable that the delicate negotiations of a union contract are carried on only by the members of top administration. There is usually an air of secrecy surrounding the negotiations, which often take place in a hotel room or at a lawyer's office.

Since a committee of employees is participating in these negotiations, there exists a fast line of communication with the other employees of the hospital but not necessarily with the supervisor. The latter often runs the danger of being less well informed about the course of negotiations than his subordinates are. Therefore, the administrator must make it his business to keep the supervisor fully advised as to the progress and the direction which the negotiations are taking. In addition, he should give the supervisor an opportunity to express his opinions in reference to matters which are brought up during the negotiations. In other words, even though top management is representing the institution at the negotiating sessions, the supervisor should be able to express his views through them because in the final analysis it is the supervisor who bears the major responsibility for fulfilling the contract provisions.

The same necessity exists whenever the annual or bi-annual re-negotiations of the labor agreement take place. At that time, top administration should consult with the supervisor as to how specific provisions in the contract have worked out and what changes in the contract the supervisor would like to have made. It is essential for both the administrator and the supervisor to realize that although the latter does not actually sit at the negotiating table, he has a great deal to do with the nature of the negotiations. Many of the demands that the union brings up during the negotiations have their origin in the day-to-day operations of the department. Many of the difficult questions which must be solved in the bargaining process stem from the relationship that the supervisor has with the employees in his department.

Therefore, it is obvious that there must be a great amount of checking back and forth between the administrator and the supervisor during the negotiation of a labor agreement. In order to supply valuable information, the supervisor must know what has been going on in his department and he must have facts to substantiate his statements. This points to the value of documentation, of keeping good records of disciplinary incidents, of productivity, leaves, promotions, etc. The supervisor should also be alert to problem situations which he can call to the administrator's attention so that in the next set of negotiations these matters may be worked out more satisfactorily. It is in the interest of both the union and the institution to have as small a number of unresolved problems as possible. But if problems do arise, it is the supervisor's responsibility to see that the administrator is aware of them at the time of contract negotiations.

THE SUPERVISOR AND THE CONTENT OF THE AGREEMENT

Once the administration and the union have agreed upon a labor contract, this agreement will be the document on the basis of which both parties have to operate. Since the supervisor now has the obligation to manage his department within the over-all framework of this labor agreement, it is of prime necessity that he have complete knowledge of its provisions and how they are to be interpreted. The supervisor in his daily relations with his employees has the responsibility for carrying out the provisions of the contract. He is the one who can cause disagreements between the union and the hospital by failing to live up to its terms. Thus, the content of the union contract must be fully explained to and understood by the supervisor.

A good way to present such explanations is at a meeting arranged for himself and all the supervisors, and probably including the personnel director. The purpose of the meeting would be to brief the supervisors on the content of the labor contract, giving them an opportunity to ask questions about any part which they do not understand. Copies of the contract and clarification of the various clauses must be furnished to the supervisors so that they may study them in advance. Since no two contracts are alike, however, it is impossible to pinpoint specific provisions which the supervisor should check into. Normally, all contracts deal with matters of pay, such as hourly rates, bonus rates, conditions and hours of work, overtime, vacations, leaves of absences, promotions, and similar matters. Almost certainly there will also be provisions covering complaint and grievance procedures. But in addition to these there may be many other provisions which are peculiar to each institution in question.

It is not only necessary for the administrator to familiarize the supervisors with the exact provisions of the contract, it is just as important to explain to them the thinking and philosophy of top administration in reference to general relations with the union. The supervisors should understand that it is the intention of the administration to maintain harmonious working conditions with the union so that hospital objectives are achieved in the most ideal fashion. The administrator should clarify the fact that the only way to create harmonious relations in a hospital or any other large institution is by effective contract administration. Of course, the experts in the personnel department or the labor relations department will have a great deal to do with effective contract administration, but much will still depend upon the way in which the supervisor handles the contract on a day-to-day basis.

It is important for the supervisor to bear in mind that the negotiated contract was carefully and thoughtfully worked out and finally agreed upon by both parties. Thus, it is not in the interest of successful contract administration for the supervisor to try to "beat the contract," even though he may think he is doing the institution a favor. The administrator must make it clear that in order to achieve harmonious cooperation the supervisor may not construct his own contractual clauses as he thinks they should be, nor can he re-interpret clauses in his own way. Once the agreement has been reached the supervisor should not attempt to change or circumvent it.

If the administrator should fail to familiarize his supervisors with the provisions and the spirit of the agreement, the supervisor should insist on briefing sessions and explanations before he applies the clauses of the contract in the daily working situation of his department. The advent of the labor contract does not change the supervisor's job as a manager. He must still perform the managerial functions of planning, organizing, staffing, influencing, and controlling. There is no change in the authority delegated to him by the administrator or in the responsibility which he has accepted. The significant change which does take place is that he must now perform his managerial duties within the framework of the union agreement. He still has the right to require his subordinates to carry out his orders; he still has the obligation to get the job done within his department. But there are likely to be certain provisions within the union agreement which influence and even delineate his activities, especially within the areas of disciplinary action and dismissal. Undoubtedly, in many instances these provisions of the contract will make it more challenging for the supervisor to be a good manager. But the only way for him to meet the challenge is to improve his own managerial faculties as well as his knowledge and techniques of good labor relations.

THE SUPERVISOR AND CONTRACT ADMINISTRATION

It is in the daily administration of the labor agreement that the real importance of the supervisor's contribution shows up. The manner in which he handles the day-to-day problems within the framework of the union contract will make the difference between harmonious labor-management relations and a situation filled with unnecessary tensions and bad feelings. At best, a union contract can only set forth the broad outline of labor-management relations. To make it a positive instrument of constructive relations, the contract must be filled in with appropriate and intelligent supervisory decisions. It is the supervisor who interprets the administrator's intent by his everyday actions. In the final analysis, it is the supervisor who, with his decisions and actions and attitudes, really gives the contract meaning and life.

In many instances, it is true that the supervisor for all practical purposes often "rewrites" some of the provisions of the contract when he interprets and applies them to specific situations. In so doing, the supervisor sets precedents to which arbitrators pay heed when deciding grievances that come before them. It is impossible for the administrator and the union to draw up a contract which anticipates every possible situation that could occur in employee relations and which specifies exact directives for dealing with them. Therefore, the individual judgment of the supervisor becomes very important in deciding each particular situation. This again illustrates the vast significance of the supervisor's influence on the interpretation of the labor agreement. Since the supervisor represents administration, any error in his decisions is the administration's error. It is the immediate supervisor on whom the greatest responsibility falls to see to it that the clauses of the agreement are carried out appropriately. It is, therefore, necessary for the administrator to realize how significant a role the supervisor plays in the contract administration, and it is just as essential for the supervisor to realize how far-reaching his decisions are.

Areas of Difficulty in Contract Administration

There are usually two broad areas in which the supervisor is likely to run into difficulties in the administration of a labor agreement. The first broad area of difficulty covers the vast number of complaints which are concerned with single issues. These would include grievances involving a particular disciplinary action, a particular assignment of work, the distribution of overtime, as well as questions of promotion, transfer, or downgrading. In each of these situations, the personal judgment of the supervisor is of great importance and he should feel free to deal with such grievances as he sees fit so long as he is sure that he is clear on the contract provisions and that he is complying with them. Of course, the supervisor must make certain that his actions are consistent and logical even though they are made on the basis of personal judgment rather than hard and fast rules.

The second broad area of difficulty in contract administration covers those grievances and problems in which the supervisor is called upon to interpret a clause of the contract. The supervisor is placed in a situation where he must attempt to carry out the generalized statement of the contract but he finds that it is subject to varying interpretations. In such instances, it would be wrong for the supervisor to handle the problem without consulting higher management first. Whenever an interpretation of the contract is at issue, any decision is likely to be long-lasting. Such a decision may set a precedent which the hospital, the union, or even an arbitrator would want to make use of in the future. Therefore, as we said, if interpretation of a clause is in doubt, the question should be brought to the attention of higher management, the administrator, and possibly the personnel director. Although the supervisor may have been well indoctrinated in the meaning, the philosophy, and the clauses of the contract, his perspective is probably not broad enough to make a potentially precedent-setting interpretation.

The Supervisor's Right to Decide

In non precedent-setting situations, however, and in the daily administration of the labor agreement, the supervisor must bear in mind the fact that as a member of management he has the right and even the duty to make a decision. The supervisor must realize that the union contract does not abrogate management's right to decide; it is still management's prerogative to do so. However, the union has a right to protest the decision.

For instance, it is the supervisor's job to maintain discipline and if he should see that disciplinary action is necessary, he should take such action without first discussing it with the union's representative. The supervisor should understand that usually there is no co-determination clause and he should not set any precedent of determining together with the union what the supervisor's rights are in a particular disciplinary case. Of course, before he takes any disciplinary measures every wise supervisor will see to it that he has examined all the facts in the case, has taken all preliminary steps, and has thought through the appropriateness of his action.

In a few cases, the union contract will call for consultation or advance notice before the supervisor can proceed. However, advance notice or consultation does not necessarily mean agreement on the final decision. Repercussions or protests from the union can still occur although prior communication on anticipated action can avoid some of them. In any event, the right to decide on day-to-day issues of contract administration still rests with the supervisor and not with the union.

The Supervisor and the Shop Steward

The supervisor will probably have the most union contact with the shop steward who is the first line official of the union and who is sometimes referred to as shop committeeman or departmental chairman. The shop steward, of course, is still an employee of the hospital or related health care facility and he is expected to put in a full day's work for his employers regardless of the fact that he has been selected by his fellow workers to be their official spokesman both with the institution and with the union. This, obviously, is a difficult position since the steward has to serve two masters. As an employee, he has to follow his supervisor's orders and directives; as a union official, he has responsibilities to his co-workers who selected him as their representative.

Just as individuals vary in their approach to their jobs, so do stewards vary in their approach to their position. Some are unassuming; others are overbearing. Some are helpful and courteous, while others are difficult. But unless there are special provisions, the steward's rights are merely those of any other union member. Moreover, he is subject to the same regulations regarding workmanship and conduct as every other employee of the department. However, certain privileges may be specified in the union contract such as how much hospital time the steward can devote to union business or other matters, whether or not solicitation of membership or collection of dues, may be carried on during working hours, and other questions of this type.

As stated above, the role of the shop steward will depend considerably upon the makeup of the individual. There are those who will take advantage of their position to do as little work as possible, whereas others will perform a good day's work. The supervisor should always remember that the steward is an employee of the hospital and should be treated as such. But he should also remember that the steward is the representative of the other employees and that in this capacity he learns quickly what the other employees are thinking and what is going on in the "grapevine." Thus, the supervisor will come to understand and take advantage of the fact that the dual role of the steward can make him a good link between management and employees.

The supervisor should also understand, however, that the most important responsibility of the steward is probably in relation to complaints and grievances coming from the employees. It is the steward's job to bring such complaints and grievances before the supervisor and it is the supervisor's job to settle them to the best of his ability, using the grievance procedures that are described in great detail in every union contract. Naturally, throughout these procedures which we shall discuss more fully in the next chapter, the supervisor represents management whereas the steward represents the employees for the union. In most cases, the steward is sincerely trying to redress an aggrieved employee by winning a favorable ruling for him. At times, however, the supervisor may be under the impression that the steward is out looking for grievances merely in order to stay busy. This may be partly true since the steward does have a political assignment and since it is necessary to assure the employees that the union is working in their behalf. Indeed, the steward must be able to convince the employees that they can rely on him, and through him on the union, to protect them. On the other hand, an experienced steward knows that there is normally a sufficient number of real grievances to be settled and that there is no need to look for complaints which do not have a valid background and which would rightfully be turned down by the supervisor.

Of course, the union will see to it that the shop steward is well trained to present the complaints and grievances so that they can be carried to a successful conclusion. The steward should be given a clear understanding of the content of the contract, of management's obligations, and of employees' rights. Before presenting a grievance, he should determine such matters as whether or not the contract has been violated, whether the hospital acted unfairly, whether the employee's health or safety has been put in jeopardy, etc. In grievance matters, the union is usually on the offensive and the supervisor is on the defensive. The shop steward will challenge the management decision or action and the supervisor must justify what he has done.

Obviously, the shop steward's interest is in the union and at times he may antagonize the supervisor. In some instances, it will be difficult for the supervisor to keep a sense of humor and to keep his temper. Often it is also difficult for the supervisor to discuss a grievance with a shop steward on an equal footing since the steward is, within the normal working situation, a subordinate in the department. But whenever he wears the hat of a shop steward his position as the representative of the union members gives him equal standing. The supervisor should always bear in mind that the steward's job is a political one and as such it carries certain weight. At the same time, he should understand that a good shop steward will keep any supervisor on his toes and force him to be a better manager.

SUMMARY

The supervisor's role in the union relations of a hospital or related health care facility cannot be minimized. Although the supervisor is not normally a member of the management team which sits down with union negotiators to settle the terms of the labor contract, he does play an important indirect role in this meeting. Many of the difficulties and problems discussed at a negotiating meeting can be traced back to the daily activities of the supervisor. But, at best, the union contract which results from the negotiations can set forth only the broad outline of labor-management relationships. It is the day-to-day application and administration of the agreement which will make the difference between harmonious labor relations and a situation filled with unnecessary tensions and bad feelings. The supervisor is the person who, through his daily decisions and actions, gives the contract real meaning. He must therefore be thoroughly familiar with the contents of the contract and with the general philosophy of the hospital administration toward the union. He must understand the important role of the union steward who serves in a dual capacity as one of the regular employees and at the same time as the representative of the union members. In grievance cases, the supervisor must learn to regard the steward as an equal, as one who is trained to present the complaints of union members as effectively as possible. The supervisor should always remember that a good shop steward can only serve to make him a better manager.

CHAPTER 25

Adjusting Grievances

The foregoing discussion points to the necessity for the supervisor to be well qualified in handling complaints and settling grievances. Indeed, in a unionized setting one of the supervisor's main duties is to make certain that most complaints and grievances are properly disposed of during the first step of the grievance procedure. Of course, by discussing this responsibility in relation to the supervisor we are assuming that the administration of the health care institution has not conferred functional staff authority to settle grievances (as outlined in Chapter 8) upon someone in the personnel department. In other words, the following discussion is based upon an organizational arrangement where the personnel department is strictly in a staff position within the hospital. This means that the supervisor can and should freely draw on the advice and counsel of the personnel director or of a labor relations specialist within the personnel department whenever he is confronted with a grievance. But the authority to handle and hopefully settle the grievance belongs clearly to the line supervisor.

In every unionized organization, the line supervisor knows that the handling of grievances is part of his regular day's work and that it takes judgment, tact, and often more patience than comes naturally. The supervisor may frequently feel that too much of his time is taken up in discussing complaints and grievances instead of getting the job done in his department. Or he may feel that he has to be more of a labor lawyer than a supervisor. But he should also realize that higher management regards his skill in handling grievances to be an important index of his supervisory ability, and the number of grievances that come up within his department is considered a good indication of the state of employee-management relations.

It should be pointed out before we go on that although a fine distinction can be made between the terms complaint and grievance, from the supervisor's point of view a grievance simply means a complaint which has been formally presented either to him as a management representative or to the shop steward, or to any other union official. Normally, a grievance is a complaint resulting from a mis-understanding, misinterpretation, or violation of the provisions of the labor agreement. The supervisor must learn to distinguish, however, between those grievances which are admissible and those which are gripes and merely indicate that the employee is unhappy or dissatisfied. In the latter case, the supervisor should by all means listen to what the employee has to say in order to learn what is bothering him and to decide what action he can take other than grievance procedure, to correct the situation. Grievance procedure, as we have said, must be reserved solely for a misunderstanding, misinterpretation, or violation of the union contract.

THE STEWARD'S ROLE IN GRIEVANCE PROCEDURES

The steward is usually the spokesman for the employee in a grievance procedure. He is familiar with the labor agreement and has been well indoctrinated as to how to present the employee's side of the grievance. A good shop steward is eager to get the credit for settling a grievance. Therefore, the question arises as to what the supervisor should do if an employee approaches him without the shop steward or without having consulted the shop steward. In such a case, it is appropriate for the supervisor to listen to the employee's story to see whether or not the case he submits is of interest to the union and whether or not the union is involved at all. If the indications are that the contract or the union are involved, then the supervisor should by all means call in the shop steward to listen to the employee's presentation. Although it is unlikely that a union member would present a grievance without the shop steward, the supervisor will do well to notify the steward if this should happen.

Similarly, if the steward submits a grievance by himself, the supervisor should also listen to him sympathetically and carefully. However, it is always best to listen to complaints when both the steward and the complaining employee are present. But if the steward does not bring the employee along, it still is necessary to listen to what the steward has to say. There is nothing to keep the supervisor from speaking directly to the employee later on either with or without the steward. In the latter case, the supervisor should take great care not to give the impression that he is undermining the steward's authority or the steward's relationship with the union members. There should always be free and easy communication between the supervisor and the shop steward in spite of the fact that it is the steward's job to represent employees and to fight hard to win their cases.

THE SUPERVISOR'S ROLE IN ADJUSTING GRIEVANCES

It is one of the supervisor's prime functions to dispose of all grievances at the first step of the grievance procedure. This means that it is part of the supervisor's job, often with help from staff people in the personnel department, to fully explore the details of the grievance, to deal with the problems brought out, and to try to settle them. The supervisor will quickly learn that it pays to settle grievances early, before they grow from molehills into mountains. There may occasionally be some unusual grievance cases which will go beyond the first step and which will have to be referred to higher levels of management. But normally if many grievances go beyond this step, it may indicate that the supervisor is not carrying out his duties properly. Unless circumstances are beyond the supervisor's control, he should make all efforts to handle grievances brought to his attention within reasonable time limits and to bring them to a successful conclusion. In order to achieve satisfactory adjustments of grievances at this early stage, the supervisor will do well to observe the following check list.

Be Available

The supervisor must see to it that he is readily available to the shop steward and to the aggrieved employee. Availability does not only mean being physically around. It also means being approachable and ready to listen with an open mind. The supervisor must not make it difficult for a complaining employee to see him and to sound off.

Learn How to Listen

Everything which has been stated in the chapters on communication and interviewing is applicable to this situation also. When a complaint is brought to the supervisor, the steward and the employee should be given the opportunity to present their case fully. Sympathetic listening by the supervisor is likely to minimize hostilities and tensions during the settlement of the case. The supervisor must know how to listen well. He must give the steward and the employee a chance to say whatever they have on their chests. If they gain the impression that the supervisor is truly listening to them and that he will give them fair treatment, the complaint will not loom as large to them as it did. It may even happen that halfway through the story the complaining employee realizes that he does not have a true complaint at all. Indeed, sympathetic listening can often produce this result. Or it may sometimes happen that the more a person talks the more likely he is to make contradictory and inconsistent remarks, thus weakening his own argument. But only if the supervisor is an effective listener, will he be able to catch these inconsistencies and use them to help resolve the case.

Do Not Get Angry

The supervisor must take great caution not to get angry at the shop steward or the employee. He must understand that it is the steward's job to represent the employee even in those cases where the steward himself knows and feels that the grievance is not valid. In such a situation, it is the supervisor's job to objectively point out that there are no merits in the grievance. The supervisor cannot expect the shop steward to do this for him as he must serve as the employees' spokesman at all times.

Sometimes, for particular reasons, a union deliberately creates grievances to keep things stirred up. But even this type of situation must not arouse the anger of the supervisor. If he does not know how to handle such occurrences successfully, then the supervisor should discuss the matter with higher management and experts in the labor relations or personnel department. But by no means must he get upset even if a grievance is phony.

Define the Problem

In order to determine whether a grievance is valid under the contract, it is necessary to precisely define the employee's complaint and the extent of the problem. Often the shop steward and the employee are not sufficiently clear in their presentations. It is then the supervisor's job to summarize what has been presented in explicit layman's language, and to make certain that everyone understands the real problem which the complaint is trying to solve. Sometimes the complaint merely deals with the symptoms, whereas the real problem lies much deeper. The supervisor must know how deeply to delve in order to get at the root of the situation. He knows that once the real problem is clarified and dealt with, it is not likely that grievances of the same type will come up again.

Get the Facts

In order to arrive at a solution of the problem and a successful adjustment of the grievance, it is necessary to get all the facts as quickly as possible. The supervisor can get the facts by asking the complaining employee pertinent questions which may bring out inconsistencies. In so doing, the supervisor should be objective and should try not to confuse either the shop steward or the employee. The supervisor must ascertain who, what, when, where, and why. In other words, he must find out who or what caused the grievance, where and when it happened, whether there was unfair treatment, intentionally, deliberately, or not. He must also determine whether there is any connection between the current gievance and other grievances. Although the supervisor may sometimes be inclined to hide behind the excuse of searching for more facts, he must not do so. He must decide on the basis of those facts which he has available and which he can quickly obtain.

Frequently, however, it is impossible to gather all the information at once, and therefore it will not be feasible to settle the grievance right away. Under those conditions, it is necessary to tell the complaining employee and the shop steward about this. If they see that the supervisor is working on the problem, they are likely to be reasonable and wait for an answer.

Know the Contract

After having determined the facts, it is now essential for the supervisor to ascertain whether or not this is a legitimate grievance in the context of the contract. As we have said, a grievance is usually not a grievance in the legal sense unless provisions of the labor contract have been violated or administered inconsistently. Therefore, it is necessary to check the provisions in the contract when any reference to a violation of it is made. If the supervisor has any question about this, it would be wise for him to get advice from his own boss or from the personnel department as to how to handle the problem at issue. It may be that changes have been made in the contract, and the supervisor must acquaint himself with their intent and meaning and how they are to be interpreted.

Do Not Delay

The supervisor must see to it that all grievances are settled as promptly and justly as possible. Postponing an adjustment in the hope that the complaint may disappear is courting trouble and more grievances. Moreover, an unnecessary postponement is unfair because the employee and the steward are entitled to know the supervisor's position as quickly as he can get the facts.

Speed is definitely important in the settlement of grievances, but not if it will result in unsound decisions. As we have said, if it is impossible for the supervisor to obtain the necessary facts at once, he must let the aggrieved parties know about this instead of leaving them under the impression that he is giving them the run-around. Waiting for a decision is bothersome to everybody concerned, but if a delay cannot be avoided the grievance should be reduced to writing and signed by the steward and/or the employee so they do not forget what is involved.

Adjust Grievances at an Early Stage

It is part of the supervisor's job to see that all grievances are properly adjusted at the first step of the grievance procedure. This, as we have already pointed out, is part of the managerial aspects of the supervisory function. The only cases which should be referred to higher levels of management are those which are of an unusual nature, which require additional interpretation of the meaning of the union contract, which contain problems that have not shown up heretofore, or which involve broad policy considerations.

Be Consistent

In the adjustment of grievances, the supervisor must make certain that he protects the rights of the administration and follows the policies and precedents of the hospital. If the circumstances are such that he must deviate from previous adjustments, it is necessary for him to explain the reason for this to the employee and the shop steward. He must make certain that both of them understand that this exception does not set a precedent. In such cases, of course, it is always wise for the supervisor to check with higher levels of administration or with the personnel department.

Give A Clear Answer

The supervisor must answer the grievance in a straightforward, reasonable manner, in a way which is perfectly clear to the aggrieved parties. The supervisor's answer must not be phrased in language which the aggrieved parties cannot understand, regardless of whether or not the adjustment is in favor of the employee. If the supervisor rules against the employee, the latter is that much more entitled to a clear and straightforward reply. Although the employee may disagree with such a reply, at least he will understand it.

Clarity is even more necessary if the supervisor has to reply to the grievance in writing. In that case, he must restrict his answer to the specific complaints involved and must make certain that the words he uses are appropriate and that any reference to a particular provision of the labor agreement or to plant rules is clearly cited. Unless a supervisor is forced to, however, he should not render a written reply. But if such a reply is required by the labor agreement, then it is appropriate for the supervisor to discuss all the implications with higher management or with the personnel department so that when he has to write his answer to the employee a standard set of replies are at his fingertips.

Consider the Consequences of the Settlement

Since the supervisor's decision often becomes precedent, he must consider not only what effect the adjustment will have in this particular instance, but also its implications for the future. He must bear in mind that whenever he settles a grievance there is the possibility that his settlement will show up as part of the labor contract in following years. It is therefore advisable for the supervisor to keep track of past settlements and to check with them to make certain that the current decision is consistent with what he has done before, with the institution's policy, and with the labor agreement.

Keep Records

It is, as we just pointed out, essential for the supervisor to keep records whenever he makes a decision. If he satisfied the employee's request, his decision will probaby become a precedent. If he cannot settle the complaint, there is a likelihood that this grievance will go further, possibly to arbitration. It will certainly go to higher levels of management and it is not wise for the supervisor to defend his actions by depending on his memory. Rather, he should have diligent records of the facts, of his reasoning, and of his decisions. With this documentation at hand, he will be able to substantiate his actions whenever he is asked to. Indeed, good records are an absolute necessity because the burden of proof is usually on the supervisor. It is correct to state that management has the right to decide, but that the union has the right to grieve. Whenever the employee or the union maintains that the supervisor has violated the agreement or has administered its provisions in an unfair or inconsistent manner, the supervisor must defend his action, and without good records this will often be difficult, if not impossible.

The supervisor should familiarize himself with all of the twelve foregoing points as aids in handling grievances. No doubt the supervisor's decisions and actions will have a heavy impact on employee-union relations at his hospital or related health care facility. In order for this impact to be favorable, the supervisor must not only be familiar with the above-mentioned points, but he must also apply them during honest face-to-face discussions with employees and the shop steward whenever grievances do arise.

SUMMARY

The labor agreement sets forth only a broad, general outline of labor-management relationships. This broad outline must be filled in with intelligent supervisory decisions. Occasions to make such decisions arise mainly in the settlement of complaints and grievances. Indeed, the proper adjustment of grievances is one of the important components of the supervisory position. Whenever the supervisor settles grievances, he applies and interprets the labor contract and his settlements have far-reaching implications due to the fact that they set precedents. Much of what the union will discuss at the next contract negotiations has its origin in day-to-day supervisory decisions. And if a grievance should go to arbitration, the impartial arbitrator will also attach great importance to precedents set by the supervisor. Often it is not so much what the contract says that counts, but how it has been interpreted by management's front line representative, namely, the supervisor. This shows how important a role the supervisor actually plays in the adjustment of grievances and how necessary it is for him to gain considerable skill in the use of adjustment techniques.

In order to apply adjustment techniques appropriately, the supervisor will do well to always be available and to listen, without losing his temper, even if the grievance is a "phony" one. He must learn to define the problem, get the facts, and then draw on his thorough knowledge of the contract. It is also important to avoid unnecessary delays and to settle grievances at an early stage. Moreover, the supervisor must be fair in his decisions, protecting the rights of the institution and respecting the content and spirit of the agreement; he must keep good records, give clear replies, and above all, remain consistent.

APPENDIX

Job Descriptions
Departmental Charts

APPENDIX

The purpose of the following Appendix is to provide the reader with sample job descriptions and organizational charts illustrating many of the positions found in a typical hospital. The material in these pages is taken from *Job Descriptions and Organizational Analysis for Hospitals and Related Health Services,* U.S. Department of Labor, revised edition 1971, published by the U.S. Government Printing Office. All the information in this document was compiled from a number of different sources and the results therefore show a composite picture. Naturally, the job descriptions "cannot be expected to coincide exactly with any single position in a specific institution. Therefore, usually it will be necessary to adapt descriptions to fit individual organization patterns and jobs before they can be used with complete accuracy."* In other words, the following information must be adjusted to accommodate local needs and peculiarities of a particular hospital.

In deciding which of the many activities of a hospital to illustrate, the author of this book wanted to cite some examples which are directly involved in patient care and some which merely support patient care. As examples of the first, the reader will find information on nursing service, the dietary department, and the radiology department. Housekeeping and laundry were chosen as examples of supportive activities. In addition to this, some information is given for a few over-all administrative activities; the executive job of the administrator and the activities of the personnel department are examples of the latter. Of course, the choice of these activities at the exclusion of many others should not be construed to indicate that they are more important. In a hospital no activity can exist alone. All are needed and vital in patient care.

For each of the above specified activities, the reader will find a short description of the functions, goals, and objectives of that particular department. Following this, there will be an organization chart for each of the selected departments. These charts are merely for illustrative purposes and should not necessarily be considered a recommended pattern of organization. Again, they are only a composite picture of what is often found. In addition, there are examples of job descriptions of the supervisory position in each department. However, in order to show descriptions of all the jobs in at least one particular department, the author has chosen the nursing service for this pur-

*p. 2 of the above cited U.S. Government publication.

SUGGESTED ORGANIZATION CHART FOR A TYPICAL LARGE GENERAL HOSPITAL BY DEPARTMENTS*

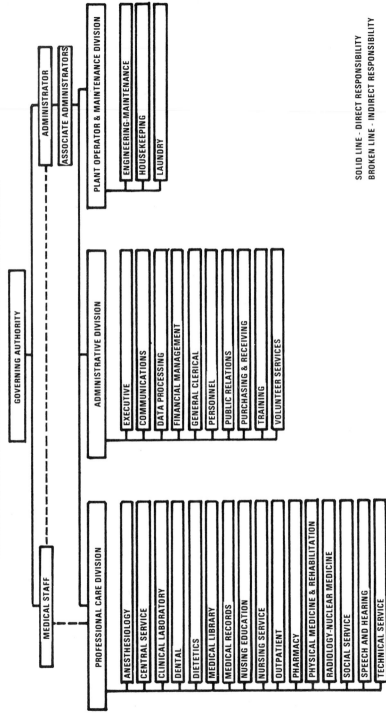

SOLID LINE - DIRECT RESPONSIBILITY
BROKEN LINE - INDIRECT RESPONSIBILITY

NOTE: This chart is for illustrative purposes only and should not be considered a recommended pattern of organization.

*Job Descriptions and Organizational Analysis for Hospitals and Related Health Services, U.S. Department of Labor, Manpower Administration, Revised Edition 1971, Washington, D.C., p. 15.

pose. Again, this was not done to indicate that this department has greater importance over the others. It was done simply because roughly half or even more of all hospital employees usually work in the nursing service.

The author wants once more to point out that the material in this Appendix should not be taken as "gospel." It must be adjusted to the idiosyncrasies of a particular job in a particular hospital. It is added with the hope that it will give the reader of the book many additional examples and greater clarification of the material discussed in the text.

EXECUTIVE DEPARTMENT*

PURPOSE: Direct all functions of the hospital in keeping with over-all policies established by the governing board, in order that objectives of health care, advancement of knowledge, and over-all contribution to community welfare may be achieved most effectively, economically, and to the satisfaction of patients, employees, and medical staff.

RESPONSIBILITY: Interpreting and administering policies of governing board, and acting as technical advisor and liaison officer in matters involving formulation of these policies. To execute these functions properly, the department is responsible for management and supervision of all aspects of hospital activities, including planning and direction, public relations, budget and finance, personnel administration, volunteer services, purchase and supply, plant maintenance, housekeeping, general administrative services, and coordination of medical staff activities into the patient care program.

More specifically, responsibilities of the Executive Department include:

1. Transmitting, interpreting, and implementing policies, rules, and regulations affecting all hospital activities and personnel; establishing procedures for systematic performance of hospital duties; and coordinating activities of all departments.

2. Acting as liaison among governing board, medical staff, and hospital personnel, and encouraging maintenance of professional and medical standards through insistence on an organized medical staff prepared to adhere to prescribed quality standards. The ADMINISTRATOR is the chief executive officer of the board. In cooperation with medical staff and governing board, the Executive Department contracts for services of members of medical staff who are licensed to practice in the State.

3. Providing for equipment and facilities consistent with community needs and goals of the hospital, and insuring that high professional standards are maintained for health care. The Executive Department has primary responsibility for the safety and protection of hospital patients.

4. Formulating and maintaining an effective program of public relations. This involves explaining hospital costs and functions to the public, interpreting purpose and importance of the hospital in relation to community welfare, and participating in community affairs.

5. Maintaining sound financial structure, including establishing fee schedules, providing for careful, economical, and safe administration of funds, and maintaining accurate records of hospital finances. In cooperation with all departments, the Executive Department prepares a budget for approval by the board and drafts recommendations covering future operations of the hospital.

*Ibid., pp. 19-21.

6. Formulating sound personnel policies and disseminating these policies to all hospital employees, developing an organizational structure with clearly defined lines of authority and areas of responsibility which will enable the employees to work together toward common objectives, selecting and training qualified department heads, coordinating all department activities, and establishing lines of communication between administrative and line employees.

7. Supervising maintenance and protection of buildings and grounds, giving final approval on equipment and supplies, and contracting for new construction.

8. Keeping up to date with advances in management techniques and business methods, technological changes, and economic and political trends, and broadening the perspective and scope of hospital services to meet expanding needs of the community.

9. Preparing periodic reports to the governing board covering progress and programs, as well as the activities of, and projected plans for, the hospital.

10. Maintaining liaison with local, State, and regional hospital and government health councils and planning agencies.

AUTHORITY: The ADMINISTRATOR reports directly to the governing authority, known as the Board of Directors, Board of Governors, or Trustees, and responsibility is delegated to him for carrying out established rules and regulations of the board. The guiding and directing force for administration comes from the governing authority as the primary policymaking body, and it specifically expresses the aims and goals to be achieved. The ADMINISTRATOR assists the governing authority in policy determination and initiates action on many matters which require an expressed policy. He develops statements of policy for consideration and approval by the governing authority. At the same time, constant review and periodic modification of policies are essential. After policies are adopted, the ADMINISTRATOR is delegated full authority to conduct activities of the hospital to achieve desired results. The ADMINISTRATOR, in turn, delegates to department heads authority over their respective departments.

INTERRELATIONSHIPS AND INTRARELATIONSHIPS: Ultimate responsibility for all hospital activities rests with the ADMINISTRATOR. Coordination of various sections or departments is a major function of the Executive Department. To accomplish this the Executive Department maintains effective communication with all departments of the hospital.

The personal contacts between the ADMINISTRATOR and governing authority, medical staff, department heads, auxiliaries, patients, public health officials, civic organizations, and numerous other groups and individuals typify interrelationships in activities of the Executive Department.

EXECUTIVE DEPARTMENT *

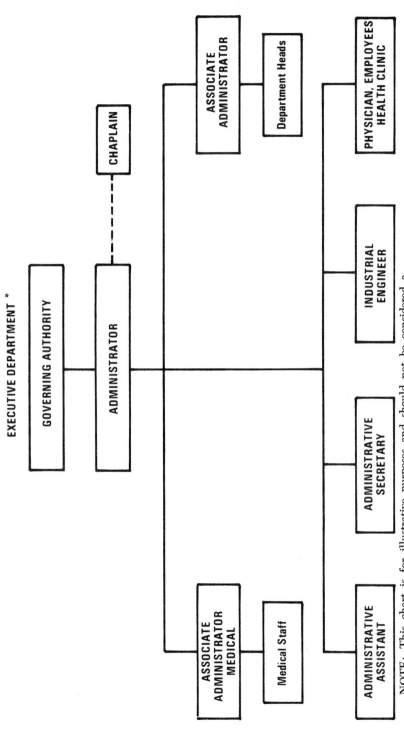

NOTE: This chart is for illustrative purposes and should not be considered a recommended pattern of organization.

*Ibid., p. 22.

The education and training functions of the hospital require careful organization and followup of all programs to insure that standards are achieved and maintained.

STANDARDS: Certain minimum standards for medical and professional care established by the Joint Commission on Accreditation of Hospitals, the American College of Surgeons, American Medical Association, American Hospital Association, American Osteopathic Hospital Association, and other accrediting and licensing agencies are obligatory for the hospital. All standards must be thoroughly understood to insure conformance.

In addition, the American College of Hospital Administrators promotes increasing efficiency of hospital administration by encouraging programs for the continuing education of hospital administrators.

STAFFING: Staffing of the Executive Department will vary in accordance with size, type, and activities of the hospital. In the large hospital, the ADMINISTRATOR may have one or more assistants in several primary administrative areas. In a small institution the ADMINISTRATOR may attend to details in many functional areas.

Executive Department   Superintendent, Hospital 187.118

ADMINISTRATOR*

executice director
executive vice president
hospital administrator

JOB DUTIES

Administers, directs, and coordinates all activities of the hospital to carry out its objectives in the provision of health care, furtherance of education and research, and participation in community health programs:

Is responsible for the operation of the hospital, for the application and implementation of established policies, and for liaison among the governing authority, the medical staff, and the departments of the hospital.

Organizes the functions of the hospital through appropriate departmentalization and the delegation of duties. Establishes formal means of accountability from those to whom he has assigned duties. Regularly schedules interdepartmental and departmental meetings, where appropriate, to maintain liaison between the medical staff and other departments. Names appropriate departmental representatives to the multidisciplinary committee of the hospital.

Prepares reports for, and attends meetings with, the governing body regarding the total activities of the institution as well as governmental developments which affect health care. Provides for personnel policies and practices that adequately support sound patient care and maintain accurate and complete personnel records.

Reviews and acts upon the reports of authorized inspecting agencies.

Implements the control and effective utilization of the physical and financial resources of the hospital. Employs a system of responsible accounting, including budget and internal controls.

*Ibid., pp. 23-25.

Participates, or is represented, in community, State, and national hospital associations and professional activities which define the delivery of health care services and aid in short- and long-range planning of health services and facilities. Provides an acceptable public relations program.

Pursues a continuing program of formal and informal education in health care, administrative, and management areas to maintain, strengthen, and broaden his concepts, philosophy, and ability as a health care administrator.

Delegates administrative responsibilities to ASSOCIATE ADMINISTRATORS and to department heads.

MACHINES, TOOLS, EQUIPMENT, AND WORK AIDS
None.

EDUCATION, TRAINING, AND EXPERIENCE

Graduation from an accredited college or university, with graduate work in an accredited program in hospital administration.

Education and experience requirements may vary according to individual background, size of hospital, and section of the country. However, a minimum of 3 years of serving in subordinate administrative positions is required by most hospitals. Larger hospitals may require 1 year of resident or administrative internship experience.

WORKER TRAITS

Aptitudes: Verbal ability is required to express ideas and views effectively when speaking to groups, hospital directors, and personnel. Must be able to gather and analyze data contained in reports.

Numerical ability required to evaluate statistical data and to make various computations in planning hospital operations and budget.

Clerical ability is necessary to read reports and utilize data accurately for other purposes.

Interests: A preference for activities involving esteem of others is required to lead professional and nonprofessional workers and to participate in community activities.

Temperaments: Organizational ability to plan and control the total activity of the hospital and the activities of all its personnel.

Ability to relate to people in a manner so as to win confidence and establish support.

Ability to evaluate reports, research studies, and other data against both judgmental and verifiable criteria.

Flexibility to adjust to changing conditions and the various details of the job.

Physical Demands and Working Conditions: This is light work. Sits and walks throughout the working day.

Talking and hearing to converse with individual members of hospital staff and to address various groups.

Handling office equipment and supplies.

Works inside. Usually has own office.

Visual acuity to prepare and read reports.

Hours of duty may be long and irregular.

JOB RELATIONSHIPS

Workers supervised: All employees of hospital through ASSOCIATE ADMINISTRATORS and department heads.

Supervised by: Governing authority of hospital.

Promotion from: ASSOCIATE ADMINISTRATOR.

Promotion to: No formal line of promotion. This is the highest occupation level in the hospital.

PROFESSIONAL AFFILIATIONS

American College of Hospital
   Administrators
840 North Lake Shore Drive
Chicago, Illinois 60611

Association of University Programs
   in Hospital Administration
1642 East 56th Street
Chicago, Ill. 60637

Local, state, and national hospital
   associations.
Local and State civic and services
   organizations.

PERSONNEL DEPARTMENT*

PURPOSE: To coordinate the needs and interests of the institution with those of the employees in a manner so as to provide the community with efficient, economical hospital service, and to staff the hospital with qualified, productive employees.

RESPONSIBILITY: Personnel administration is characterized by the philosophy, motives, and methods of organizing and treating people so that they will consistently perform at the highest levels of which they are capable, while obtaining the greatest degree of satisfaction.

The number and kinds of functions assigned the Personnel Department will vary greatly depending upon the needs, size, and goals of the hospital.

The department is responsible within delegated authority, for planning and administering a comprehensive personnel program, including participation in development of an overall personnel policy. It is responsible for developing techniques and procedures to assist line supervisors in improving the personnel aspects of their jobs. It serves as advisor to the ADMINISTRATOR on personnel problems, proposes changes in established personnel policies, and consults with and assists supervisors on a continuing basis. The major functions of this department may be classified as (1) developing sources of qualified employees, (2) recruiting and retaining competent personnel, and (3) increasing employee productivity and job stability.

Specifically, the Personnel Department performs some or all of the following functions: Recruits and screens job applicants; inducts and orients new employees; advises on methods of training and may plan and conduct training programs; develops procedures and policies to promote employee stabilization; develops procedures for position control through job analyses and job evaluations; establishes and maintains programs of wage and salary administration, and employee benefits; assists in planning and establishing lines of communication; may take part in collective bargaining procedures; establishes health and safety programs; advises the administration on legal problems relating to employment; does research to determine causes of and solution to personnel problems; advises on hospital organization and helps establish employee budgetary controls; maintains complete personnel files on all employees; and maintains organization charts and staffing patterns.

AUTHORITY: Final authority for applying sound personnel policies rests with the ADMINISTRATOR. The PERSONNEL DIRECTOR exercises line authority only over employees in the Personnel Department. Personnel administration is a staff function. As such, it has no direct authority over operating or line supervision.

*Ibid., pp. 161-163.

PERSONNEL DEPARTMENT*

```
                    ┌─────────────────────────┐
                    │   PERSONNEL DIRECTOR    │
                    └─────────────────────────┘
         ┌───────────────────────────┬─────────────────────┐
    ┌─────────────────┐       ┌─────────────────┐
    │   EMPLOYMENT    │       │   PERSONNEL     │
    │    MANAGER      │       │   ASSISTANT     │
    └─────────────────┘       └─────────────────┘
    ┌─────────────────┐       ┌─────────────────┐
    │  INTERVIEWER    │       │  STATISTICAL    │
    │                 │       │     CLERK       │
    └─────────────────┘       └─────────────────┘
    ┌─────────────────┐
    │    TRAINING     │
    │    OFFICER      │
    └─────────────────┘
    ┌─────────────────┐
    │      JOB        │
    │   ANALYST       │
    └─────────────────┘
```

NOTE: This chart is for illustrative purposes only and should not be considered a recommended pattern of organization.

*Ibid., p. 164.

INTERRELATIONSHIPS AND INTRARELATIONSHIPS: Because administrative officials recognize the need for specialized knowledge and careful planning to insure sound personnel relations, personnel administration has become a separate department. Since the PERSONNEL DIRECTOR, as a specialist, is chief advisor to the ADMINISTRATOR on all matters involving employee relations, he should report directly to the ADMINISTRATOR. As a staff officer, he works in cooperation with each department head to secure the maximum in employee efficiency and morale within the hospital.

Sound employee relations tend to be reflected in employee contacts with the public; therefore, the Personnel Department is a key to good public relations. Through direct contacts with other departments, job applicants, employment agencies, social agencies, schools, public officials, and many other groups and individuals, the Personnel Department is in a unique position to create a favorable impression of the hospital and promote progressive public relations.

PHYSICAL FACILITIES AND STAFFING: The personnel offices should be easily accessible to job applicants and hospital personnel. They should be attractive and impress visitors favorably. Provision should be made for privacy in employment interviews and discussions with employees.

The Personnel Department is normally under the supervision of a PERSONNEL DIRECTOR, who has mature judgment, leadership, and specialized knowledge of personnel administration. No exact ratio has been established between numbers of employees in the Personnel Department and total personnel in the organization. The needs of the institution and functions assigned to the Personnel Department will affect the number of employees required. In smaller hospitals, personnel functions are often combined with other administrative responsibilities. With such combinations, there should be a clear division of time and responsibility, so that the personnel function is not subordinated to another function.

Both the professional and clerical staffs of this department are subject to combinations of job duties. Depending upon the size and organizational makeup of the particular hospital, each job shown on the organization chart may merit standing alone as described in the JOB DUTIES, or be broken into additional job titles (not shown), or be combined into any one of the job titles listed.

Personnel Department   Manager, Personnel 166.118

PERSONNEL DIRECTOR*

JOB DUTIES

Plans, coordinates, and administers policies relating to all phases of hospital personnel activities:

Plans and develops a personnel program and establishes methods for its installation and operation. Develops the techniques and procedures for and directs the activities of recruitment, induction, placement, orientation and training. He may also be responsible for the safety and security programs. Interprets hospital policies and regulations to new employees, arranges for their physical examinations, and conducts or advises on training programs. Establishes uniform employment policies and confers with department heads and supervisors to discuss improvement of working rela-

*Ibid., pp. 165-167.

tionships and conditions. Assists in development of plans and policies related to personnel and advises supervisors and administrative officials regarding specific personnel problems. Initiates and recommends policies and procedures necessary to achieve objectives of the hospital and insure maximum utilization and stability of personnel. Initiates and directs surveys related to turnover, wages, benefits, morale, and other personnel considerations. Prepares training manuals and directs job analysis program, including preparation of job descriptions and specifications. Acts as liaison between employees and administrative staff. Investigates causes of disputes and grievances and recommends corrective action. Supervises workers engagd in carrying out personnel department functions.

Plans and sets up system of recordkeeping. Devises forms relative to the personnel functions. Organizes system for maintenance of central personnel files that will provide ready analysis of all personnel management functions.

Administers benefit services and other employer-employee programs, including recreation, pension and hospitalization plans, credit union, vacation and leave policies, and others. Initiates and implements employee suggestions and performance evaluation systems.

Informs employees of hospital activities and administrative policies by means of handbooks, house organs, bulletin boards, and other media. Performs research as a basis for recommending changes in procedures and policies. Interviews all terminating employees to determine causes of termination. Represents hospital at conferences relative to personnel activities. Prepares budgets.

MACHINES, TOOLS, EQUIPMENT, AND WORK AIDS

Office supplies and equipment.

EDUCATION, TRAINING, AND EXPERIENCE

Graduation from a recognized college or university with a degree in personnel management, industrial relations, or business administration.

Courses should include tests and measurements, statistics, applied psychology, personnel and business administration, economics, labor relations, and cost accounting.

Experience as Assistant Personnel Director is recommended. Receives inservice indoctrination in hospital policies and regulations.

WORKER TRAITS

Aptitudes: Verbal ability is required to discuss personnel programs with administrative staff and employees of varying levels of verbal ability, to effectively promote the personnel program, and to explain hospital policy to individuals and groups. Capability also required to prepare manuals.

Numerical ability is required to evaluate personnel statistical data, to make various computations of departmental operations, and to prepare budgets.

Clerical ability is required to avoid and detect errors in verbal and tabular material prepared for submission to administrative personnel.

Interests: A preference for technical activities in order to develop and administer personnel policies.

A preference for activities that involve working with people in order to make the personnel policy effective and satisfactory to all hospital employees and to administrators.

Temperaments: Ability to direct and plan the activities of the entire Personnel Department.

Ability to communicate with hospital staff and outsiders as well as workers within his department, in making and carrying out personnel policies and regulations.

Must be able to make decisions.

Physical Demands and Working Conditions: Work is sedentary, requiring lifting and handling personnel records and files, seldom exceeding 10 pounds.

Frequent talking and hearing when conferring on personnel matters, interviewing, or assigning work to subordinates.

Works inside. Usually has own office.

JOB RELATIONSHIPS

Workers supervised: EMPLOYMENT MANAGER; INTERVIEWER; TRAINING OFFICER; JOB ANALYST; and clerical staff.

Supervised by: ADMINISTRATOR.

Promotion from: Assistant Personnel Director or EMPLOYMENT MANAGER.

Promotion to: No formal line of promotion. May be promoted to an ASSOCIATE ADMINISTRATOR.

PROFESSIONAL AFFILIATIONS

American Society for Personnel
    Administration
52 East Bridge Street
Berea, Ohio 44017

American Personnel and Guidance
    Association
1605 New Hampshire Avenue, NW.
Washington, D.C. 20009

Public Personnel Association
1313 East 60th Street
Chicago, Ill. 60637

American Society for Hospital
    Personnel Directors
840 North Lake Shore Drive
Chicago, Ill. 60611

State and local personnel associations and societies.

NURSING SERVICE DEPARTMENT*

PURPOSE: To provide safe, efficient, and therapeutically effective nursing care.

RESPONSIBILITY: To care for the patient. The Nursing Service Department carries out its functions according to the philosophy, objectives, and policies of the hospital established by the governing authority. Within this framework the department's functions are:

1. To provide and evaluate nursing service for patients and their families in support of medical care as directed by the medical staff.

2. To define and carry out the philosophy, objectives, policies, and standards for nursing care of patients and related nursing services.

3. To provide and implement a departmental plan of administrative authority which clearly delineates responsibilities and duties of each category of nursing personnel.

4. To coordinate the department's functions with the functions of all other hospital departments and services.

5. To estimate the department's requirements and to recommend policies and procedures to maintain an adequate and competent nursing staff.

6. To provide the means and methods by which the nursing personnel can work with other groups in interpreting the objectives of the hospital and nursing service to the patient and community.

7. To participate in the formulation of personnel policies, interpret established policies, and evaluate their effectiveness.

8. To develop and maintain an effective system of clinical and administrative nursing records and reports.

9. To estimate needs for facilities, supplies, and equipment, and to establish an evaluation and control system.

10. To participate in and adhere to the financial plan of operation of the hospital.

11. To initiate, utilize, and/or participate in studies or research projects for improving patient care and other administrative and hospital services.

12. To provide and execute a program of continuing education for all nursing personnel.

13. To participate in and/or facilitate all educational programs which include student experiences in the Nursing Service Department.

The special nursing units in the Nursing Service Department usually include medical, surgical, pediatric, obstetric, and psychiatric. In addition to the overall responsibilities and functions of nursing service, the units also carry more specific responsibilities and functions of patient care, varying with each nursing unit. The establish-

*Ibid., pp. 389-394.

ment and execution of educational programs for staff and student nurses are functions of these special nursing units.

Medical and Surgical: Nursing care is provided in medical and surgical units in accordance with physician's instructions and recognized techniques and procedures. While medical conditions are not easily divided into distinct categories, medical nursing is considered a specialty in that normal and abnormal reactions or symptoms of diagnosed diseases must be recognized and reported. The patient with a stroke or a cardiac condition requires a much different type of nursing from that given the patient with an ulcer or diabetes. Surgical patients also require special preoperative and postoperative care.

Pediatrics: This service embraces the care of children. Care of the newborn is usually in a separate unit located in the obstetric unit. The activities of the pediatric unit require understanding of the unique needs, fears, and behavior of children, which is reflected in the type and degree of nursing care given. Where illnesses require protracted convalescence, educational and occupational therapy become concerns of the nursing service. Relationships with parents pose further important responsibilities.

Obstetrics: Prenatal care, observation, and comfort of patients in labor, delivery room assistance, and care of mother after delivery, as well as nursing care of newborn, are important responsibilities of this unit. Obstetric nurses assist in instructing new mothers in postnatal care and care of the newborn. Care of the newborn, particularly the premature, requires special nursing skills dictated by their unique requirements.

Psychiatric: While most emotionally disturbed patients are treated in specialized hospitals, the general hospital also recognizes a responsibility and provides facilities for the mentally ill. Nursing care of the mentally ill requires a knowledge of their various behavior patterns and how to cope with them. Techniques must be learned for dealing with all types of problem behavior, so that skilled, therapeutic care is given to such patients. Family and community education is also an important function of the psychiatric unit.

Other special units within the Nursing Service Department are Operating Room, Recovery Room, Emergency Room, and an Intensive Care Unit.

Operating Room: This unit has primary responsibility for comforting patients in the O. R.; maintaining aseptic techniques; scheduling all operations in cooperation with surgeons; and determining that adequate personnel, space, and equipment are available. Nursing personnel assist the surgeon during operations and are part of the surgical team. Preparation for operations includes sterilization of instruments and equipment; cleaning up after operations is also part of the unit's responsibility.

Recovery Room: In many hospitals, the Recovery Room unit is an adjunct responsibility of the Operating Room unit. Special nursing attention must be given patients after an operation until they have completely recovered from the effects of anesthesia.

Emergency Room: This unit is responsible for emergency care, and for arrangements to admit the patient to the hospital, if necessary. The unit completes required records; makes reports to police and safety and health agencies; handles matters of payment, and notification of relatives; and refers patients to other services within the hospital or community, as needed.

Intensive Care: Many hospitals have an Intensive Care unit; some hospitals have several. These units usually accommodate a limited number of patients whose conditions are very critical or require specialized care and equipment such as electronic instruments for observation, signaling, recording, and measuring physiological functions. In addition to providing continuous recording of cardiac function, bedside systems may monitor temperature, blood pressure, respiration rate, and other measurements. More nurses are assigned per number of patients and they are continuously in the room or within sight of the patient under care. This makes it possible to give close attention to the critically ill or postoperative patient requiring intensive care, and to concentrate special equipment where it is most likely to be needed. An increasing number of specialized "teams" consists of one or more physicians and other medical specialists, nurses, and ancillary personnel who respond to emergency situations. They are known by the specialized function they perform such as "cardiac team" or "kidney failure team."

AUTHORITY: At the head of the department is a DIRECTOR, NURSING SERVICE, who reports to the ADMINISTRATOR, and as a part of top management, is delegated authority to provide a nursing service in accordance with overall hospital policies. Although professional nursing practices are developed cooperatively with the medical and other professional staffs, the DIRECTOR, NURSING SERVICE retains authority over nursing practice.

The ASSISTANT DIRECTOR, NURSING SERVICE, assists in planning and directing all hospital nursing service activities.

Each of the special units described earlier is usually headed by a nurse supervisor who reports to the ASSISTANT DIRECTOR, NURSING SERVICE. Nurses and ancillary workers assigned to each unit are supervised by the unit supervisor, who is delegated authority for accomplishing the unit's functions.

A single composite job description has been prepared for NURSE, SUPERVISOR, one for NURSE, HEAD, and one for NURSE, STAFF. Nurses within each of these three categories perform essentially the same duties and have the same responsibilities.

The variations and additional duties depend upon the specialized nursing unit to which the nurse is assigned or in which she has specialized. Nursing positions have been treated in this manner to eliminate repetition and simplify presentation of the jobs in the Nursing Service Department.

INTERRELATIONSHIPS AND INTRARELATIONSHIPS: The relationships between the Nursing Service Department and other hospital departments are complex and numerous.

Smooth operation of hospital services and patient care and treatment depend upon coordinated activities of all hospital departments. The Nursing Service Department is the hub around which many of the activities of direct patient care are centered. The department should participate in the development of administrative policies and procedures affecting nursing as well as other hospital services. Relationships with other departments such as dietary, housekeeping, laundry, laboratories, and medical records and the importance of each in the care of a patient should be mutually understood and appreciated. A definite program of conferences to work out common problems helps in developing more effective work relationships. Manuals of standard techniques, procedures, and policies to accomplish this objective should be written and periodically reviewed, discussed, and revised.

Nursing personnel have closer contact with patients over longer periods of time than any other group of hospital personnel. The nurses' attitudes are vitally important to the emotional and physical well-being of patients. The nurse-patient relationship cannot be given too much emphasis. The Nursing Service Department plays an important role in the development of good public relations for hospitals.

STANDARDS: Standards for this department have been defined by the American Nurses' Association, National League for Nursing, and the Joint Commission for Accreditation of Hospitals. Registered Nurses must be licensed by their State; most States also require the licensing of practical nursing personnel.

PHYSICAL FACILITIES AND STAFFING: The physical facilities of the Nursing Service Department will depend upon, among other factors, the size and type of hospital. Certain special facilities have already been mentioned. In addition to patient care facilities, the department will need administrative offices, conference rooms, and dressing rooms for personnel.

Ancillary workers, such as NURSING AIDES, ORDERLIES, clerical workers, and others, assume many of the nonprofessional responsibilities associated with care of the patient.

An inservice training program should be set up for both professional and nonprofessional workers. All members of the Nursing Service Department should be included in order to develop and main-

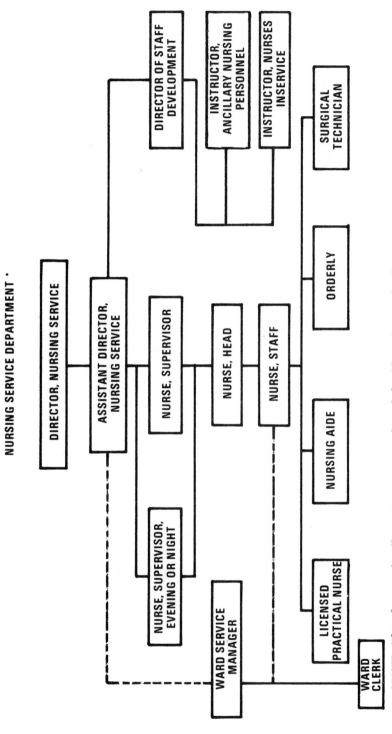

NURSING SERVICE DEPARTMENT *

NOTE: This chart is for illustrative purposes only and should not be considered a recommended pattern of organization.

*Ibid., p. 395.

tain an esprit de corps, foster new ideas, improve technical and professional skills of the individual, and provide a means of group expression.

Certain special demands on nursing service personnel exist because of their relationship with the patients they care for. They must be able to work with the realization that incompetence and errors may have serious consequences for the patient. Understanding, patience, and tact enhance the emotional well-being of patients. These qualities are needed, also, in dealing with patients' visitors and relatives. Nursing service personnel must be alert in recognizing symptoms and skillful in applying techniques and procedures in which they have been trained, in treating unusual, unfavorable, and often unpleasant conditions. Resourcefulness and the ability to think clearly in emergencies are also needed.

GENERAL WORKING CONDITIONS: Although nursing service personnel may be subject to various physical strains in caring for patients who are wholly or partially unable to move themselves, this hazard, as well as danger to the patient, can be minimized by following proper lifting techniques and using various devices and equipment designed for this purpose.

There is also the possibility of exposure to communicable disease or infections. When these conditions are suspected or become known, special isolation and asepsis procedures are followed to prevent spreading of the condition to self and others.

Some patients undergo radiological treatments which require the presence of nursing personnel or may bear radiological materials as a result of certain treatments. Where the possibility of exposure to dangerous amounts of radioactivity exists, personnel wear film badges which are periodically analyzed, as well as following specified procedures in caring for such patients.

Traditionally, nursing service personnel wear distinctive clothing on duty. In special units, such as operating room, nursery, or in rooms isolated due to presence of communicable disease, special (often sterile) clothing is usually required. Special clothing is worn to prevent the spread of disease or other contamination. In the operating room, clothing is sterile to prevent contamination.

Nursing Service Department   Director, Nursing Service 075.118

DIRECTOR, NURSING SERVICE*

JOB DUTIES

Organizes and administers the department of nursing:

Establishes objectives for the department of nursing and the organizational structure for achieving these objectives. Interprets and puts into effect administrative

*Ibid., pp. 396-397.

policies established by the governing authority. Assists in preparing and administering budget for the department. Selects and recommends appointment of nursing staff.

Directs and delegates management of professional and ancillary nursing personnel. Plans and conducts conferences and discussions with administrative and professional nursing staff to encourage participation in formulating departmental policies and procedures, promote initiative, solve problems, and interpret new policies and procedures. Coordinates activities of various nursing units, promoting and maintaining harmonious relationships among nursing personnel and with medical staff, patients, and public. Plans and directs orientation and inservice training programs for professional and nonprofessional nursing staff. Analyzes and evaluates nursing and related services rendered to improve quality of patient care and plan better utilization of staff time and activities. Participates in community educational health programs.

MACHINES, TOOLS, EQUIPMENT, AND WORK AIDS

Office equipment.

EDUCATION, TRAINING, AND EXPERIENCE

Graduation from an accredited school of nursing with a bachelor's degree preferred, and a master's degree desirable. Current licensure by State Board of Nursing required, and demonstrated administrative ability.

Five to 10 years' nursing experience, including satisfactory experience as instructor or supervisor, or as assistant director in a school of nursing.

WORKER TRAITS

Aptitudes: Verbal ability is required to express ideas and views effectively when speaking to groups, hospital directors, and personnel, and to gather and analyze data and prepare reports.

Numerical ability is required to evaluate statistical data and to make various computations in planning departmental operations and budget.

Interests: A preference for contacts with people, such as organizing and planning programs, developing staff, and assigning personnel.

Temperaments: Organizational ability to plan and control the entire activities of the Nursing Service Department and personnel activities.

Ability to relate to people to win their confidence and establish support for programs.

Ability to evaluate reports, programs, and other data against both judgmental and verifiable criteria.

Physical Demands and Working Conditions: Work is sedentary. Occasional walking about office and to and from various hospital areas.

Talking and hearing when supervising and conferring with others.

Works inside.

JOB RELATIONSHIPS

Workers supervised: General supervision of all nursing personnel in the hospital.
Supervised by: ADMINISTRATOR.
Promotion from: ASSISTANT DIRECTOR, NURSING SERVICE.
Promotion to: No formal line of promotion.

PROFESSIONAL AFFILIATIONS

American Nurses' Association
10 Columbus Circle
New York, N.Y. 10019

American Society for Nursing
Service Administrators
840 North Lake Shore Drive
Chicago, Ill. 60611

National League for Nursing
10 Columbus Circle
New York, N.Y. 10019
State and local nursing associations.

Nursing Service Department   Director, Nursing Service 075.118

ASSISTANT DIRECTOR, NURSING SERVICE*

JOB DUTIES

Assists in organizing and administering the department of nursing; assumes responsibilities delegated by DIRECTOR, NURSING SERVICE:

Conducts conferences and discussions with personnel to encourage participation in formulating departmental policies, promote initiative, solve problems, and present new policies and procedures.

Analyzes nursing and auxiliary services to improve quality of patient care and to obtain maximum utilization of staff time and abilities. Coordinates activities of the nursing service units to achieve and maintain efficient and competent nursing service and to promote and maintain harmonious relationships among personnel supervised, medical staff, patients, and others. Assists in establishing lines of authority and responsibility, and defining the duties of nursing service personnel, consistent with good administrative techniques, to assure that department objectives are accomplished.

Assists in review and evaluation of budget requests against current and projected needs of nursing service.

Interviews applicants and recommends appointment of staff personnel, outlining their duties, scope of authority, and responsibilities. Participates in establishing and administering orientation and inservice training programs for both professional and nonprofessional personnel. Insures proper and economical use of equipment, supplies, and facilities for maintaining patient care. Maintains personnel and other records, and directs maintenance of patient care records.

Cooperates with medical staff performing research projects or studies as they affect nursing. Works with other agencies and groups in the community to promote the growth and broaden knowledges and skills of professional staff, and improve quality of hospital services.

MACHINES, TOOLS, EQUIPMENT, AND WORK AIDS

Office equipment.

EDUCATION, TRAINING, AND EXPERIENCE

Graduation from an accredited school of nursing with bachelor's degree preferred, and master's degree desirable. Current licensure by State Board of Nursing required, and demonstrated administrative ability.

Experience in a supervisory capacity with demonstrated executive ability and leadership.

*Ibid., pp. 398-399.

WORKER TRAITS

Aptitudes: Verbal ability is necessary to understand and present oral and written material in communicating with superiors and subordinates.

Numerical ability is required to evaluate statistical data and to make various computations in planning departmental operations and budget.

Clerical ability is necessary to read reports and utilize data accurately for other purposes.

Interests: A preference for contacts with people, implemented in organizing and planning programs and assigning personnel to provide nursing service for patients.

Temperaments: Ability to plan and direct hospital nursing service program, coordinating it with activities of other departments.

Ability to confer and cooperate with other department heads, personnel of outside agencies, and supervisors.

Physical Demands and Working Conditions: Work is sedentary; occasional walking about office and to and from various hospital areas.

Talking and hearing are involved in supervising and conferring with others.

Works inside.

JOB RELATIONSHIPS

Workers supervised: Direct supervision of NURSE, SUPERVISORS and indirect supervision of all professional and ancillary nursing staff in the department.

Supervised by: DIRECTOR, NURSING SERVICE.

Promotion from: May be promoted from a nursing position in which administrative ability has been demonstrated.

Promotion to: DIRECTOR, NURSING SERVICE.

PROFESSIONAL AFFILIATIONS

American Nurses' Association
10 Columbus Circle
New York, N.Y. 10019
State and local nursing associations.

National League for Nursing
10 Columbus Circle
New York, N.Y. 10019

Nursing Service Department   Nurse, Supervisor 075.128

NURSE, SUPERVISOR*

JOB DUTIES

Supervises and coordinates activities of nursing personnel engaged in specific nursing services, such as obstetrics, pediatrics, or surgery, or for two or more patient care units:

Supervises Head Nurses in carrying out their responsibilities in the management of nursing care. Evaluates performance of Head Nurse and nursing care as a whole and suggests modifications. Inspects unit areas to verify that patient needs are met.

Participates in planning work of own units and coordinates activities with other patient care units and with those of related departments.

Consults with NURSE, HEAD, on specific nursing problems and interpretation of hospital policies. Supervises maintenance of personnel and nursing records.

Plans and organizes orientation and inservice training for unit staff members and participates in guidance and educational programs. Interviews prescreened applicants and makes recommendations for employing or for terminating personnel. Assists

*Ibid., pp. 400-401.

DIRECTOR, NURSING SERVICE in formulating unit budget. Engages in studies and investigations related to improved nursing care.

NURSE, SUPERVISOR is usually known by name of nursing section to which assigned or in which she has specialized, such as NURSE, SUPERVISOR, MEDICAL AND SURGICAL or NURSE, SUPERVISOR, PEDIATRICS. Specialized duties will be required by the specialized section.

MACHINES, TOOLS, EQUIPMENT, AND WORK AIDS

Manuals, patient charts, nursing care plans, records, and work schedules.

EDUCATION, TRAINING, AND EXPERIENCE

Graduation from an accredited school of nursing and current licensure by State Board of Nursing. Advanced education desirable. Experience as NURSE, HEAD in which administrative, supervisory, and teaching abilities have been demonstrated.

WORKER TRAITS

Aptitudes: Verbal ability is necessary to present information and ideas essential to supervisory duties, to understand advanced nursing theory and practice, and to maintain good working relationships with staff and medical personnel.

Clerical perception is necessary to prepare records and charts and to organize training programs.

Interests: A preference for contacts with people, as in supervising and instructing nursing personnel.

A preference for scientific and technical activities for understanding and responding to medical problems and concepts.

Temperaments: Ability to plan, supervise, and coordinate activities.

Ability to interpret operating policies and procedures and to review work performance in determining conformance to recognized standards.

Able to make decisions regarding performance methods.

Physical Demands and Working Conditions: Work is of medium demand; walking and standing most of the time on duty.

Frequent reaching, handling, and fingering of instruments, equipment, records, and reports.

Talking and hearing essential to instruct and supervise nursing personnel.

Near-visual acuity required to detect changes in patients' condition.

Color vision for perceiving changes in patients' skin color and colors of medicines and solutions.

Works inside.

JOB RELATIONSHIPS

Workers supervised: NURSES, HEAD directly, and indirectly other professional and nursing personnel.

Supervised by: ASSISTANT DIRECTOR, NURSING SERVICE.

Promotion from: NURSE, HEAD.

Promotion to: ASSISTANT DIRECTOR, NURSING SERVICE.

PROFESSIONAL AFFILIATIONS

American Nurses' Association
10 Columbus Circle
New York, N.Y. 10019

National League for Nursing
10 Columbus Circle
New York, N.Y. 10019

State and local nursing associations.

NURSE, SUPERVISOR, EVENING OR NIGHT*
assistant director of nursing, evening or night

JOB DUTIES

Supervises and coordinates activities of nursing personnel on evening or night tour to maintain continuity for around-the-clock nursing care:

Visits nursing units to oversee nursing care and to ascertain condition of patients. Advises and assists nurses in administering new or unusual treatments. Gives advice for treatments, medications, and narcotics, in accordance with medical staff policies, in absence of physician. Arranges for emergency operations and reallocates personnel during emergencies. Admits or delegates admissions of new patients. Arranges for services of private-duty nurses. Determines necessity of calling physician. May perform some bedside nursing services.

Delegates preparation of reports covering such items as critically ill patients, new admissions, discharges or deaths, emergency situations encountered, and private-duty nurses employed. Informs supervisory personnel on ensuing tour of duty of patients' condition and hospital services rendered during work period.

Interprets hospital policies and regulations to staff members, patients, and visitors, and insures conformance. Evaluates work performance and assists in preparing performance reports for nursing staff. Participates in staff education and conferences for formulating policies and program plans and for integration of various nursing services.

MACHINES, TOOLS, EQUIPMENT, AND WORK AIDS

Manuals, patient charts, nursing care plans, records, and work schedules.

EDUCATION, TRAINING, AND EXPERIENCE

Graduation from an accredited school of nursing and current licensure by State Board of Nursing. Experience desirable as NURSE, SUPERVISOR, during which executive ability has been demonstrated.

WORKER TRAITS

Aptitudes: Verbal ability is necessary to present information and ideas essential to supervisory duties.

Numerical ability is required to evaluate statistical data and to make various computations in planning operations and budgets for units.

Clerical perception is necessary for the preparation of records and charts.

Interests: A preference for business contacts with people, for supervising and instructing nursing personnel.

A preference for scientific and technical activities, for understanding and responding to medical problems and concepts.

Temperaments: Ability to plan, supervise, and coordinate activities of nursing personnel on night duty.

Ability to interpret operating policies and procedures and to review work performance in determining conformance to recognized standards.

Ability to make decisions regarding work performance of nursing personnel.

Physical Demands and Working Conditions: Work is of medium demand; walking and standing most of the time on duty.

Frequent reaching, handling, and fingering of instruments, equipment, records, and reports, and in caring for patients' needs.

Talking and hearing essential to instruct and supervise nursing personnel.

*Ibid., pp. 402-403.

Near-visual acuity required to detect changes in patients' condition.

Color vision for perceiving changes in patients' skin color and colors of medicines and solutions.

Works inside.

JOB RELATIONSHIPS

Workers supervised: Professional and ancillary nursing personnel assigned to evening or night service.

Supervised by: DIRECTOR, NURSING SERVICE or ASSISTANT DIRECTOR, NURSING SERVICE.

Promotion from: NURSE, SUPERVISOR.

Promotion to: DIRECTOR, NURSING SERVICE.

PROFESSIONAL AFFILIATIONS

American Nurses' Association	National League for Nursing
10 Columbus Circle	10 Columbus Circle
New York, N.Y. 10019	New York, N.Y. 10019
State and local nursing associations.	

Nursing Service Department   Nurse Head 075.128

NURSE, HEAD*

JOB DUTIES

Directs nursing service activities including the preparation of nursing care plans, and instructs nurses in an organized hospital patient care unit:

Assigns duties to professional and ancillary nursing personnel based on patients' needs, available staff, and unit needs. Supervises and evaluates work performance in terms of patient care, staff relations, and efficiency of service. Provides for nursing care in unit and cooperates with other members of medical care team in coordinating patients' total needs. Identifies and studies nursing service problems and assists in their solution. Observes nursing care and visits patient to insure that nursing care is carried out as directed and treatment is administered in accordance with physicians' instructions and to ascertain need for additional or modified services. Maintains a safe environment for patients. Operates or supervises operation of specialized equipment assigned to unit and provides assistance and guidance to nursing team as required.

Accompanies physician on rounds to answer questions, receive instructions, and note patients' care requirements. Reports to replacement on next tour on condition of patients or of any unusual actions taken. May render professional nursing care and instruct patients and members of their families in techniques and methods of home care after discharge.

Directs preparation and maintenance of patients' clinical records, including nursing and medical treatments and related services provided by NURSE, STAFF. Compiles daily reports on staff hours worked and care and condition of patients. Investigates and adjusts complaints or refers them to supervisor.

Insures established inventory standards for medicines, solutions, supplies, and equipment. Accounts for narcotics. Provides orientation for new personnel to job requirements, equipment, and unit personnel. Instructs unit personnel in new nursing care techniques, procedures, and equipment. Presides over unit personnel meetings to discuss patient care needs. Evaluates individual work performance through observation, spot-checking work completed, and conferences. Promotes individual staff development.

*Ibid., pp. 404-406.

Attends meetings of supervisory and administrative staff to discuss unit operation and staff training needs and to formulate programs to improve these areas. May assist in developing and administering budget for nursing unit to which assigned. Assists with studies related to improvement of nursing care.

NURSE, HEAD is usually known by the nursing unit to which assigned or in which she has specialized, such as NURSE, HEAD, MEDICAL AND SURGICAL or NURSE, HEAD, PEDIATRICS. Specialized duties will be required by the specialized unit.

In smaller hospitals, duties and responsibilities of this job may be combined with those of NURSE, SUPERVISOR.

MACHINES, TOOLS, EQUIPMENT, AND WORK AIDS

Medical equipment, patient charts, nursing care plans, records and reports, and work schedules.

EDUCATION, TRAINING, AND EXPERIENCE

Graduation from an accredited school of nursing and current licensure by State Board of Nursing. Advanced preparation in the clinical specialty, ward management, principles of supervision, and teaching is preferred.

Experience as a professional nurse in which potential administrative and supervisory competence has been demonstrated.

WORKER TRAITS

Aptitudes: Verbal ability is necessary to present information and ideas essential to supervisory duties and to understand general nursing theory and practice.

Motor coordination and manual dexterity are required to coordinate hands, eyes, and fingers in administering medications and treatments, using clinical instruments, and handling patients.

Some clerical ability is necessary to prepare and review records and charts.

Interests: A preference for business contacts with people, for supervising and instructing nursing personnel.

A preference for performing services that will benefit and help people. A preference for scientific and technical activities to understand and work with medical concepts while performing nursing duties.

Temperaments: Ability to direct activities of a single nursing unit.

Capable of dealing with people in actual job duties. Works intimately with patients, family members, and medical staff.

A sense of discipline to work in accordance with accepted nursing and medical standards.

Physical Demands and Working Conditions: Work is of medium demand; walking and standing most of time on duty.

Reaches for, handles, and fingers reports and charts, instruments, and equipment.

Talking and hearing essential in instructing and supervising nursing personnel and in receiving doctors' orders and patients' requests.

Near-visual acuity required to work with charts and records and to observe patients.

Color vision to perceive changes in patients' skin color and colors of medicines and solutions.

Works inside.

JOB RELATIONSHIPS

Workers supervised: NURSES, STAFF and ancillary nursing personnel assigned to the unit.

Supervised by: NURSE, SUPERVISOR, assigned unit.

Promotion from: NURSE, STAFF.

Promotion to: NURSE, SUPERVISOR.

PROFESSIONAL AFFILIATIONS

American Nurses' Association
10 Columbus Circle
New York, N.Y. 10019
State and local nursing associations.

National League for Nursing
10 Columbus Circle
New York, N.Y. 10019

Nursing Service Department   Nurse, General Duty 075.378

NURSE, STAFF*

JOB DUTIES

Renders professional nursing care to patients within an assigned unit of a hospital, in support of medical care as directed by medical staff and pursuant to objectives and policies of the hospital:

Performs nursing techniques for the comfort and well-being of the patient. Prepares equipment and assists physician during treatments and examinations of patients. Administers prescribed medications, orally and by injections; provides treatments using therapeutic equipment; observes patients' reactions to medications and treatments; observes progress of intravenous infusions and subcutaneous infiltrations; changes or assists physician in changing dressing and cleaning wounds or incisions; takes temperature, pulse, respiration rate, blood pressure, and heart beat to detect deviations from normal. and gage progress of patient, following physician's orders and approved nursing care plan. Observes, records, and reports to supervisor or physician patients' condition and reaction to drugs, treatments, and significant incidents.

Maintains patients' medical records on nursing observations and actions taken such as medications and treatments given, reactions, tests, intake and emission of liquids and solids, temperature, pulse, and respiration rate. Records nursing needs of patients on nursing care plan to assure continuity of care.

Observes emotional stability of patients, expresses interest in their progress, and prepares them for continuing care after discharge. Explains procedures and treatments ordered to gain patients' cooperation and allay apprehension.

Rotates on day, evening, and night tours of duty and may be asked to rotate among various clinical and nursing services of institution. Each service will have sepcialized duties and NURSE, STAFF may be known by the section to which assigned such as NURSE, STAFF, OBSTETRICS or NURSE, STAFF, PEDIATRICS. May serve as a team leader for a group of personnel rendering nursing care to a number of patients.

Assists in planning, supervising, and instructing LICENSED PRACTICAL NURSES, NURSING AIDES, ORDERLIES, and students. Demonstrates nursing techniques and procedures, and assists nonprofessional nursing care personnel in rendering nursing care in unit.

May assist with operations and deliveries by preparing rooms; sterilizing instruments, equipment, and supplies; and handing them, in order of use, to surgeon or other medical specialist.

MACHINES, TOOLS, EQUIPMENT, AND WORK AIDS

Medical and nursing equipment and supplies.

EDUCATION, TRAINING, AND EXPERIENCE

Graduation from an accredited school of nursing and current licensure by State Board of Nursing.

Orientation training in specific unit only; no experience required beyond that obtained in school of nursing.

*Ibid., pp. 407-408.

WORKER TRAITS

Aptitudes: Verbal ability is necessary to understand patients' charts, doctors' orders, nursing care plan, and medication orders and to communicate with patients and staff.

Motor coordination and manual dexterity are necessary to coordinate hands, eyes, and fingers in administering medications and treatments, using clinical instruments, and handling patients.

Some clerical perception is required to prepare records and charts.

Interests: A preference for performing services of benefit and help.

A preference for scientific and technical activities, for understanding and responding to medical problems and concepts.

Temperaments: Ability to perform of variety of duties characterized by frequent change as work schedules will change on a daily basis.

Able to work intimately with patients, doctors, nursing staff, and families of patients.

Capable of working to prescribed hospital and nursing standards.

Physical Demands and Working Conditions: Work is of medium demand; walking and standing most of time on duty.

Occasional lifting of patients with assistance.

Frequent reaching, handling, and fingering of instruments and equipment, and caring for patients' needs.

Hearing to distinguish differences in heartbeat and breathing of patient.

Near-visual acuity to read gages and dials on equipment.

Color vision for perceiving changes in patients' skin color and colors of medicines and solutions.

Works inside.

JOB RELATIONSHIPS

Workers supervised: May supervise ancillary nursing personnel of unit.
Supervised by: NURSE, HEAD.
Promotion from: No formal line of promotion.
Promotion to: NURSE, HEAD.

PROFESSIONAL AFFILIATIONS

American Nurses' Association
10 Columbus Circle
New York, N.Y. 10019
State and local nursing associations.

National League for Nursing
10 Columbus Circle
New York, N.Y. 10019

Nursing Service Department   Nurse, Licensed, Practical 079.378

LICENSED PRACTICAL NURSE*

licensed vocational nurse

JOB DUTIES

Performs a wide variety of patient care activities and accommodative services for assigned hospital patients, as directed by the Head Nurse and/or team leader:

Performs assigned nursing procedures for the comfort and well-being of patients such as assisting in admission of new patients, bathing and feeding patients, making beds, helping patients into and out of bed. Takes patients' temperature, blood pressure, pulse, and respiration, and records results on patients' charts. Collects specimens, such as sputum and urine, in containers, labels containers, and sends to laboratory for analysis. Dresses wounds, administers prescribed procedures, such as enemas, douches, alcohol rubs, and massages. Applies compresses, ice bags, and hot water bottles. Ob-

*Ibid., pp. 415-416.

serves patients for reaction to drugs, treatment, cyanosis, weak pulse, excessive respiratory rate, or any other unusual condition, and reports adverse reactions to NURSE, HEAD or NURSE, STAFF. Administers specified medication, and notes time and amount on patients' charts. Assembles and uses such equipment as catheters, tracheotomy tubes, and oxygen supplies. Drapes or gowns patients for various types of examinations. Assists patients to walk about unit as permitted, or transports patient by wheelchair to various departments. Records food and fluid intake and emission. Sterilizes equipment and supplies, using germicides, sterilizer, or autoclave. Answers patients' call signals, and assists NURSE, STAFF or physician in advanced medical treatments. Assists in the care of deceased persons.

May specialize in work of a particular patient care unit and be known by the name of that unit, such as LICENSED PRACTICAL NURSE, RECOVERY ROOM or LICENSED PRACTICAL NURSE, PSYCHIATRICS.

May be required to work rotating shifts.

MACHINES, TOOLS, EQUIPMENT, AND WORK AIDS

Nursing supplies and equipment such as blood-pressure device, thermometer, and surgical dressings.

EDUCATION, TRAINING, AND EXPERIENCE

High school graduation plus graduation from a recognized 1-year practical nurse program. Must pass State Board of Nursing licensing examination.

WORKER TRAITS

Aptitudes: Verbal ability is necessary to understand instructions, limited medical terminology, and concepts; to communicate with patients and hospital staff; and to keep accurate records.

Form perception is necessary to observe pertinent detail when reading thermometers and blood-pressure devices and to observe patients' condition.

Manual dexterity is necessary for easy and skillful use of the hands when working with patients or equipment.

Interests: A preference for performing services of benefit and help.

A preference for people and communication of ideas in caring for patients.

Temperaments: Ability to perform a variety of activities characterized by change and short duration in caring for patients.

Adapted to working with ill people who may be difficult in carrying out job duties.

Physical Demands and Working Conditions: Work is of medium demand. Standing and walking most of time on duty.

Occasionally lifts patients with assistance.

Frequent reaching and handling of instruments and equipment when attending to patients' needs.

Fingering when changing dressings and bandages.

Talking and hearing for discussions with patients and supervisors.

Near-visual acuity for accurate reading of gages and thermometers and for recording on patients' charts.

Works inside.

JOB RELATIONSHIPS

Workers supervised: None

Supervised by: A member of professional nursing staff, depending upon organization of the hospital and nursing unit to which assigned.

Promotion from: No formal line of promotion.

Promotion to: No formal line of promotion.

PROFESSIONAL AFFILIATIONS

National Federation of Licensed
   Practical Nurses
250 West 57th Street
New York, N.Y. 10019

National Association for Practical
   Nurse Education and Service, Inc.
535 Fifth Avenue
New York, N.Y. 10017

Nursing Service Department   Surgical Technician 079.378

SURGICAL TECHNICIAN*

scrub technician

JOB DUTIES

Performs a variety of duties in an operating room to assist the surgical team:
Assists surgical team during operative procedure. Changes into operative clothing,
scrubs hands and arms, puts on sterile gown and gloves. Arranges sterile setup for
operation. Passes instruments, sponges, and sutures to surgeon and surgical assistants.
Assists circulating nurse to prepare patient for surgery. May assist in positioning patient
in prescribed position for type of surgery to be performed. May assist in preparation
of operative area of patient. May assist the ANESTHESIOLOGIST during administration of anesthetic. Adjusts light and other equipment as directed. Assists other team
members, upon completion of surgery, in moving patient onto wheeled stretcher for
delivery to the recovery room. Assists in cleanup of operating theater following operation including disposal of used linen, gloves, instruments, utensils, equipment, and
waste.

May count sponges, needles, and instruments used during operation. May prepare operative specimens, place in preservative solution, and deliver to laboratory
for analysis. May record data on patients' record data sheets.

May be required to work rotating shifts.

MACHINES, TOOLS, EQUIPMENT, AND WORK AIDS

Instruments and operating room equipment.

EDUCATION, TRAINING, AND EXPERIENCE

High school graduation or equivalent. Some employers prefer graduation from a
recognized 1-year practical nurse program.

Hospital-conducted on-the-job training in operating room techniques.

WORKER TRAITS

Aptitudes: Verbal ability is required to use and understand medical terminology to
fulfill quickly and accurately surgeons' and nurses' instructions.

Motor coordination is required for rapid and accurate movements of body and
hands in response to visual and audio stimuli.

Interests: A preference for performing services of benefit and help.

A preference for working with scientific objects used to aid people.

Temperaments: Ability to perform a variety of duties in the operating room
under supervision.

Capable of attaining set standards of asepsis and antisepsis techniques.

Physical Demands and Working Conditions: Work is of medium demand. Standing and walking during tour of duty.

Assists in lifting patients onto operating table and carrying instruments and
supplies.

Reaching, handling, and fingering instruments during surgery and in sterilizing
equipment.

*Ibid., pp. 421-422.

Hearing to understand verbal instructions.

Near-visual acuity to distinguish between different instruments.

Works inside. While certain anesthetics are explosive, they are not critical because of safety measures taken.

JOB RELATIONSHIPS

Workers supervised: None.

Supervised by: NURSE,STAFF.

Promotion from: No formal line of promotion.

Promotion to: No formal line of promotion.

PROFESSIONAL AFFILIATIONS

None.

Nursing Service Department   Nurse Aid 355.878

NURSING AIDE*

nurse aide

nursing assistant

JOB DUTIES

Performs various patient care activities and related nonprofessional services necessary in caring for the personal needs and comfort of patients:

Answers signal lights and bells to determine patients' needs. Bathes, dresses, and undresses patients and assists with personal hygiene to increase their comfort and well-being. May serve and collect food trays, feed patients requiring help, and provide between-meal nourishment and fresh drinking water, when indicated. Transports patients to treatment units, using wheelchair or wheeled carriage, or assists them to walk. Drapes patients for examinations and treatments; remains with patients, performing such duties as holding instruments and adjusting lights. Takes and records temperatures, pulse, respiration rates, and food intake and output, as directed. May apply ice bags and hot water bottles. Gives alcohol rubs. Reports all unusual conditions or reactions to nurse in charge. May assemble equipment and supplies in preparation for various diagnostic or treatment procedures performed by physicians or nurses.

Tidies patients' rooms and cares for flowers. Changes bed linen, runs errands, directs visitors, and answers telephone. Collects charts, records, and reports, delivers them to authorized personnel. Collects and bags soiled linen and stores clean linen. May clean, sterilize, store, and prepare treatment trays and other supplies used in the unit. May be known by unit or section of hospital to which assigned, such as NURSING AIDE, PSYSHIATRIC or NURSING AIDE, NURSERY, where special duties required by patients are performed.

May be required to work rotating shifts.

MACHINES, TOOLS, EQUIPMENT, AND WORK AIDS

Nursing supplies and equipment.

EDUCATION, TRAINING, AND EXPERIENCE

High school graduation preferred.

Hospital-conducted on-the-job training programs. To work in some departments, additional training is given.

WORKER TRAITS

Aptitudes: Verbal ability is required to communicate with patients and to understand instructions received from nursing staff.

*Ibid., pp. 417-418.

Manual dexterity is required to move and use hands easily and skillfully while aiding patients and giving treatments.

Interests: A preference for performing services of benefit and help.

Temperaments: Able to perform a variety of activities characterized by change and short duration in caring for patients.

Adapted to working with ill people in carrying out job duties.

Physical Demands and Working Conditions: Work is of medium demand. Standing and walking most of time on duty.

Lifting and pushing patients, carts, and wheelchairs.

Handling, reaching, and feeling when distributing supplies and equipment and checking patients.

Talking and hearing to converse with patients and staff members.

Near-visual acuity for accurate reading of gages and thermometers and for recordings on patients' charts.

Works inside.

JOB RELATIONSHIPS

Workers supervised: None.

Supervised by: A member of nursing staff, depending on organization of hospital and unit to which assigned.

Promotion from: This is an entry job in the department of nursing.

Promotion to: No formal line of promotion.

PROFESSIONAL AFFILIATIONS

None.

Nursing Service Department   Orderly 355.878

ORDERLY*

nursing assistant, male

JOB DUTIES

Assists nursing service personnel by performing a variety of duties for patients (usually male) and certain heavy duties in the care of the physically or mentally ill and the mentally retarded:

Performs same job duties as NURSING AIDE.

MACHINES, TOOLS, EQUIPMENT, AND WORK AIDS

Nursing supplies and equipment.

EDUCATION, TRAINING, AND EXPERIENCE

High school graduation preferred.

Hospital-conducted on-the-job training programs. For work in some departments, additional training is given.

WORKER TRAITS

Aptitudes: Verbal ability is required to communicate with patients and to understand instructions received from nurse.

Manual dexterity is necessary to move hands easily and rapidly when working with small equipment and in aiding patient with personal care.

Interests: A preference for performing services of benefit and help.

A preference for routine and organized activities and working under direct supervision to aid and assist patients.

Temperaments: Ability to perform a variety of repetitive duties involving aid to patients.

*Ibid., pp. 419-420.

Adapted to working with ill people in performing job duties.
Physical Demands and Working Conditions: Work is heavy.
Standing and walking most of time on duty.
Lifting and carrying equipment, supplies, and patients.
Pushing and pulling wheelchairs, wheeled bed, or stretcher.
Reaching, handling, and fingering equipment and supplies when assisting patient.
Talking and hearing for conversing with patients and supervisors.
Works inside. May be member of a team. Care must be exercised when lifting or assisting patients.

JOB RELATIONSHIPS

Workers supervised: None.
Supervised by: A member of nursing staff, depending on organization of hospital and unit to which assigned.
Promotion from: This is usually an entry job in the department of nursing.
Promotion to: No formal line of promotion.

PROFESSIONAL AFFILIATIONS

None.

Nursing Service Department   Ward Service Manager 187.—T

WARD SERVICE MANAGER*

unit manager
ward supervisor

JOB DUTIES

Supervises and coordinates administrative management functions for one or more patient care units:

Supervises clerical staff and assures accomplishment of administrative functions on a 24-hour basis by scheduling working hours and arranging for coverage of nursing care unit by nonnursing personnel. Performs personnel-management tasks by orienting and training new personnel. Evaluates performance of assigned workers by checking for quality and quantity.

Inventories and stores patients' personal effects either within the unit or in the hospital vault.

Establishes and maintains an adequate inventory of drugs and supplies for the unit.

Coordinates with other departments such as housekeeping and maintenance to maintain a unit that is hygenically safe and functional. Checks for cleanliness of the units and reports discrepancies to the appropriate supervisor. Performs daily maintenance inspection, and through proper channels initiates minor facility improvement projects.

Maintains close contact with medical and surgical reservations in regard to admissions, transfers, discharges, and other services. Serves as liaison between the specific patient care unit and other departments. Reviews special tests at the end of shift.

Insures that the medical record is completed in accordance with the standards of the Joint Commission on Accreditation of Hospitals. Insures hospital compliance with Medicare requirements insofar as certification and related administrative matters are concerned. Checks charts of patients scheduled for surgery or other special procedures to verify completeness of orders of consents, preparation orders, and lab results, and for necessary signatures.

Greets, directs, and gives nonprofessional factual information to patients, visitors, and personnel from other departments.

*Ibid., pp. 425-426.

Participates in projects, surveys, and other information-gathering activities approved by hospital management.

MACHINES, TOOLS, EQUIPMENT, AND WORK AIDS

Nursing Service supplies, medications, and records.

EDUCATION, TRAINING, AND EXPERIENCE

One year of college or equivalent.

A minimum of 1 year's supervisory experience.

On-the-job training in coordinating nonnursing services for the assigned nursing units.

WORKER TRAITS

Aptitudes: Verbal ability is required to schedule, assign, and supervise workers and to communicate with personnel from other departments.

Numerical ability is required to verify quantities of incoming items and prepare reports of stock on hand.

Interests: A preference for activities involving contact with subordinates and other hospital employees.

Temperaments: Ability to perform a wide variety of duties when supervising the nonnursing personnel of the units.

Able to plan, control, and direct the work activities of the nonnursing personnel of one or more nursing units.

Capable of dealing with subordinates, department heads,, and nursing personnel.

Physical Demands and Working Conditions: Work is light. Lifts and carries supplies weighing from 5 to 10 pounds.

Reaches for and handles supplies, records, and equipment.

Talking and hearing for communicating with other personnel of the department and other departments.

Near-visual acuity for reading reports and records.

Works inside.

JOB RELATIONSHIPS

Workers supervised: WARD CLERK and other nonnursing personnel assigned to the unit.

Supervised by: ASSISTANT DIRECTOR, NURSING SERVICE or ADMINISTRATOR.

Promotion from: No formal line of promotion.

Promotion to: No formal line of promotion.

PROFESSIONAL AFFILIATIONS

None.

Nursing Service Department   Ward Clerk 219.388

WARD CLERK*

floor clerk
nursing station assistant

JOB DUTIES

Performs general clerical duties by preparing, compiling, and maintaining records in a hospital nursing unit:

*Ibid., pp. 423-424.

Records name of patient, address, and name of attending physician on medical record forms. Copies information, such as patients' temperature, pulse rate, and blood pressure, from nurses' records. Writes requisitions for laboratory tests and procedures such as basal metabolism, X-ray, EKG, blood examinations, and urinalysis. Under supervision, plots temperature, pulse rate, and other data on appropriate graph charts. Copies and computes other data, as directed, and enters on patients' charts. May record diet instructions. Keeps file of medical records on patients in unit. Routes charts when patients are transferred or dismissed, following specified procedures. May compile census of patients.

Keeps record of absences and hours worked by unit personnel. Types various records, schedules, and reports and delivers them to appropriate office. May maintain records of special monetary charges to patient and forward them to the business office. May verify stock supplies on unit and prepare requisitions to maintain established inventories. Dispatches messages to other departments or to persons in other departments and makes appointments for patients' services in other departments as requested by nursing staff. Makes posthospitalization appointments with patients' physicians. Delivers mail, newspapers, and flowers to patients.

MACHINES, TOOLS, EQUIPMENT, AND WORK AIDS

Office supplies and equipment.

EDUCATION, TRAINING, AND EXPERIENCE

High school graduation or equivalent, including courses in English, typing, spelling, and arithmetic, or high school graduation supplemented by commercial school course in subjects indicated.

No previous experience is required.

On-the-job training in practices and procedures of the hospital and certain medical terminology.

WORKER TRAITS

Aptitudes: Verbal ability is necessary for understanding procedure routines and instructions.

Numerical ability is needed to make accurate computations of patients' and other data.

Clerical perception is necessary to perceive and maintain detail in entering data on patients' charts and to avoid errors in arithmetic.

Interests: A preference for established routine in keeping patients' charts, preparing schedules, and verifying supplies.

Temperaments: Ability to carry out repetitive operations, under specific instructions and in accordance with established procedures.

Physical Demands and Working Conditions: Work is sedentary. Occasionally walks about ward and to and from other departments.

Reaching for and handling charts, reports, and other office supplies.

Talking and hearing when receiving instructions and conversing on telephone.

Near-visual acuity to record information accurately.

Works inside.

JOB RELATIONSHIPS

Workers supervised: None.

Supervised by: WARD SERVICE MANAGER or nurse in charge of unit or ward in which work is performed.

Promotion from: This is usually an entry job.

Promotion to: No formal line of promotion. May be promoted to higher grade clerical job for which ability is demonstrated.

PROFESSIONAL AFFILIATIONS

None.

Nursing Service Department   Director of Staff Development 075.118

DIRECTOR OF STAFF DEVELOPMENT*

inservice-education coordinator

JOB DUTIES

Plans, develops, and directs program of education for all hospital nursing service personnel, and coordinates staff development with nursing service program:

Develops, schedules, and directs orientation program for professional and auxiliary nursing service personnel. Develops instructional materials to assist new personnel in becoming oriented to hospital operational techniques. If not scheduled by Personnel Department, schedules hospital tours and addresses by administrative staff to acquaint new personnel with over-all operation and interrelationship of hospital services. Determines effectiveness of orientation materials and procedures through practice sessions. Sets up demonstrations of nursing service equipment to acquaint hospital staff with new equipment and make them more familiar with established equipment.

Plans, coordinates, and conducts regular and special inservice training sessions for hospital nursing staff to acquaint them with new procedures and policies and new trends and developments in patient care techniques; and to provide opportunity for individual members to develop to their full potential.

Keeps current on latest developments by attending professional seminars, institutes, and reading professional journals. Assists Supervisors and Head Nurses in planning and implementing staff development programs in their units. Keeps bulletin boards current by listing information on seminars and institutes and promotes appropriate staff attendance at these professional meetings. Plans training sessions for supervisory staff members.

May participate with committees in writing and maintaining policies and procedures manuals and nursing service forms. Reviews suggestions submitted by nursing service staff for changes or clarification in policies and procedures.

Writes annual reports on activities and prepares plans for future activities. Prepares budget requests.

MACHINES, TOOLS, EQUIPMENT, AND WORK AIDS

Nursing supplies and equipment for demonstration purposes, manuals and clerical forms, and audiovisual equipment.

EDUCATION, TRAINING, AND EXPERIENCE

Graduation from an accredited school of nursing and current licensure by State Board of Nursing; graduation from a recognized college or university with specialization in education; bachelor's degree required. Experience as NURSE, HEAD; NURSE, SUPERVISOR; or Nurse, Educator.

WORKER TRAITS

Aptitudes: Verbal ability is necessary in communicating and in compiling written reports; must be able to understand and use medical terminology.

Clerical perception is necessary to organize materials for program and to proofread technical materials.

Interests: A preference for activities dealing with scientific and technical materials.

A preference for activities dealing with the communication of technical ideas and concepts.

Temperaments: Ability to plan and direct a nursing development program.

Capable of dealing with people in actual job duties in developing nursing policies and procedures.

*Ibid., pp. 409-410.

Physical Demands and Working Conditions: Work is sedentary.
Reaching for and handling reports, forms, and equipment.
Talking and hearing while discussing procedures and instructing nursing staff.
Near-visual acuity for demonstrating techniques and reviewing manuals.
Works inside.

JOB RELATIONSHIPS

Workers supervised: Supervises other training personnel in Nursing Service Department.

Supervised by: ASSISTANT DIRECTOR, NURSING SERVICE or Head of Training Department.

Promotion from: NURSE, SUPERVISOR or NURSE, HEAD.

Promotion to: No formal line of promotion.

PROFESSIONAL AFFILIATIONS

American Nurses' Association
10 Columbus Circle
New York, N.Y. 10019
State and local nursing associations.

National League for Nursing
10 Columbus Circle
New York, N.Y. 10019

Nursing Service Department   Nurse Instructor 075.128

INSTRUCTOR, ANCILLARY NURSING PERSONNEL*

JOB DUTIES

Plans, coordinates, and carries out educational programs (theoretical and practical aspects of nursing) to train ancillary nursing personnel:

Prepares and issues trainee manuals (which describe duties and responsibilities of nursing assistants) to be used as training guides. Familiarizes new employees with physical layout of hospital and hospital policies and procedures, organizational structure, hospital etiquette, and employee benefits. Plans educational program and schedules classes in basic patient care procedures, such as bedmaking, blood-pressure and temperature taking, and feeding of patients. Teaches NURSING AIDES and ORDERLIES nursing procedures by demonstration in classrooms and clinical units and by lectures in classrooms, using such aids as motion pictures, charts, and slides. Observes trainees in practical application of procedures. Secures cooperation of Supervisors and Head Nurses to assist in teaching their specialty; coordinates training with all nursing service units to maintain consistency in practice and establish relationships, to give scope to program, and to point out variations of duties required by different units and on different shifts.

Prepares, administers, and scores examinations to determine trainees' suitability for the job. Makes recommendations to nursing service regarding placement of trainees according to test scores and practical application performance. Evaluates trainees' progress following training period and submits report to nursing service for further processing. Conducts meetings with trainees and with supervisors to discuss problems and ideas for improving nursing service training program.

MACHINES, TOOLS, EQUIPMENT, AND WORK AIDS

Teaching aids such as movies and charts, nursing supplies, and equipment for demonstration purposes.

EDUCATION, TRAINING, AND EXPERIENCE

Graduation from an accredited school of nursing and current licensure by State Board of Nursing; advanced training in teaching methods and supervision.

One year's experience as NURSE, HEAD or NURSE, SUPERVISOR.

*Ibid., pp. 411-412.

WORKER TRAITS

Aptitudes: Verbal ability is necessary to present ideas and subject matter to trainees, to express clearly new ideas and techniques, to understand medical terminology, and to prepare manuals.

Some clerical ability is necessary to prepare, administer, and score performance tests, and to prepare course content.

Interests: A preference for scientific and technical materials and a desire to teach these to others.

A preference for people and communication of ideas to instruct trainees and to communicate with fellow staff members.

Temperaments: Ability to organize and direct course content and classroom and clinical instruction for a class of nonprofessional nursing personnel.

Able to deal with people in actual job duties in training new employees.

Equipped to make decisions when evaluating trainees' achievement and potential.

Physical Demands and Working Conditions: Work is light. Considerable walking and standing while instructing and observing students.

Reaching, handling, and fingering instruments, supplies, and teaching aids.

Talking and hearing when conducting classes.

Near-visual acuity to demonstrate techniques and keep records.

Works inside.

JOB RELATIONSHIPS

Workers supervised: Trainees during training period.
Supervised by: DIRECTOR OF STAFF DEVELOPMENT.
Promotion from: NURSE, HEAD or NURSE, SUPERVISOR.
Promotion to: DIRECTOR OF STAFF DEVELOPMENT.

PROFESSIONAL AFFILIATIONS

American Nurses' Association
10 Columbus Circle
New York, N.Y. 10019
State and local nursing associations.

National League for Nursing
10 Columbus Circle
New York, N.Y. 10019

Nursing Service Department   Nurse, Instructor 075.128

INSTRUCTOR, NURSES, INSERVICE*

JOB DUTIES

Plans, directs, and coordinates inservice orientation and educational program for professional nursing personnel:

Assists DIRECTOR OF STAFF DEVELOPMENT in planning and carrying out program of staff development. Confers with DIRECTOR OF STAFF DEVELOPMENT to schedule training programs for professional nurses already on the staff, according to departmental work requirements. Lectures to nurses and demonstrates improved methods of nursing service. Lectures and demonstrates procedures, using motion pictures, charts, and slides.

Orients new staff members and provides inservice refresher training for professional nurses returning to hospital nursing service.

Instructs volunteer workers in routine procedures such as aseptic practices and blood-pressure and temperature taking.

MACHINES, TOOLS, EQUIPMENT, AND WORK AIDS

Teaching aids such as movies and charts, nursing supplies, and equipment for demonstration purposes.

*Ibid., pp. 413-414.

EDUCATION, TRAINING, AND EXPERIENCE

Graduation from an accredited school of nursing and current licensure by State Board of Nursing; advanced training in teaching methods and supervision.

One year's experience as NURSE, HEAD or NURSE, SUPERVISOR.

WORKER TRAITS

Aptitudes: Verbal ability is necessary to present ideas and subject matter to trainees, express clearly new ideas and techniques, and understand medical terminology.

Some clerical ability is necessary to prepare, administer, and score performance tests and to prepare course content.

Interests: A preference for scientific and technical materials and a desire to teach and explain these to others.

A preference for people and communication of ideas to instruct nurses and to communicate with fellow staff members.

Temperaments: Ability to organize and direct course content and classroom and clinical instruction for professional nursing personnel.

Able to deal with people in actual job duties in training nursing personnel.

Ability to make decisions when evaluating nurses' achievements and potentials.

Physical Demands and Working Conditions: Work is light. Considerable walking and standing while instructing and observing nurses' performance.

Reaching, handling, and fingering instruments, supplies, and teaching aids.

Talking and hearing when conducting classes.

Near-visual acuity to demonstrate techniques and keep records.

Works inside.

JOB RELATIONSHIPS

Workers supervised: None.

Supervised by: DIRECTOR OF STAFF DEVELOPMENT.

Promotion from: NURSE, HEAD or NURSE, SUPERVISOR.

Promotion to: DIRECTOR OF STAFF DEVELOPMENT.

PROFESSIONAL AFFILIATIONS

American Nurses' Association
10 Columbus Circle
New York, N.Y. 10019
State and local nursing associations.

National League for Nursing
10 Columbus Circle
New York, N.Y. 10019

DIETETIC DEPARTMENT*

PURPOSE: To provide complete dietetic treatment to all patients, including patient therapy and education, and to plan, prepare, and serve nutritious and appetizing food for patients, personnel, and visitors. To train dietetic and other hospital personnel and to maintain close working relationships with other hospital activities and community agencies.

RESPONSIBILITY: To plan, organize, and direct all phases of the dietetic operation which includes menu planning; food preparation and service; budget estimates; cost control and administrative record-keeping; patient therapy and education; analysis and appraisal of personnel requirements; and safety and sanitation programs. The department is responsible for keeping informed of advancements and changes in equipment and food for possible application.

It is a responsibility of the Dietetic Department to specify quantity and quality of food through use of commodity specifications. Meals must supply basic physiological needs and also have aesthetic appeal to the patient. For efficiency in operations, all diets can be built around general diets by additions and modifications.

Files of recipes for quantity cooking are maintained to facilitate preparation and cost control. The recipes should contain formulas to be followed and indicate yields in terms of number and size of servings, and costs of both total recipe and single servings. A diet manual, prepared or recommended by the department and approved by the medical staff, must be available for use by physicians and nurses.

Food preparation and service constitute a large part of the work of the Dietetic Department. All foods should be prepared under strictly sanitary conditions in accordance with local and State public health regulations. Foods should be prepared preserving full color, flavor, and nutritional value; meals should be attractively served. Trays must be inspected so that patients on modified diets will receive proper meals. Dishwashing and housekeeping in main kitchen, floor kitchen, and other dietetic areas usually are also functions of this department.

Another function is that of formal and informal education. Dietetic interns are trained in many hospitals. Nurses, medical and dental students, and interns and residents are instructed in principles of nutrition and diet therapy. The department is also responsible for teaching patients and their families nutrition and modified diet requirements.

Infant formulas may be prepared by the Dietetic Department or preprepared formulas purchased from vendors.

Other dietetic services include visiting patients in nursing units to determine their food preferences both as to type of food and man-

*Ibid., pp. 317-319.

ner in which it is prepared; advising patients with special dietetic problems prior to their discharge from the hospital, or as referred from the outpatient clinic; cooperating with medical staff in planning, preparing, and serving metabolic research diets.

Dietetics is an important aspect of hospital medical care. To be effective, the Dietetic Department must develop a planned program, efficient organization and administration, and close coordination with other hospital activities. The program must be flexible enough to take advantage of current developments in medicine, dietetics, and the food-service industry.

AUTHORITY: The Dietetic Department is under the direction of a DIRECTOR, FOOD SERVICE, who reports directly to the ADMINISTRATOR or to an ASSOCIATE ADMINISTRATOR. Administrative policies, budgetary controls, and procedures for carrying out the dietetic program are determined by the ADMINISTRATOR in cooperation with the DIRECTOR, FOOD SERVICE and heads of other departments involved such as Nursing, Housekeeping, or Laundry. The DIRECTOR, FOOD SERVICE is then delegated full authority for implementing the dietetic program.

INTERRELATIONSHIPS AND INTRARELATIONSHIPS: The Dietetic Department maintains operating relationships with most of the medical care and administrative activities of the hospital. Close relationships are maintained with the medical staff on special dietetic needs of patients, with nursing services on provisions of regular and modified diets and between-meal nourishment, and with the ADMINISTRATOR on management matters. The department usually takes an active part in formal and informal educational programs of the hospital and works closely with physicians, interns, residents, nurses, student nurses, dietetic interns, and other employees. The department may have an opportunity to conduct instructive courses in dietetics for the general public.

STANDARDS: The Joint Commission on Accreditation of Hospitals has developed minimum standards for Dietetic Departments in hospitals, which include standards on organization, facilities, personnel, foodhandling practices, records, and policies.

The American Dietetic Association has developed standards for the education of dietetic interns and has established specified educational requirements for qualified dietitians.

In most States, it is required by law that those involved with food service shall be subject to physical examinations to determine that they are free of communicable diseases. Local or State Health Departments require that the premises and personnel conform to ordinances and regulations. All employees must wear hair nets and/or caps when handling and preparing food.

PHYSICAL FACILITIES AND STAFFING: Modern food service in a hospital requires not only the necessary space for main and area kitchens, storage, refrigeration, modified diet preparation, infant for-

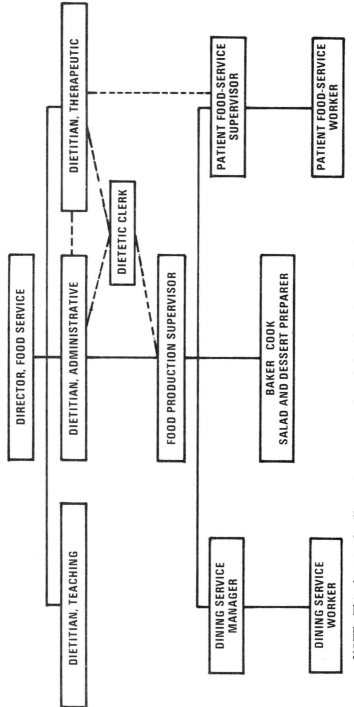

DIETETIC DEPARTMENT *

NOTE: This chart is for illustrative purposes only and should not be considered a recommended pattern of organization.

*Ibid., p. 320.

mula room, dining room for employees and visitors but also should take into consideration such factors as location, utilities, transportation of food, garbage disposal, dishwashing, and general cleaning. Employee locker rooms and restroom facilities are also necessary. Careful consideration should be given to laborsaving devices and to location and arrangement of equipment.

A DIRECTOR, FOOD SERVICE heads the department and must possess requisite qualifications. The number of staff is determined by such factors as average number of hospital patients, number of modified diets, type of service, number of personnel served, extent of educational programs, and physical capacities of the department.

GENERAL WORKING CONDITIONS: Workers may be subject to cuts, burns, muscle sprains, and falls. Handtrucks are available for moving heavy food supplies, garbage, and trash cans. Much of the work in the department is interchangeable, and personnel work according to an assigned schedule.

Dietetic Department   Dietitian, Chief 077.118

DIRECTOR, FOOD SERVICE*
chief dietitian
director, dietetics

JOB DUTIES

Plans, directs, and coordinates activities of Dietetic Department to provide dietetic services for patients and hospital employees:

Establishes departmental regulations and procedures, in conformance with administrative policies, and develops standards for organization and supervision of dietetic service. Determines quality and quantity of food required, plans menus, and controls food costs. Reviews regular diet menus as to cost and suitability to type of hospital, and standardized recipes for menu requirements. Makes frequent inspections of all work, storage, and serving areas to determine that regulations and directions governing dietetic activities are followed. Recommends or institutes changes in techniques or procedures for more efficient operation. Develops and prepares policies and procedures governing handling and storage of supplies and equipment, sanitation, and for records and compiling reports. Prepares job descriptions, organization charts, manuals, and guidebooks covering all phases of departmental operations for use by employees. Makes final determination of kinds and amounts of supplies and equipment needed.

Interviews and makes final selection of applicants for employment. Reviews work schedules for personnel and job performance ratings.

Selects, upon recommendation, personnel for transfer, promotion, and special training to insure most effective utilization of individual skills and employee development.

Reviews records and reports covering number and kinds of regular and therapeutic diets prepared, nutritional and caloric analyses of meals, costs of raw food and labor, computation of daily ration cost, inventory of equipment and supplies. Develops and directs cost control system. Prepares and submits department budget.

Confers with other department heads regarding technical and administrative aspects of dietetic service. Establishes effective relationships with medical staff,

*Ibid., pp. 321-323.

nursing, and other patient care services. Attends hospital staff conferences and transmits information to department staff regarding new developments and trends.

Delegates authority to supervisory staff for task details to facilitate smooth flow of materials and services.

Attends professional meetings and conferences to keep informed of current practices and trends in fields of dietetics and nutrition. May prepare articles for publication in professional journals and lecture on various aspects of dietetic operations. May discuss dietetic problems with patients or their families and explain diet therapy for specific case.

In smaller hospitals the duties of DIETITIAN, ADMINISTRATIVE and/or DIETITIAN, THERAPEUTIC may be combined with this job.

MACHINES, TOOLS, EQUIPMENT, AND WORK AIDS

Dietetic personnel records, inventory records, purchase requisitions, recipes, other records and reports, and work schedules.

EDUCATION, TRAINING, AND EXPERIENCE

Bachelor's or advanced degree from an accredited institution, with major in foods, nutrition, or food-service administration.

May have completed an internship in hospital offering dietetic internship approved by The American Dietetic Association or have met necessary experience requirements.

Varied experience in dietetics and administration is required.

WORKER TRAITS

Aptitudes: Verbal ability required to understand medical and scientific terminology in order to communicate with professional staff regarding technical aspects of the department; ability to understand policies, principles, and procedures of dietetics and hospital administration; ability to communicate with personnel of all levels; and ability to solve problems.

Numerical ability required to evaluate and prepare statistical material for budget, cost control, and other purposes.

Interests: A preference for contacts with people to confer with administrative personnel regarding department activities and to direct work of department personnel.

Temperaments: Suitability to direct, control, and plan all activities in the department.

Able to deal with people, for conferring with other department heads, supervisors, and patients.

Physical Demands and Working Conditions: Work is light.

Talking and hearing essential to consult with departmental personnel and applicants, to confer with other hospital department heads, and to represent department in hospital staff meetings.

Works inside.

JOB RELATIONSHIPS

Workers supervised: All employees assigned to the department.

Supervised by: ADMINISTRATOR or an ASSOCIATE ADMINISTRATOR.

Promotion from: DIETITIAN, ADMINISTRATIVE; DIETITIAN, TEACHING, or DIETITIAN, THERAPEUTIC.

Promotion to: No formal line of promotion. May be promoted to an ASSOCIATE ADMINISTRATOR.

PROFESSIONAL AFFILIATIONS

American Society for Hospital Food
    Service Administrators
840 North Lake Shore Drive
Chicago, Ill. 60611

The American Dietetic Association
620 North Michigan Avenue
Chicago, Ill. 60611

DIETITIAN, ADMINISTRATIVE*
assistant director, food service
food production manager

JOB DUTIES

Directs and supervises hospital personnel concerned with planning, preparing, and serving food to patients, staff, and visitors:

Plans basic menus considering such factors as variety, season of the year, availability of foods, known food preferences of the group, nutritional and caloric content, and food costs. Estimates number of people to be served and computes quantity of food to be prepared to insure that individual portions will be in conformance with dietetic standards. Prepares daily menus and portion specification orders for guidance of the staff and inspects prepared food to insure adherence to specifications, observing appearance, quantity, and temperature, and sampling the food to estimate its palatability.

Develops and implements work standards, sanitation procedures, and personal hygiene requirements consistent with institutional rules; local, State and Federal regulations; and foodhandling principles. Inspects food preparation and serving areas, equipment, and storage facilities, observes the appearance and personal habits of the staff to detect deviations and violations of current health regulations, and orders corrective measures as necessary.

Prepares daily work schedules and assigns duties and responsibilities, through supervisors, to dietetic staff. Employs dietetic personnel, directs orientation and training, and initiates, recommends, and approves personnel actions, such as transfers, promotions, and separations, according to procedures established by hospital administration.

Responsible for records and reports concerning technical and administrative operations, such as number of meals served, menus, analyses of diets, food costs, supplies issued, repairs to dietetic equipment, maintenance service and costs, personnel data, and continuous inventory of supplies on hand. Suggests revisions or adaptations of procedures for more efficient performance of department and for training of employees.

Reviews technical publications, studies journals, and confers with food industry representatives regarding new developments in food packing and processing, new and modified equipment, and new nutritional concepts. Selects those with merit for possible incorporation into the hospital programs.

Depending on the size and organization of the Dietetic Department, may directly supervise the food preparation personnel, overseeing the cooking, serving, and cleaning tasks. May also supervise all dietetic personnel not specifically assigned to patient food service or modified diet preparation. May direct the employee food-service activity.

In smaller hospitals, the duties of DIRECTOR, FOOD SERVICE or DIETITIAN, THERAPEUTIC may be combined with this job.

MACHINES, TOOLS, EQUIPMENT, AND WORK AIDS

Food preparation reports, inventory records, menus, personnel records, recipes, work schedules, and all institutional kitchen equipment.

EDUCATION, TRAINING, AND EXPERIENCE

Bachelor's or advanced degree from an accredited college or university with major in foods, nutrition, or food-service administration.

May have completed a dietetic internship approved by The American Dietetic Association or have met necessary experience requirements.

Varied experience in dietetics and administration is required.

*Ibid., pp. 324-325.

WORKER TRAITS

Aptitudes: Verbal ability required to direct work activities and to utilize hospital and dietetic terminologies.

Numerical ability required to calculate nutritional values of foods, plan work schedules, develop requisitions, and estimate food purchasing requirements.

Form perception required to judge adherence to portion-size specifications.

Interests: A preference for contacts with people, to direct departmental personnel and their activities and to resolve problems related to departmental activities.

Temperaments: Capable of the direction, control, and planning of the food production activities of the department.

Able to deal with people, for supervising staff, conducting on-the-job training, and conferring with associates.

Physical Demands and Working Conditions: Work is light. Stands and walks much of working day.

Talking and hearing essential to give assignments and work instructions to subordinates and to resolve dietary matters with associates. Works inside.

JOB RELATIONSHIPS

Workers supervised: All employees of food production unit.

Supervised by: DIRECTOR, FOOD SERVICE.

Promotion from: No formal line of promotion. May be promoted from staff level position.

Promotion to: DIRECTOR, FOOD SERVICE.

PROFESSIONAL AFFILIATIONS

American Society for Hospital Food
    Service Administrators
840 North Lake Shore Drive
Chicago, Ill. 60611

The American Dietetic Association
620 North Michigan Avenue
Chicago, Ill. 60611

Dietetic Department   Dietitian, Teaching 077.128

DIETITIAN, TEACHING*

assistant director, dietetic education

JOB DUTIES

Plans, organizes, and conducts dietetic educational programs for nurses, medical and dental interns, medical residents, dietetic interns, and other personnel:

Plans schedule of instruction and on-the-job training. May conduct classes in subjects such as nutrition, diet therapy, sanitation, infant nutrition, marketing, menu planning, food procurement, food cost control, and supervisory techniques. Arranges for additional lectures by medical staff, teachers of dietetic subjects in colleges and universities, and members of professional associations. Supervises dietitians in any teaching or training functions they may perform in connection with the program for teaching in the area of dietetics.

May recommend and supervise procedures in orientation and on-the-job training of food-preparation and food-service workers: Institutes orientation program to acquaint employees with work assignments, schedules, and required performance standards.

Selects textbooks and reference materials for subjects to be presented in classroom and prepares course outlines. Prepares manuals and guidebooks for use in on-the-job training. Prepares and presents visual aids to supplement textbook information and to portray on-the-job methods.

*Ibid., pp. 326-327.

Requests, from accredited colleges, universities, and professional associations, literature on trends and practices in fields of dietetics and nutrition.

Participates in meetings of professional associations.

In smaller hospitals the duties of this job may be combined with those of DIETITIAN, ADMINISTRATIVE; DIETITIAN, THERAPEUTIC; or DIRECTOR, FOOD SERVICE.

MACHINES, TOOLS, EQUIPMENT, AND WORK AIDS

Course outlines, dietetic literature, files, manuals, visual aids, textbooks, and written examinations.

EDUCATION, TRAINING, AND EXPERIENCE

Bachelor's and master's degrees from accredited institution with major in foods, nutrition, or food service management. Completion of courses in methods and principles of teaching required.

May have completed an internship in hospital offering dietetic internship approved by The American Dietetic Association or equivalent approved experience. At least 1 year's experience as instructor in one or more phases of dietetics in a college or institution is preferred.

WORKER TRAITS

Aptitudes: Verbal ability required to read and comprehend complex principles of dietetics and to be able to develop and prepare course outlines, conduct class lectures, prepare examinations, and rate student performance.

Interests: A preference for working with people and the communication of ideas to conduct educational program.

A preference for scientific and technical activities to present such subject matter as nutrition, sanitation, and diet therapy.

Temperaments: Leadership required to plan, control, and direct all phases of the educational program relating to dietetics.

Capable of guiding students in their opinions, attitudes, and judgments in teaching dietetics.

Physical Demands and Working Conditions: Work is light. Intermittent standing, walking, and sitting to conduct classes and observe activities of students.

Talking and hearing essential in lecturing to students and answering questions. Works inside.

JOB RELATIONSHIPS

Workers supervised: All trainees and dietetic personnel who take part in training activities.

Supervised by: DIRECTOR, FOOD SERVICE.

Promotion from: No formal line of promotion. May be promoted from staff level position.

Promotion to: No formal line of promotion. May be promoted to DIRECTOR, FOOD SERVICE.

PROFESSIONAL AFFILIATIONS

The American Dietetic Association
620 North Michigan Avenue
Chicago, Ill. 60611

DIETITIAN, THERAPEUTIC*

assistant director, therapeutic dietetics

JOB DUTIES

Plans and directs preparation of modified diets prescribed by medical staff for patients with therapeutic diet needs:

Reviews medical orders for modified diets required for patients. May interview patients to obtain information regarding food habits and preferences for guidance in planning diets. Advises on types and quantities of foods and methods of preparation for therapeutic diets. May instruct personnel regarding type and quantity of food to be prepared and any special techniques to be employed. May inspect meal assembly so that trays conform to prescribed diet and meet standards and directions as to quality, quantity, temperature, and appearance. May instruct patients and/or their relatives, regarding diet therapy to be applied during and subsequent to hospitalization. Initiates referral of specific patients to community agencies for follow-up, with physician's approval.

Is responsible for records and reports concerning technical and administrative operations, such as number of meals served, menus, analyses of modified diets, and food costs.

In smaller hospitals, the duties of this job may be combined with those of DIETITIAN, ADMINISTRATIVE or DIRECTOR, FOOD SERVICE.

MACHINES, TOOLS, EQUIPMENT, AND WORK AIDS

Diet manuals, diet lists, diet orders, menus, and related reference and research publications.

EDUCATION, TRAINING, AND EXPERIENCE

Bachelor's or advanced degree from accredited institution with a major in foods and nutrition.

May have completed an internship in hospital offering dietetic internship approved by The American Dietetic Association or have had equivalent approved experience.

WORKER TRAITS

Aptitudes: Verbal ability required to comprehend dietetic course work, practices, principles, and theories; to communicate effectively with medical personnel and staff; and to explain dietetic restrictions to patients.

Numerical ability required to compute dietetic values of food and to work with dietetic chemical formulas.

Interests: A preference for dealing with people and the communication of ideas, to instruct patients and/or their relatives regarding diet therapy to be followed after hospitalization.

A preference for scientific and technical activities to perform duties requiring a knowledge of chemistry, caloric values, and physical properties of foodstuffs, as well as understanding the medical basis for dietetic restrictions.

Temperaments: Capable of the direction, control, and planning of duties of personnel concerned with meals served in the modified diet unit.

Ability to deal with people to explain dietetic restrictions to patients and the necessity for following such restrictions.

Physical Demands and Working Conditions: Work is light.

Talking and hearing essential to discuss food preparation with cooking personnel and section staff, to explain dietetic restrictions to patients, and to discuss diet plans with supervisor or attending medical personnel.

Works inside.

*Ibid., pp. 328-329.

JOB RELATIONSHIPS

Workers supervised: All employees of therapeutic or modified diet unit.

Supervised by: DIRECTOR, FOOD SERVICE.

Promotion from: No formal line of promotion. May be promoted from a staff level position.

Promotion to: No formal line of promotion. May be promoted to DIRECTOR, FOOD SERVICE.

PROFESSIONAL AFFILIATIONS

The American Dietetic Association
620 North Michigan Avenue
Chicago, Ill. 60611

Dietetic Department

Executive Chef 313.168
Kitchen Supervisor 310.138

FOOD PRODUCTION SUPERVISOR*

chef
chief cook
first cook
head cook

JOB DUTIES

Supervises and coordinates activities of kitchen workers preparing and cooking foods for hospital patients, staff, and visitors:

Plans or participates in planning menus and utilization of foodstuffs and leftovers, taking into consideration number and types of meals to be served, marketing conditions, and recency of menus. Estimates food consumption and requirements to determine type and quantity of meats, vegetables, and other foods to be prepared. Supervises cooking personnel and coordinates their assignments to insure economical and timely food preparation. Reviews menus and determines food quantities, labor, and overhead costs in cooperation with the DIETITIAN, ADMINISTRATIVE. Observes methods of food preparation, cooking, and sizes of portions to insure food is prepared in prescribed manner. Tests cooked foods by tasting and smelling. May develop and standardize recipes.

May inspect trays for attractiveness, palatability, and temperature of food.

Inspects purchased foods for standards of quality.

May train new food service employees. Keeps records of work assignments and hours worked of personnel under his supervision.

MACHINES, TOOLS, EQUIPMENT, AND WORK AIDS

Various types of food preparation equipment, menus, work schedules, and records and reports.

EDUCATION, TRAINING, AND EXPERIENCE

High school education. In addition, may have completed a special 1-year course which includes such subjects as sanitation, hygiene, quantity food preparation, supervisory techniques, estimating requirements, purchasing food, and managing kitchen and storeroom.

WORKER TRAITS

Aptitudes: Verbal ability is required to read and comprehend menus and to issue clear and concise instructions when supervising kitchen employees.

*Ibid., pp. 330-331.

Numerical ability is required in estimating daily food requirements and in calculating amount of foodstuffs to be purchased to augment existing stocks or for replenishment.

Manual dexterity is required to demonstrate easily and skillfully food preparation and cooking techniques.

Color discrimination is required to recognize freshness from appearance of meats and other foods; also to determine the accepted degree of palatability from color shadings of cooked foodstuffs.

Interests: A preference for managerial activities for the direction and supervision of personnel involved with cooking.

A preference for multiple operations in order to produce satisfactorily finished, palatable meals.

Temperaments: Versatility to adapt to frequent changes in job duties covering a broad range of kitchen occupations, including supervisory responsibility as well as actual preparation and cooking of foods.

A sense of responsibility for the planning and control of an extensive program for feeding a large number of hospital patients, in an expeditious manner, and according to set procedures and stringent sanitation conditions.

Physical Demands and Working Conditions: This work is light.

Stands and walks short distances most of working day.

Stoops, reaches for, and lifts kitchen equipment.

Handles and uses kitchen utensils.

Tastes and smells food to determine its quality and palatability.

Talking and hearing for supervising staff.

Near-visual acuity and color discrimination for examining cooked and stored foods to determine quality.

Works inside. Work area may be warm and humid.

JOB RELATIONSHIPS

Workers supervised: Employees concerned with preparation of food.

Supervised by: DIETITIAN, ADMINISTRATIVE or DIETITIAN, THERAPEUTIC.

Promotion from: COOK or BAKER.

Promotion to: No formal line of promotion.

PROFESSIONAL AFFILIATIONS

None.

Dietetic Department   Food Service Supervisor 319.138

DINING SERVICE MANAGER*

cafeteria food-service supervisor
counter service manager
manager, cafeteria

JOB DUTIES

Supervises and coordinates activities of dietetic personnel who serve meals in a cafeteria, dining room, or coffee shop:

Assigns tasks to employees and arranges work schedules. Sees that service is prompt and courteous, and makes adjustments following complaints.

Directs the setup of tables in the dining room and the preparation and serving of food for regular and special luncheons and dinners. Inspects cafeteria, dining room, coffee shop, and equipment for cleanliness.

*Ibid., pp. 338-339.

Interviews and recommends employment of new workers, assigns them to various duties, and instructs them in work procedures. Maintains record of meals served. Keeps cost records and makes periodic reports of operating expenses. Orders food, supplies, and equipment; assists in menu planning.

MACHINES, TOOLS, EQUIPMENT, AND WORK AIDS

Menus, order books, time records, work schedules.

EDUCATION, TRAINING, AND EXPERIENCE

High school graduation preferred. Some college education is desirable but not essential. Courses in foods and nutrition and personnel management or supervisory training are desirable.

Six months to 1 year of supervisory experience in a hospital department of dietetics, as manager of a cafeteria or dining room of a hotel or restaurant.

One to 3 months' on-the-job training provided to learn policies and procedures of the establishment.

WORKER TRAITS

Aptitudes: Verbal ability is required in supervising and explaining job duties to workers.

Numerical ability at level of simple arithmetic in order to work out time schedules and prepare inventory control.

Clerical perception for the maintenance of records and reports.

Interests: A preference for contact with people.

Temperaments: Capability to direct, control, and coordinate the activities of dietetic personnel engaged in serving food.

Cooperative, to work with staff, associates, and supervisors in resolving food-service problems.

Physical Demands and Working Conditions: Work is light. Constant walking and standing.

Reaches for and handles dishes, utensils, and other equipment to inspect for cleanliness and to demonstrate work methods.

Talking and hearing to communicate with employees and supervisors.

Visual acuity and color discrimination for judging appearance, condition, and attractiveness of foods and displays.

Works inside.

JOB RELATIONSHIPS

Workers supervised: All workers engaged in serving meals in the cafeteria, dining room, or coffee shop.

Supervised by: FOOD PRODUCTION SUPERVISOR or DIETITIAN, ADMINISTRATIVE.

Promotion from: Qualified worker in the department.

Promotion to: No formal line of promotion.

PROFESSIONAL AFFILIATIONS

None.

PATIENT FOOD-SERVICE SUPERVISOR*
kitchen steward
patient tray-line supervisor
sanitation supervisor

JOB DUTIES

Trains and supervises personnel who serve trays to patients and maintain cleanliness of food service areas and equipment, and otherwise assists DIETITIAN, THERAPEUTIC, as directed:

Instructs workers in methods of performing duties and assigns and coordinates work of employees to promote efficiency of operations.

Observes filled trays to assure that foods are properly apportioned and attractively garnished and arranged on trays. Directs workers in loading trays on carts or in automatic conveyor units, in dispatching to nursing stations, and in serving food trays to patients.

Interviews and recommends employment of new workers. Visits patients to learn of food preferences. Calculates routine modified diets.

MACHINES, TOOLS, EQUIPMENT, AND WORK AIDS

Menus, time records, work schedules.

EDUCATION, TRAINING, AND EXPERIENCE

High school graduation preferred. Some college education is desirable but not essential. Courses in foods, nutrition, and personnel management, or supervisory training are desirable.

Six months to 1 year of supervisory experience in a hospital food preparation unit.

One to 3 months' on-the-job training is provided to learn policies and procedures of the establishment.

WORKER TRAITS

Aptitudes: Verbal ability is required in supervising and explaining job duties to workers.

Numerical ability at the level of simple arithmetic is required in order to work out time schedules and prepare inventory control.

Clerical perception for the maintenance of records and reports.

Interests: A preference for contact with workers, in preparing and serving meals to patients.

Temperaments: Capability to direct, control, and coordinate the activities of dietetic personnel engaged in preparing and serving food.

Deals with staff, associates, and supervisors in resolving food-service problems.

Physical Demands and Working Conditions: The work is light. Constant walking and standing.

Reaches for and handles dishes, utensils, and other equipment to inspect for cleanliness and to demonstrate work methods.

Talking and hearing to communicate with subordinates and supervisors.

Near-visual acuity and color discrimination for judging appearance, condition, and attractiveness of foods and displays.

Works inside.

JOB RELATIONSHIPS

Workers supervised: PATIENT FOOD-SERVICE WORKERS.

Supervised by: FOOD PRODUCTION SUPERVISOR or DIETITIAN, THERAPEUTIC.

*Ibid., pp. 342-343.

Promotion from: PATIENT FOOD-SERVICE WORKER.
Promotion to: No formal line of promotion.

PROFESSIONAL AFFILIATIONS

None.

RADIOLOGY — NUCLEAR MEDICINE DEPARTMENT*

PURPOSE: To provide an adjunct diagnostic and therapeutic radiology service as required in examination, care, and treatment of hospital patients.

RESPONSIBILITY: Taking, processing, examining, and interpreting radiographs and fluorographs. Radiographs may be taken for diagnostic purposes or to study physiological processes. Fluoroscoping may be done to study action of internal physiological processes, localize foreign bodies, or for related medical purposes. Radioisotopes are used to indicate the course of compounds introduced into the human body. Radiographs and fluorographs must be examined, and the extent and significance of their pathology or deviation from the normal interpreted. Roentgenotherapy and therapy by radium and radioactive substances are also a responsibility of this department. In large research or teaching hospitals there may be a separate Department of Nuclear Medicine concerned with medical diagnosis and therapy through the use of radioisotopes, as well as research in radiochemical analysis, radiation biology research, instrumentation and monitoring techniques, radioactive waste disposal, control and reduction of occupational and environmental exposures, and special health problems of nuclear propulsion.

In addition to these functions, the department is responsible for planning and carrying out policies and procedures to insure protection to all hospital personnel in contact with radiation modalities; providing consultation and advice to clinicians in interpreting diagnostic roentgenological findings; planning diagnostic X-ray procedures and other pertinent matters; administering therapeutic treatment; participating in research programs; presenting films at autopsies and making additional post mortem examinations as required to complete records; participating in hospital's educational program; and maintaining accurate and complete records.

AUTHORITY: The authority for the radiological services of the hospital rests with a DIRECTOR OF RADIOLOGY or RADIOLOGIST (depending upon the size of the department) who reports to the administration on administrative matters and to the Chief of the Medical Staff on professional practices. The DIRECTOR is delegated authority for organization, operation, and training of personnel so that an effective organization is established and maintained. While standardizing agencies recommend medical supervision, the administrative functions may be assigned to the RADIOLOGIC TECHNOLOGIST, CHIEF.

In those hospitals where nuclear medicine has evolved as a separate department, the CHIEF OF NUCLEAR MEDICINE is

*Ibid., pp. 487-490.

delegated authority for those workers concerned with theory, research, techniques, and procedures of nuclear medicine. However, few hospitals have developed this separate department with its own staff. The reasons given for this lack of evolution in more hospitals are: (1) Complexity of new techniques, procedures, and equipment; (2) cost of the equipment; (3) necessity for a highly trained staff skilled in the use of these procedures, techniques, and equipment; (4) a relatively small number of cases that require such radiologic services. This is a fast-changing and rapidly advancing segment of medical science. What is written today may well be outmoded tomorrow.

In this study, because of similarity of purpose, responsibility, equipment, and techniques, and since both processes utilize the properties of radioactive substances, nuclear medicine has been combined with radiology.

INTERRELATIONSHIPS AND INTRARELATIONSHIPS: An effective diagnostic and therapeutic radiological program is accomplished through sound planning of the program and its supporting policies and procedures, efficient internal administration and organization, and cooperation and liaison with other hospital activities. The department serves inpatients, and outpatients, and hospital personnel. There must be close coordination between activities of this department and all clinical activities of the hospital. Contact and cooperation with Outpatient Department, nursing service, and medical staff are essential. The DIRECTOR or RADIOLOGIST serves as a member of the medical staff as well as an administrative department head. This department participates in the total hospital program of patient care, research, education, and community health programs.

STANDARDS: The American College of Surgeons and American College of Radiology have cooperated in establishing minimum standards for hospital roentgenological service. To meet the minimum standards, the radiology program should have adequate space and equipment, qualified personnel, proper records and reports, and sufficient authority and personnel to carry out an acceptable program.

The American Registry of Radiologic Technologists and Council of Medical Education and Hospitals of the American Medical Association have formulated standards for technologists and it is recommended that hospitals adopt these standards, which also constitute qualifications for registry by the accrediting agency. Many hospitals conduct their own schools for training RADIOLOGIC TECHNOLOGISTS and other technical workers in the department. These schools are under the direction of a RADIOLOGIST and must meet standards formulated by the Council on Medical Education of the American Medical Association, in conjunction with the American Registry of Radiologic Technologists and American College of Radiology. The Committee on Hospitals of the Bureau of Professional Education of the American Osteopathic Association has established minimum standards of similar scope for hospital roentgenological services.

RADIOLOGY - NUCLEAR MEDICINE DEPARTMENT **

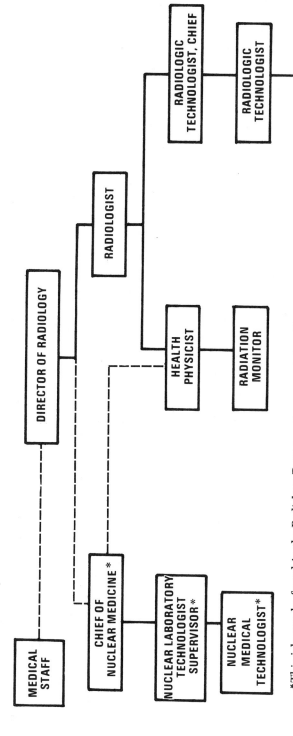
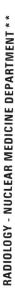

*This job may be found in the Radiology Department or separate in a Department of Nuclear Medicine.

NOTE: This chart is for illustrative purposes only and should not be considered a recommended pattern of organization.

**Ibid., p. 491.

PHYSICAL FACILITIES AND STAFFING: The Radiology Department usually consists of therapeutic radiology, physics, and diagnostic radiology sections. All three provide specialized services to the clinical activities of the hospital.

With the growth of the department's functions, in most instances, it is necessary to provide offices for the DIRECTOR OF RADIOLOGY, RADIOLOGIST, CHIEF OF NUCLEAR MEDICINE, and possibly one for the HEALTH PHYSICIST, who is responsible for protecting the workers in the department by monitoring programs and controlling radiation hazards. Space should be provided for a viewing room; a waiting room; dressing rooms; a dark room; a file room; roentgenography, roentgenoscopy, and roentgenotherapy (one or more rooms); and storage and usage of radioactive materials. In the smaller hospital these rooms may be variously combined. Equipment may be located in a single convenient area or may be dispersed in operating rooms and near outpatient clinics. Portable units can be brought to bedside. Technical equipment should be modern and paced to technological advances but will vary with type and activity of the hospital.

The problems of contamination and exposure to radiation are, of course, present but safety regulations are enforced. All radiology employees wear badges to measure the exact amount of radiation to which they are exposed. Fluoroscopy treatment offers the greatest radiation hazard, and lead aprons and gloves are worn to protect the worker. The badges are checked monthly by the RADIATION MONITOR and resulting information recorded in the Radiology Department records. Radiation hazards can be reduced to a minimum as a result of safety precautions. The Atomic Energy Commission has specific regulations for those workers in nuclear medicine who handle radioisotopes and other radioactive substances.

Responsibility for all radiological examinations, diagnosis, and treatment rests with the department head who may be DIRECTOR OF RADIOLOGY assisted by RADIOLOGIST and CHIEF OF NUCLEAR MEDICINE. All three should hold a degree of Doctor of Medicine or Osteopathy from an accredited medical school or school of osteopathy and have qualifications in radiology acceptable to the Council on Medical Education and Hospitals of the American Medical Association or the Committee on Hospitals of the Bureau of Professional Education of the American Osteopathic Association. A part-time RADIOLOGIST who periodically visits the hospital and makes necessary interpretations of X-ray films is the usual practice followed in the small hospital, although this does not preclude the study and interpretation of films by a qualified attending staff physician. If a member of the medical staff with fundamental training in radiology is assigned to supervise the service, a RADIOLOGIST should be engaged and called upon to interpret obscure findings. RADIOLOGIC

TECHNOLOGISTS and NUCLEAR MEDICAL TECHNOLOGISTS operate radiologic equipment for diagnosis and therapy. The films are processed by the DARKROOM ATTENDANT.

Radiology—Nuclear Medicine Department

Director of Radiology
070.118 T

DIRECTOR OF RADIOLOGY*

chief of radiology

JOB DUTIES

Administers radiology programs and directs and coordinates department activities in accordance with accepted national standards and administrative policies:

Plans scope, emphasis, and objectives of the radiology programs, conferring with administrators, directors of other departments, and medical staff to ascertain hospital needs. Participates with personnel of other departments in planning joint administrative and technical programs and recommends methods and procedures for coordinating radiological services with other patient care services. Investigates and studies trends and developments in radiologic practices and techniques and develops operation manuals, outlining methods, procedures, and techniques reflecting applicable advances in the field to guide professional and technical staff. Establishes and enforces, through subordinate supervisors, safety regulations for the department to insure that both patients and hospital personnel receive maximum protection from the hazardous effects of roentgen rays and radioactive materials used in diagnosis and therapy.

Prepares budget estimates of personnel, supplies, and equipment and prepares narrative and statistical reports of activities and expenditures. Recommends and approves personnel actions, such as hirings, transfers, and promotions, usually interviewing and hiring the professional applicants. Resolves problems requiring administrative authority or professional knowledge, and outlines policies, procedures, and methods for resolving lesser problems by subordinate personnel.

Instructs students and interns in theory and practice of radiology, lecturing, conducting diagnostic seminars, or providing individual instruction and on-the-job training.

The director's actual involvement in providing diagnostc and therapeutic radiology service for patients depends on the size of the radiology staff and hospital organization. He may, in small hospitals, be a director in name only, having responsibility for the department's activities, aspects of which are required by law, and advising the staff on technical matters but delegating actual administrative duties to the RADIOLOGIC TECHNOLOGIST, CHIEF, so that he may devote his time to performing the duties of a RADIOLOGIST. He may, in large hospitals, confine his clinical activities to a single specialty, such as radiation therapy, nuclear medicine, or diagnosis. He may limit his activities to those furthering a specific research project or act solely as a consultant to assist staff radiologists and the medical staff with unusual or complex cases. His services as consultant, adviser, and coordinator may, in some communities, extend to other hospitals, especially if the other hospitals have limited radiological services. His research activities are also determined by the size and kind of hospital as well as by his own interests and abilities. He may, in a large hospital, determine the nature of research to be performed and assign specific projects to staff members.

MACHINES, TOOLS, EQUIPMENT, AND WORK AIDS

The administrative duties of this occupation do not require any machines, tools, equipment, or work aids. However, if he is performing any diagnostic or therapeutic

*Ibid., pp. 492-494.

radiology, he will use what the specific procedure requires, such as X-rays and an X-ray viewer for diagnostic work.

EDUCATION, TRAINING, AND EXPERIENCE

Graduation from a medical school recognized by the Council on Medical Education and Hospitals of the American Medical Association or Committee on Hospitals of the Bureau of Professional Education of the American Osteopathic Association. License to practice medicine or osteopathy in State where located.

For certification by the American Board of Radiology, applicant must have 3 years' special training in radiology in clinics, hospitals, or dispensaries recognized and approved by the Board and by the Council on Medical Education and Hospitals of the American Medical Association.

Four to 6 years' radiology specialization, 1 or more of which was in supervisory or administrative capacity.

WORKER TRAITS

Aptitudes: Verbal ability is required to read and understand professional and technical radiologic and medical material; to communicate with administrative and medical personnel; to write administrative reports and technical manuals; and to lecture to students.

Numerical ability is required to prepare budget estimates and statistical reports of department activities.

Interests: A preference for business contacts with people, in coordinating department services with other departments for the best patient care services.

A preference for communicating ideas, in planning emphasis and objectives of radiology programs, preparing manuals, and lecturing to students.

Temperaments: Ability to plan and control activities and personnel of the radiology department.

Ability to deal with people in planning and coordinating work programs and in making diagnostic recommendations based on measurable and verifiable criteria.

Physical Demands and Working Conditions: Work is sedentary.

Reaching for and handling X-rays and reports.

Talking and hearing when lecturing, interviewing applicants, and attending patients.

Near-visual acuity, depth perception, and accommodation in reading radiographs and conducting examinations and therapy treatments.

Works inside. Radiation hazards are fewer for this worker than for others in the department, since exposure is less frequent.

JOB RELATIONSHIPS

Workers supervised: All persons assigned to Radiology Department (professional, technical, clerical, and paramedical).

Supervised by: ASSOCIATE ADMINISTRATOR for administrative purposes, and Chief of Medical Staff for professional practice.

Promotion from: RADIOLOGIST.

Promotion to: No formal line of promotion.

PROFESSIONAL AFFILIATIONS

American Medical Association
535 North Dearborn Street
Chicago, Ill. 60610
American Osteopathic Association
212 East Ohio Street
Chicago, Ill. 60611

American College of Radiology
20 North Wacker Drive
Chicago, Ill. 60606

RADIOLOGIC TECHNOLOGIST, CHIEF*

chief X-ray technologist

JOB DUTIES

Plans, directs, and supervises all technical aspects of the department in regard to services, programs, and evaluations of such programs:

Maintains radiologic services in accordance with standards established by the hospital and with State, local, and Federal standards which may apply. Is responsible for the technical aspect of radiologic safety in the hospital, recommending programing, monitoring, and location of warning or identifying devices in carrying out recommendations of the radiation safety officer.

Recommends equipment modification, new equipment, and essential construction within the department. Is responsible for existing equipment and such contractual services as may be required. Coordinates departmental purchasing and is responsible for stock level, storage, and utilization.

Administers preparation of reports, documents, payroll records, statistical surveys, and other data required. Provides for recruitment, selection, training, supervision, and other personnel matters in the department. Makes work assignments and coordinates requests for radiologic service with hospital routine. Evaluates accuracy and technical quality of X-rays; demonstrates and explains difficult or new techniques and procedures to the technical staff. Delegates responsibilities to designated staff.

Assists RADIOLOGIST with difficult radiologic procedures and performs general technical duties when workload is heavy.

MACHINES, TOOLS, EQUIPMENT, AND WORK AIDS

Diagnostic and therapeutic radiographic units, reports and records, and protective garments.

EDUCATION, TRAINING, AND EXPERIENCE

High school graduation or equivalent. Satisfactory completion of formal radiologic technology training in an AMA-approved school and able to meet the requirements for registry by the American Registry of Radiologic Technologists (ARRT).

At least 5 years' experience with appropriate broad experience within the department to be familiar with all aspects of departmental policy and administrative procedures.

WORKER TRAITS

Aptitudes: Verbal ability is necessary to read and understand medical and technical materials and instructions; to communicate with medical, technical, and clerical personnel as well as hospital administrators and patients; and to lecture to students.

Numerical ability is necessary to compile statistical data and prepare reports relating to operating costs, purchases, and services rendered.

Clerical perception is necessary to detect errors in written material and statistical data and when writing and proofreading records and reports.

Spatial perception is necessary to visualize relationships of internal organs in relation to X-ray tube and film in order to obtain radiographs of diagnostic value.

Form perception is necessary to perceive detail in X-rays to determine acceptability of exposure.

Manual dexterity is necessary to adjust machine controls and arrange, attach, and adjust supportive devices.

Interests: A preference for scientific and technical activities to master principles, techniques, and procedures of radiology.

*Ibid., pp. 508-510.

A preference for processes, machines, and techniques to direct RADIOLOGIC TECHNOLOGIST in obtaining radiographs, developing X-ray film, and performing diagnostic tests using radioisotopes.

A preference for people and for communicating ideas in supervising department personnel and assisting them in solving technical problems.

Temperaments: Ability to direct, control, and plan an entire activity and activities of others in the Radiology Department.

Able to evaluate processed X-rays against measurable and verifiable criteria.

Physical Demands and Working Conditions: Work is of medium demand. Stands when supervising technologists and sits when preparing reports.

Reaching for and handling machine controls and setting up equipment.

Talking and hearing to converse with patients and staff and to conduct training classes.

Near-visual acuity, accommodation, and depth perception for setting up X-ray equipment, and preparing and maintaining radiologic records and reports.

Works inside. Electrical and radiant energy hazards are present. Wears protective gloves and apron during certain procedures. May wear film badge and have periodic blood counts to detect effects of radiation.

JOB RELATIONSHIPS

Workers supervised: DARKROOM ATTENDANT, RADIOLOGIC TECHNOLOGIST, NUCLEAR MEDICAL TECHNOLOGIST, clerical assistants, and student technologists.

Supervised by: RADIOLOGIST.

Promotion from: RADIOLOGIC TECHNOLOGIST, NUCLEAR MEDICAL TECHNOLOGIST.

Promotion to: No formal line of promotion.

PROFESSIONAL AFFILIATIONS

American Society of Radiologic
  Technologists
645 North Michigan Avenue
Chicago, Ill. 60611

American Registry of Radiologic
  Technologists
2600 Wayzata Boulevard
Minneapolis, Minn. 55404

Radiology—Nuclear Medicine Department

Chief of Nuclear Medicine
070.118T

CHIEF OF NUCLEAR MEDICINE*
director of radioisotope laboratory

JOB DUTIES

Coordinates and directs activities of radioisotope laboratory; instructs students and interns in theory and techniques of nuclear medicine; serves as specialist in diagnosis, internal, and nuclear medicine; and performs nuclear medical research:

Interviews, selects, and hires staff for radioisotope laboratory. Participates in hospital staff meetings to maintain liaison between department and medical staff and to recommend methods and procedures for coordinating functions of the Nuclear Medical Department with other patient care services. Prepares budgets indicating estimated cost of new equipment, maintenance, and personnel costs. Formulates and directs policies and procedures to be followed by staff personnel to provide best possible patient care. Establishes and enforces, through subordinate supervisors, safety regulations for the department to insure that patients and hospital personnel receive maximum protection from the hazardous effects of roentgen rays and radioactive materials used in diagnosis and therapy.

*Ibid., pp. 511-513.

Formulates and conducts teaching program, conferences, and seminars on nuclear medicine for students and interns. Studies technical and trade journals; attends local and national nuclear medicine seminars and medical conferences to acquire and contribute knowledge of procedures and methods.

Examines new patients and discusses diagnoses with attending physicians to determine courses of treatment. Reads medical charts and reports of examinations and tests (made in own department and in other departments) and makes recommendations for treatment plan according to organs or tissues involved and type of radioisotope applicable. Writes instructions on patients' charts to be followed by technologist or technician. Studies scans (X-ray type pictures of a malfunctioning organ or area reproduced in small squares on film plate by the Magna-Scanner and utilizing gamma rays emanating from radioisotopes injected into the patient's body) and X-rays, interprets findings, and records data for hospital records and information of referring physician. Is available to other physicians for discussions, conferences, and advice to benefit patients and to further knowledge of nuclear medicine.

Conducts research in nuclear medicine to discover ways and means of utilizing radioisotopes in diagnosis and treatment of disease. Studies current unsolved medical problems or observes patients' needs and notes area of medicine needing research to select a project in which use of radioisotopes could be applied. Studies similar research projects and reviews known information to become familiar with related aspects of the proposed research. Studies properties of all available isotopes, considering source, half-life (a measure of the rate of decay), and expense to select the one which is specifically adaptable to proposed research. Considers function of organ or tissue involved to select a carrier (an agent — chemical or natural — selected according to its affinity for the involved organ and to, or with, which the isotope is bound or combined to introduce it to the area to be scanned), if one is needed. Assembles all information and writes a protocol to present to the research reviewing board for approval. Delegates authority to technologist or technician to carry out technical aspects of the project according to plan. Writes final report at completion of research and publishes results in medical journals, prepares paper for presentation at seminars, and adapts data obtained to practical use for benefit of patients.

MACHINES, TOOLS, EQUIPMENT, AND WORK AIDS

Radioactive compounds and research laboratory equipment and apparatus.

EDUCATION, TRAINING, AND EXPERIENCE

Graduation from a medical school recognized by the Council on Medical Education and Hospitals of the American Medical Association or Committee on Hospitals of the Bureau of Professional Education of the American Osteopathic Association. License to practice medicine or osteopathy from State where located.

For certification by the American Board of Radiology, applicant must have 3 years' special training in radiology in clinics, hospitals, or dispensaries recognized and approved by the Board and by the Council on Medical Education and Hospitals of the American Medical Association.

Four to 6 years' specialization in nuclear medicine or radiology, of which 1 or more years was in supervisory or administrative capacity.

WORKER TRAITS

Aptitudes: Verbal ability is required to read and understand professional and technical radiologic and nuclear medical materials; to communicate with administrative and medical personnel; to write administrative reports and technical research papers; and to lecture to students.

Numerical ability is required to prepare budget estimates and to apply mathematical formulas in computing radioactive materials.

Manual and finger dexterity is needed to use laboratory instruments and apparatus for research.

Interests: A preference for contacts with people, in coordinating department services with other departments for the best patient care services.

A preference for scientific and technical activities to conduct research to discover ways and means of combating disease with radioactive materials.

Temperaments: Ability to plan, direct, and control activities of the nuclear medical laboratory and its personnel.

Ability to deal with people in planning and coordinating work programs and in making diagnostic recommendations based on measurable and verifiable criteria.

Capable of working to exact tolerances and standards when performing nuclear medical research.

Physical Demands and Working Conditions: Work is light. Standing and walking when lecturing to students and supervising activities of the department.

Reaching for and handling equipment when performing research.

Talking and hearing when lecturing, interviewing applicants, and attending patients.

Near-visual acuity, depth perception, and accommodation in conducting examinations and in performing research.

Works inside. Rigid adherence to established laboratory techniques and standards prescribed by the Atomic Energy Commission is vital to minimize hazards to the worker. Must wear protective clothing.

JOB RELATIONSHIPS

Workers supervised: All persons assigned to Nuclear Medical Laboratory (professional, technical, clerical, and paramedical).

Supervised by: DIRECTOR OF RADIOLOGY and Chief of Medical Staff.

Promotion from: No formal line of promotion.

Promotion to: No formal line of promotion.

PROFESSIONAL AFFILIATIONS

American College of Radiology
20 North Wacker Drive
Chicago, Ill. 60606
American Medical Association
535 North Dearborn Street
Chicago, Ill. 60610

American Osteopathic Association
212 East Ohio Street
Chicago, Ill. 60611

Radiology—Nuclear Medicine Department

Nuclear Laboratory
Technologist Supervisor 078.221T

NUCLEAR LABORATORY TECHNOLOGIST SUPERVISOR*

radioisotope laboratory supervisor

JOB DUTIES

Supervises and directs activities of personnel engaged in diagnostic laboratory testing, instructs medical students in nuclear medical technology, and performs the technical aspects of nuclear medical research:

Assigns work schedules, explains duties, and interprets policies and regulations. Reviews appointment schedules, suggesting or effecting changes necessary to provide for maximum use of facilities and staff and most efficient service to patients and physicians. Demonstrates and explains procedures and techniques involved in using radioisotopes in diagnostic studies, such as how to compute doses, operate equipment, and minimize the possibility of excessive radiation exposure, for the purpose of training new technologists and improving work performance of regular staff.

*Ibid., pp. 514-516.

Evaluates work performance of staff and makes recommendations for promotions, transfers, or other personnel actions.

Instructs medical students in procedures and techniques in nuclear medical technology, demonstrating laboratory machines and equipment and following a course designed to supplement theoretical instruction.

Performs assigned phases of nuclear research, under direction of CHIEF OF NUCLEAR MEDICINE, concerned with isotopes, carriers, and organs to be studied in terms of research objectives. Injects test doses into the test subject (usually a rabbit); counts and traces the radioactivity, using spectrometer and Magna-Scanner; and records all pertinent data in specified report form.

Insures a sufficient stock of radioisotopes at all times by weekly review of appointment schedules, listing isotope requirements for each test and using knowledge of nuclear medicine. Computes remaining radioactivity of stock on hand and, considering known rate of decay, determines supplementary isotopes needed and prepares requisition.

MACHINES, TOOLS, EQUIPMENT, AND WORK AIDS

Magna-Scanner, X-ray machine; spectrometer and laboratory equipment; and glassware, protective clothing.

EDUCATION, TRAINING, AND EXPERIENCE

High school graduation or equivalent. Satisfactory completion of formal radiologic technology training in an AMA-approved school and ability to meet requirements for registry by the American Registry of Radiologic Technologists (ARRT).

WORKER TRAITS

Aptitudes: Verbal ability is needed to give training and work instructions to subordinate personnel, lecture to medical students, and discuss nuclear medical technology with professional medical personnel.

Numerical ability is needed to apply mathematical formulas in computing radioactivity of radioisotopes and dosages.

Spatial ability is needed to visualize spatial relationships of internal organs for proper focus of X-ray machine and to adjust detector head of scanner.

Manual and finger dexterity is needed to adjust machine controls and to use small laboratory instruments for research.

Interests: A preference for scientific and technical activities to master principles of radiology and elements of radiologic procedures, and to perform research in nuclear medicine.

A preference for processes, machines, and techniques of handling radioisotopes in performing diagnostic tests and research.

Temperaments: Ability to direct and control activities of technologists.

Able to evaluate work performance of staff against measurable and verifiable criteria.

Qualified to work to exact tolerances and standards when performing nuclear medical research.

Physical Demands and Working Conditions: Work is light. Standing and walking when demonstrating equipment, lecturing to students, and supervising department activities.

Reaching for, handling, and fingering laboratory glassware and machine dials.

Talking and hearing to instruct students and subordinates, to supervise, and to converse with medical staff.

Visual acuity and depth perception to read machine dials and to distinguish markings on scans.

Works inside.

Exposed to radioactivity while preparing doses to be administered to patients and while handling body products containing isotopes. Protective lead shielding and constant monitoring of laboratory by Geiger counter to safeguard work surroundings. Sensitized film badges are worn by all isotope personnel to measure cumulative radiological exposures. Worker wears disposable gloves and uses metal tongs when preparing isotope doses. Rigid adherence to established laboratory techniques and standards prescribed by the Atomic Energy Commission to minimize hazards to the worker.

JOB RELATIONSHIPS

Workers supervised: NUCLEAR MEDICAL TECHNOLOGISTS.
Supervised by: CHIEF OF NUCLEAR MEDICINE.
Promotion from: NUCLEAR MEDICAL TECHNOLOGIST.
Promotion to: No formal line of promotion.

PROFESSIONAL AFFILIATIONS

Registry of Medical Technologists
P.O. Box 2544
Muncie, Ind. 47304
American Society of Radiologic
   Technologists
645 North Michigan Avenue
Chicago, Ill. 60611

American Registry of Radiologic
   Technologists
2600 Wayzata Boulevard
Minneapolis, Minn. 55405

HOUSEKEEPING DEPARTMENT*

PURPOSE: To maintain the hospital facilities in a clean, sanitary, orderly, and attractive condition, to provide a suitable environment for the care of patients and for the work of the hospital staff and employees.

RESPONSIBILITY: Clean, sanitary, pleasant environment and facilities are essential to medical and nursing care of patients, and to hospital staff. The responsibility for providing such surroundings in as economic a manner as possible falls in a large measure upon the housekeeping staff of the hospital. Housekeeping is a complex activity requiring constant attention to many different details and to an over-all plan which provides for the utilization of personnel, procedures, and material in an efficient and effective manner.

More specifically, responsibilities of the Housekeeping Department include:

1. Establish and maintain a regularly scheduled cleaning program throughout the hospital complex. Patient-care areas, intensive-care units, surgical suites, and other specialized areas require that a high level of sanitation and sterilization be maintained.

2. Recruit, select, and train personnel for this purpose.

3. Study new techniques for improving housekeeping services; evaluate, select, and provide proper equipment and supplies for efficient and economical operation of the housekeeping services.

4. Provide qualified supervision and direction to scheduled work activities in the most effective utilization of manpower.

5. Establish and maintain procedures which will insure acceptable standards of quality. This includes routine cleaning of windows, walls, floors, fixtures, and furnishings as well as responsibility for disposal of ordinary and contaminated refuse; disinfection of contaminated areas; pest and rodent control; taking bacteriological surface samplings; and carrying out pertinent infection-control procedures.

6. Utilize good interior design principles with regard to decorating and choice of furniture and furnishings, and attend to furniture repairs, refinishing, and upholstering or replacement of equipment and supplies. May move and relocate furniture.

7. Maintain linen selection, distribution, control, and repair.

8. Be aware of common safety precautions and correct or report safety hazards to the correct authority.

9. Coordinate department activities with those of all other departments.

10. Report building repair needs to the Engineering and Maintenance Department.

The Housekeeping Department may also be responsible for the following services: Hospital security; elevator operation; operation

*Ibid., pp. 649-650.

HOUSEKEEPING DEPARTMENT*

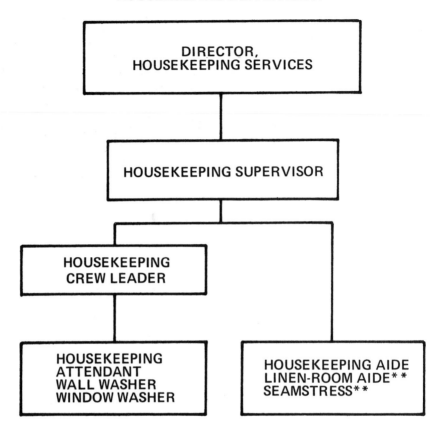

**This job may be assigned to the Laundry Department.

NOTE: This chart is for illustrative purposes only and should not be considered a recommended pattern of organization.

of the laundry; and control of service contracts for services provided by nonhospital personnel.

AUTHORITY: While the housekeeping function is performed within every department of the hospital, it should be the sole responsibility of the DIRECTOR, HOUSEKEEPING SERVICES who reports to an ASSOCIATE ADMINISTRATOR.

INTERRELATIONSHIPS AND INTRARELATIONSHIPS: Cleanliness, sanitation, and pleasant appearance of facilities are vital to the well-being and safety of patients. Housekeeping services must be coordinated with activities of other departments so that minimal disturbance is caused to patients, staff, and employees.

Functions of the Housekeeping Department must be clearly identified and understood by other departments to avoid duplication of services or misunderstanding resulting in loss of services to patients and staff.

*Ibid., p. 651.

PHYSICAL FACILITIES AND STAFFING: The Housekeeping Department requires adequate space and facilities according to the functions under its jurisdiction. An office should be provided for the head of the department, clerical and supporting staff, and housekeeping supervisors. A central storeroom for supplies and equipment is required as well as supply rooms and closets with sinks, shelving, and storage space on every floor and near strategic areas. There should be locker rooms for all personnel, sewing repair rooms, and workrooms of various kinds.

The department is headed by a DIRECTOR, HOUSEKEEPING SERVICES who may have a number of assistants and supervisors as well as a clerical staff. Work must be planned and carefully allocated to prevent overlapping and unbalanced distribution. The DIRECTOR is responsible for training and supervision of all departmental personnel and advises personnel in other departments who may necessarily perform housekeeping duties.

Housekeeping Department   Executive Housekeeper 187.168

DIRECTOR, HOUSEKEEPING SERVICES*

administrative housekeeper

director, environmental services

executive housekeeper

JOB DUTIES

Directs and administers the housekeeping program to maintain the hospital environment in a sanitary, attractive, and orderly condition:

Establishes standards and work procedures for the housekeeping staff in accordance with the establishd policies of the hospital. Plans work schedules and assigns hours and areas of work to insure adequate service for all areas of the hospital. Interviews, selects, hires, evaluates, and terminates personnel and is responsible for their training and supervision.

Inspects and evaluates the physical condition of the hospital; recommends painting, repairs, furnishings and refurnishing, relocation of equipment, and reallocation of space to improve sanitation, appearance, and efficiency. Reports any unsafe conditions. Conducts research to improve housekeeping technology. Investigates and evaluates new housekeeping supplies and equipment. Takes, processes, and analyzes microbiological samples of air and surfaces to evaluate housekeeping methods and materials.

Conducts staff meetings and meets with members of other departments to coordinate housekeeping activities with those of other departments. Serves on the Infection Control Committee and other committees as requested.

Prepares budgets, work reports, and other administrative guides. Inventories housekeeping supplies and equipment, and selects and requisitions new or replacement supplies and equipment. Is responsible for maintaining the records of the Housekeeping Department.

MACHINES, TOOLS, EQUIPMENT, AND WORK AIDS

Records and reports.

*Ibid., pp. 652-653.

EDUCATION, TRAINING, AND EXPERIENCE

A high school education is the minimum formal education required; a college degree is desirable. In addition, special courses in housekeeping or institutional management are desirable.

Experience as a Housekeeping Supervisor or as an Assistant Director of Housekeeping is required.

WORKER TRAITS

Aptitudes: Verbal ability is needed to comprehend and communicate with housekeeping personnel and to prepare reports in concise, understandable language.

Numerical ability is required to perform arithmetic operations in keeping work records, preparing budgets, in requisitioning supplies, and in preparing and balancing workloads.

Color discrimination is needed in the preparation of decorative recommendations.

Interests: A preference for working with people in order to supervise them and to coordinate housekeeping activities with those of other departments.

A preference for activities resulting in the satisfaction of maintaining the hospital in a clean, orderly, attractive, and safe condition.

Temperaments: Ability to direct, control, and plan the total activity of the entire housekeeping department.

Able to communicate with people beyond giving instructions, as in coordinating activities with other department heads and staff.

Physical Demands and Working Conditions: Work is light. There is extensive walking and standing.

Frequent talking and hearing when giving instructions and explanations and in receiving oral information.

Color vision is necessary for determining harmonious color schemes.

Works inside.

JOB RELATIONSHIPS

Workers supervised: All personnel assigned to the Housekeeping Department either directly or through supervisors.

Supervised by: ASSOCIATE ADMINISTRATOR or ADMINISTRATOR.

Promotion from: HOUSEKEEPING SUPERVISOR.

Promotion to: ASSOCIATE ADMINISTRATOR.

PROFESSIONAL AFFILIATIONS

Institute of Sanitation Management
1710 Drew Street
Clearwater, Fla. 33515

National Executive Housekeepers
Association
204 Business and Professional
Building
Second Avenue
Gallipolis, Ohio 45631

Housekeeping Department   Housekeeper 321.138

HOUSEKEEPING SUPERVISOR*

assistant housekeeper

housekeeper

JOB DUTIES

Supervises work activities of cleaning personnel to ensure clean, orderly, and attractive conditions in the hospital:

*Ibid., pp. 660-661.

Prepares daily assignment schedules to include established routine duties, as well as special areas to be cleaned to maintain adequate service at all times to all areas. Tours hospital periodically, covering each assigned area to observe cleaning crews at work and to determine that instructions are followed and safety rules are observed. Inspects hospital premises to determine next assignments such as preparation of vacated rooms for next patient, and to insure that trash and garbage disposal meet safety, health, and sanitation regulations. Occasionally, takes cultures from bed linens, floors, beds, or other equipment and submits them for laboratory analysis.

Introduces and instructs personnel in use of new equipment and cleaning methods to provide most efficient and economical methods of maintaining hospital. Trains new employees, assigns them to tasks, and closely supervises them until fully trained. Recommends personnel actions, such as employing, transfering. or termination.

Maintains an inventory of cleaning materials, supplies, and equipment, and prepares requisitions for replacement of items "used up" or in need of repair. Inspects hospital equipment and furnishings such as beds, cabinets, chairs, screens, and fans, and prepares requisition for maintenance.

Determines that collection and distribution of linen meet needs of the hospital.

Keeps records of rooms and other areas of the hospital that have been cleaned.

May be responsible for keeping a lost-and-found department for the convenience of patients, visitors, and employees. Also may keep personnel records on workers such as hour and wage data.

MACHINES, TOOLS, EQUIPMENT, AND WORK AIDS

Linens and household cleaning supplies, wheeled equipment, tools, mops, and similar items.

EDUCATION, TRAINING, AND EXPERIENCE

High school graduation is required. Courses in hospital housekeeping or institutional management are helpful.

Experience in functions to be supervised is essential, whether gained from employment or practical training. Must have demonstrated leadership potential.

WORKER TRAITS

Aptitudes: Verbal ability is needed to supervise workers.

Clerical ability is needed to keep departmental records in good order.

Interests: A preference for working with people to supervise, instruct, and maintain harmony among workers .

A preference for activities resulting in tangible, productive satisfaction, such as maintaining hospital areas in clean, orderly, and pleasant condition.

Temperaments: Ability to direct and control housekeeping activities, and evaluate cleanliness and neatness of work against established procedures.

Physical Demands and Working Conditions: Work is light. Extensive walking and standing while supervising workers or inspecting for cleanliness of area.

Bending and stooping for inspecting work areas.

Talking and hearing are required in giving and receiving instructions and explanations.

Near-visual acuity needed to inspect hospital areas for cleanliness.

Works inside.

JOB RELATIONSHIPS

Workers supervised: Supervises housekeeping personnel.

Supervised by: DIRECTOR, HOUSEKEEPING SERVICES.

Promotion from: HOUSEKEEPING AIDE.

Promotion to: DIRECTOR, HOUSEKEEPING SERVICES.

PROFESSIONAL AFFILIATIONS

Institute of Sanitation Management
1710 Drew Street
Clearwater, Fla. 33515

National Executive Housekeepers
   Association
204 Business and Professional
   Building
Second Avenue
Gallipolis, Ohio 45631

Housekeeping Department   Porter, Head 381.137

HOUSEKEEPING CREW LEADER*

group leader

head porter

lead houseman

JOB DUTIES

Supervises, coordinates activities of, and works with cleaning crews engaged in housekeeping activities:

Receives special work assignments for crew or individuals under his supervision from the DIRECTOR, HOUSEKEEPING SERVICES or the HOUSEKEEPING SUPERVISOR. Establishes daily work schedule for special and routine assignments, assigns duties, issues supplies and equipment, and inspects completed work. Leads and works with cleaning crew in housekeeping services in patient rooms, locker rooms, cast rooms, utility storage, treatment rooms, offices, storage rooms, and specialty areas such as, operating rooms, delivery rooms, and clinics. May work on ladders or scaffolding when washing walls and ceilings.

Inspects equipment used, to determine needs for new parts, repairs, overhaul, replacement, and for cleanliness before and after use. Recommends needs for equipment additions, changes, or dispositions. Inspects and takes corrective action in supply needs. Prepares cleaning and disinfectant solutions as prescribed. Enters in record book supplies, material, and equipment dispersed to workers.

Trains new employees by demonstrating use of cleaning materials and equipment; explains methods of cleaning and insures most efficient and economical use of materials and manpower. Recommends personnel actions such as promotions, demotions, transfers, or discharges.

Reviews, continuously, procedures to assure standardized work methods. Records work accomplished, schedules work for semiannual completion reports or machine-record unit cards. Completes requisitions for supplies to be issued from stock.

MACHINES, TOOLS, EQUIPMENT, AND WORK AIDS

Floor scrubbing and polishing machines; pressurized wall-washing equipment, vacuum cleaners, ladders and scaffolds; cleaning supplies such as mops, pails, and solvents.

EDUCATION, TRAINING, AND EXPERIENCE

Employers' requirements range from grammar school to high school graduation.

Up to 2 years' experience as a HOUSEKEEPING ATTENDANT in a hospital.

From 1 to 4 months' on-the-job training to become familiar with all housekeeping duties, to acquire working knowledge of cleaning procedures, record-keeping, adjustment and maintenance of power equipment.

WORKER TRAITS

Aptitudes: Verbal ability is necessary to discuss assignments with workers and supervisors, to train new workers and to demonstrate new techniques and equipment.

*Ibid., pp. 658-659.

Numerical ability is necessary to measure ingredients and to learn dilution ratios; ability to measure square area and to count out supply items.

Motor coordination is necessary to be able to operate floor scrubbing and polishing machines and to move equipment safely within the confines of patients' rooms and heavily traveled hallways.

Manual and finger dexterity is necessary to reach for, handle, lift, and carry housecleaning supplies and equipment and to finger equipment controls.

Interests: An interest in working with people to supervise, instruct, and maintain harmony among workers.

A preference for activities resulting in the satisfaction of maintaining hospital areas in clean, orderly, pleasant conditions.

Temperaments: Ability to direct and control housekeeping personnel activities, evaluating quality and quantity of work against established criteria.

Physical Demands and Working Conditions: Work is heavy, involving lifting and carrying supplies, equipment, and materials weighing up to 100 pounds.

Extensive standing and walking.

Pushing and pulling on handles of floor polishers to steer along hallways, floors, and corridors.

Stoops, kneels, and crouches to sweep floors, pick up waste and litter, and to polish fixtures and fittings.

Talking and hearing necessary to train new workers, supervise cleaning crews, and discuss work schedules with supervisor.

Visual acuity is required for inspection of surfaces and observation of procedures. Works inside.

Subject to injury from moving parts of housecleaning equipment and falls from scaffolds or ladders.

JOB RELATIONSHIPS

Workers supervised: Members of cleaning crew.

Supervised by: HOUSEKEEPING SUPERVISOR or DIRECTOR, HOUSEKEEPING SERVICES.

Promotion from: A member of the cleaning crew.

Promotion to: HOUSEKEEPING SUPERVISOR.

PROFESSIONAL AFFILIATIONS

None.

LAUNDRY DEPARTMENT*

PURPOSE: To collect and launder hospital linens, garments, and all washables in order to provide adequate supplies of clean, sanitary linens to all departments.

RESPONSIBILITY: Collecting and processing linens according to the particular system in use, checking condition of linens for worn spots or tears, and weighing for production records. Linens are then sorted on the basis of type of washing to be used and processed through washer-extractor-dryer equipment after load limits have been determined. The laundry is finished by one of two methods — dried in dry tumblers or ironed by a flatwork ironer, hothead presses, or hand iron. During these finishing processes each item of laundry will be checked for stains and damage and, where necessary, returned for rewashing or mending.

In some hospitals, the Laundry Department is assigned responsibility for storing, issuing, and inventorying all linens to maintain centralized control. In other hospitals, laundered articles are returned to the Housekeeping Department for distribution. SEAMSTRESS and LINEN-ROOM AIDE may be found in either department.

AUTHORITY: The Laundry Department is usually an independent department under the supervision of a LAUNDRY MANAGER who has full authority over laundry functions and reports to either the ADMINISTRATOR or an ASSOCIATE ADMINISTRATOR.

INTERRELATIONSHIPS AND INTRARELATIONSHIPS: Every effort should be made to emphasize the importance of clean linens in care and treatment of patients and of the coordinated effort required in providing adequate supplies. Linens are furnished to many departments and units of the hospital, necessitating close coordination between the laundry and various users of linens. Work schedules should be set up in cooperation with department heads, and consideration given to over-all requirements and daily distribution of finished laundry. The LAUNDRY MANAGER should recommend and advise on purchase of hospital linens and laundry equipment.

STANDARDS: The National Association of Institutional Laundry Managers, the American Institute of Laundering, and the Laundry Manual of the American Hospital Association recommend washing formulas and supplies. Periodic bacteriological counts are taken to test for presence of bacteria and germs in washing and pressing areas of the laundry. In some hospitals a Sanitarian periodically reviews the laundering and distribution process.

PHYSICAL FACILITIES AND STAFFING: Adequate space, equipment, and staff necessary to meet the established objectives of the laundry must be provided.

*Ibid., pp. 671-672.

LAUNDRY DEPARTMENT*

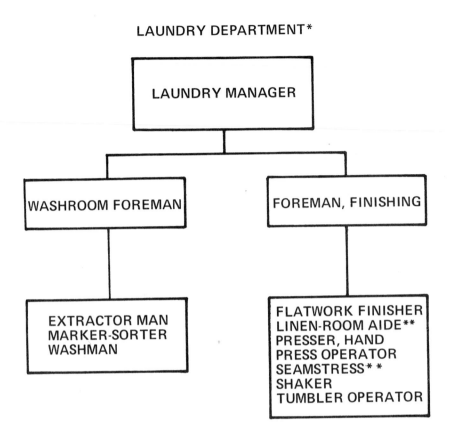

* *See Housekeeping Department.

NOTE: This chart is for illustrative purposes only and should not be considered a recommended pattern of organization.

Laundry Department   Laundry Foreman 361.138

LAUNDRY MANAGER ***

director, laundry and linen

JOB DUTIES

Supervises and coordinates activities of laundry personnel:

Determines the amount of laundry to be processed and plans daily work schedule accordingly. Schedules work loads and assigns workers to maintain even flow of work. Inspects the area periodically and observes laundry equipment in use. Ascertains that standards are being met. When repairs are needed, notifies Maintenance Department. Adjusts workflow as required.

Establishes procedures for examination of finished laundry in the interest of quality control. Arranges for distribution and storage of finished laundry to insure adequate supplies of clean laundry for all departments.

*Ibid., p. 673.

* * * Ibid., pp. 674-676.

Tests samples of water periodically to determine hardness of water and effectiveness of cleaning agents and stain removers.

Changes formulas as needed. Charts and logs quantities of laundry collected and processed on daily and monthly basis for departmental charges, and to aid in scheduling work. Prepares charts indicating quantities of detergents, soaps, bleaches, and other materials used on a daily basis to aid in maintenance of inventory. Prepares written formulas indicating quantity of washing and rinsing compounds required and posts them for use by washing section personnel. Posts temperatures and pressures required for effective operation of equipment.

Inspects and inventories supplies to estimate consumption and orders accordingly. Prepares requisitions and checks quantities delivered. May order replacements for worn linens.

Records hours worked by each laundry worker and submits report to payroll office. Maintains production records and computes operating costs. Interviews new employees to determine amount and type of experience, and assigns workers to tasks accordingly. Trains new workers to operate equipment in order to secure a maximum of transferability among workers in case of absenteeism and during peakloads. Inspects laundered articles and evaluates worker efficiency. Corrects faulty techniques by demonstration.

Investigates new equipment and procedures in laundry operations and recommends changes and additions.

May supervise workers directly or through forelady or foreman, in washing, extracting, and finishing sections. May perform any laundry operation where needed. May remove stains or handle isolation wash requiring special treatment.

MACHINES, TOOLS, EQUIPMENT, AND WORK AIDS

Washers, extractors, tumblers, ironers, laundry washing agents, and compounds.

EDUCATION, TRAINING, AND EXPERIENCE

Preference will be given to a graduate of a laundry school or to one who holds a certificate of professional laundry manager.

A minimum of 1 year's laundry supervision, or 5 years' general laundry work with ability to supervise workers is required.

A new LAUNDRY MANAGER should be given on-the-job training in procedures and practices of specific institution.

WORKER TRAITS

Aptitudes: Verbal ability is necessary to understand hospital reports and directives, prepare reports and schedules, issue oral instructions, and demonstrate processing techniques and methods and use of equipment.

Numerical ability is necessary to calculate anticipated laundry needs in personnel and supplies, keep records, and prepare administrative reports.

Manual dexterity is necessary to use hands rapidly to handle laundry and operate switches and controls of machines.

Color discrimination is necessary to determine cleanliness of laundry.

Interests: A preference for activities that follow a definite routine through the entire laundry process.

A preference for working with people, in a supervisory capacity.

Temperaments: Ability to plan and coordinate all laundry activities, using judgmental and verifiable criteria to evaluate performances of workers and equipment and various aspects of the laundry program.

Physical Demands and Working Conditions: Work is light. Considerable walking about the building, observing the performance of workers and equipment.

Reaching, handling, fingering, feeling, and stooping are required in inspecting operations.

Near-visual acuity and color vision are important for setting dials, testing water samples, and detecting stains or discolorations.

Works inside where area is noisy, hot, and humid. Exposed to hot equipment and wet floors.

JOB RELATIONSHIPS

Workers supervised: All laundry department workers.
Supervised by: ADMINISTRATOR or an ASSOCIATE ADMINISTRATOR.
Promotion from: WASHROOM FOREMAN.
Promotion to: No formal line of promotion.

PROFESSIONAL AFFILIATIONS

National Association of Institutional
 Laundry Managers
P.O. Box 11486
Philadelphia, Pa. 19111

American Institute of Laundering
Doris and Chicago Avenues
Joliet, Ill. 60434

Laundry Department   Flatwork Foreman 361.138

FOREMAN, FINISHING*

forelady, finishing

JOB DUTIES

Supervises and coordinates activities of workers engaged in shaking out, tumbling, flatwork feeding and catching, pressing, folding, packing, and distributing garments and articles for use by hospital staff and patients:

Plans work schedule based on production requirements and availability of workers. Assigns workers to routine tasks, allowing for interchanging of jobs, to relieve monotony and maintain workflow.

Orients and instructs new workers, emphasizing the importance of adhering to prescribed methods, techniques, and procedures to avoid spread of infection. Observes workers in performance of duties and demonstrates techniques to improve production and maintain workflow.

Inspects articles for cleanliness, routes those not meeting standards for rewashing and notifies supervisor of repeated washing discrepancies.

Performs any of the operations supervised, to maintain production schedule.

May perform any of the following tasks: Hire, transfer, and discharge worker; maintain linen stock, inventories, and payroll records; prepare requisitions for linen supplies for various departments.

MACHINES, TOOLS, EQUIPMENT, AND WORK AIDS

Handiron, flatwork ironer, presser machine, folding machine.

EDUCATION, TRAINING, AND EXPERIENCE

Grammar school education, with ability to understand laundry procedures.
Minimum of 1 year's experience in a laundry is preferred.
One to 3 months on the job to become proficient in supervisory methods.

WORKER TRAITS

Aptitudes: Verbal ability is necessary for discussing laundry finishing procedures and problems with supervisor and subordinates; for issuing instructions for successful performance of duties in coordination with activities of other departments.

Form perception is necessary to detect stains, tears, and other imperfections in articles.

Motor coordination and manual dexterity are necessary to coordinate eyes and hands, and move fingers and hands to manipulate articles rapidly and easily to maintain steady workflow.

Interests: A preference for activities in supervising workers in the routine process of finishing laundered articles.

*Ibid., pp. 681-682.

Temperaments: Ability to be alert to a variety of activities, such as hand or machine ironing, shaking of articles, folding and packing.

Ability to plan and direct various activities of finishing section.

Physical Demands and Working Conditions: Work is light. Standing and walking between work stations.

Talking and hearing for supervisory duties.

Reaching for, handling, fingering, feeling, stooping, and turning are all necessary for the variety of duties either performed or supervised.

Works inside. Area is hot, humid, and noisy. Subject to burns from hot equipment.

JOB RELATIONSHIPS

Workers supervised: Members of flatwork ironing crew, folders of tumbled work, and handironers and pressers.

Supervised by: LAUNDRY MANAGER.

Promotion from: Any member of the finishing section.

Promotion to: LAUNDRY MANAGER.

PROFESSIONAL AFFILIATIONS

National Association of Institutional Laundry Managers
P.O. Box 11486
Philadelphia, Pa. 19111

Laundry Department   Washroom Foreman 361.138

WASHROOM FOREMAN*

chief washman

JOB DUTIES

Supervises and coordinates activities of workers engaged in sorting and washing soiled linens, garments, drapes, and other hospital articles in electrically powered machines and extracting excess water to prepare them for the finishing operations:

Plans, in cooperation with LAUNDRY MANAGER, wash schedule and priorities, and assigns workers to duties, such as collecting soiled laundry from laundry chute areas, weighing and sorting laundry, and washing and extracting. Trains new workers in use of supplies and equipment by demonstrating use, explaining operating techiques, and assisting in actual operations.

Sorts, or directs workers to segregate, laundry according to volume, degree of stain or soil, and types of articles. Places heavily stained articles in cart for prewashing. Manually loads articles into washer or washwheel until machine is loaded to designated capacity. Sets water-level control and turns valve to admit water heated to a degree intended to reduce soil and infectious bacteria. Closes washer doors and starts machine. Adds soaps, detergents, bleach, and/or bluing through trough, according to treatment required for wash. Drains sudsy water, admits clean water after each washing cycle, and rerinses as required, adding specified washing chemicals to each step, as necessary.

Assists workers in loading and unloading washers and extractors. Observes and listens to operation of machines and makes minor adjustments, or reports malfunctioning to LAUNDRY MANAGER. Keeps records of total weight of wash processed each day for each hospital department, for budgetary charge purpose.

Inspects wash at various stages of processing for cleanliness, advises workers or recommends changes in washing and rinsing procedures to effect a clean and sanitary wash.

Is responsible for isolation wash.

May shut down all equipment at end of daily operation.

*Ibid., pp. 695-696.

Rotates workers within washroom or arranges for rotation with finishing section to relieve monotony and to maintain workflow.

MACHINES, TOOLS, EQUIPMENT, AND WORK AIDS

Semiautomatic and automatic washers and extractors; laundry solutions, such as soaps, detergents, bleaches; logbook.

EDUCATION, TRAINING, AND EXPERIENCE

Grammar school education, with ability to understand laundry procedures.

Minimum of 1 year's experience as WASHMAN is required.

One to 3 months' on-the-job training to become proficient in supervisory methods.

WORKER TRAITS

Aptitudes: Verbal ability is necessary for discussing washing procedures and problems with supervisor and subordinates; for issuing instructions for successful performance of washroom workers in coordination with activities of other departments and laundry sections.

Some numerical ability is necessary for proper measuring of such laundry agents and chemicals as soaps, detergents, bleaches.

Form perception is necessary to discern stains, tears, and other discrepancies in laundry articles when sorting or determining type of washing treatment necessary.

Motor coordination and manual dexterity are necessary to coordinate eyes and hands rapidly; sort, load, unload, and tend machines; and add detergents and other chemical solutions to wash. Must move rapidly to maintain flow of work to finishing section.

Interests: A preference for activities of supervisory workers in the routine process of loading, tending, and unloading washers and extractors.

Temperaments: Ability to plan and direct activities of washing sections.

Ability to determine type of wash necessary for different stains, materials, and colors for clean and sanitary wash.

Physical Demands and Working Conditions: Work can be heavy. Standing and walking from washer to washer, checking machine operation, and observing performance of workers.

Stooping, crouching, turning, reaching for, and lifting, in the process of handling laundry and tending machines.

Talking and hearing for supervisory duties.

Near-visual acuity and color vision are required to detect stains, and sort by color.

Works inside. Area is hot, humid, and noisy. Subject to burns from hot equipment and water, and falls due to wet floors.

JOB RELATIONSHIPS

Workers supervised: All workers assigned to washroom.

Supervised by: LAUNDRY MANAGER.

Promotion from: WASHMAN or EXTRACTOR MAN.

Promotion to: LAUNDRY MANAGER.

PROFESSIONAL AFFILIATIONS

National Association of Institutional Laundry Managers
P.O. Box 11486
Philadelphia, Pa. 19111